Y0-BRM-278

The Body in Balance

Series: Epistemologies of Healing
General Editors: David Parkin and Elisabeth Hsu: both are at ISCA, Oxford

This series publishes monographs and edited volumes on indigenous (so-called traditional) medical knowledge and practice, alternative and complementary medicine, and ethnobiological studies that relate to health and illness. The emphasis of the series is on the way indigenous epistemologies inform healing, against a background of comparison with other practices, and in recognition of the fluidity between them.

The Body in Balance

Humoral Medicines in Practice

Edited by
Peregrine Horden and Elisabeth Hsu

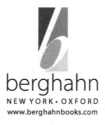

berghahn
NEW YORK · OXFORD
www.berghahnbooks.com

First published in 2013 by

Berghahn Books
www.berghahnbooks.com

©2013 Peregrine Horden and Elisabeth Hsu

All rights reserved. Except for the quotation of short passages
for the purposes of criticism and review, no part of this book
may be reproduced in any form or by any means, electronic or
mechanical, including photocopying, recording, or any information
storage and retrieval system now known or to be invented,
without written permission of the publisher.

Library of Congress Cataloging-in-Publication Data
The body in balance: humoral medicines in practice / edited by Peregrine
Horden and Elisabeth Hsu.
　　pages cm. -- (Epistemologies of healing; volume 13)
　Includes index.
　ISBN 978-0-85745-982-4 (hardback: alk. paper) -- ISBN 978-0-85745-983-1
(institutional ebook)
　1. Traditional medicine--History. 2. Holistic medicine--History. 3. Body
fluids--History. I. Horden, Peregrine. II. Hsu, Elisabeth.
　GN477.B55 2013
　306.4'6109--dc23

2013019627

British Library Cataloguing in Publication Data

A catalogue record for this book is available from the British Library

ISBN: 978-0-85745-982-4 (hardback)
ISBN: 978-0-85745-983-1 (institutional ebook)

Contents

List of Figures and Tables

Figures

Tables

Acknowledgements

The origins of this volume lie in a meeting of minds. Quite independently the two editors each conceived the idea of forming a group of scholars to compare 'humoral' medicines across world history and ethnography. Their joining forces was made possible through the intermediary of David Parkin. The first fruit of this collaboration was a conference held in May 2008 in the Osler McGovern Centre of Green College, Oxford, funded with seed monies for building up the anthropology research group at Oxford on Eastern Medicines and Religions (ArgO-EMR), and with further, indispensable financial support from the John Fell OUP Research Fund and from All Souls College, Oxford. The present collection includes papers by contributors to that conference but is much more than a set of proceedings, and includes one newly commissioned chapter. The thematic coherence that we hope the volume possesses is due above all to the patience and cooperative spirit of the contributors, who revised their chapters and then revised them again in response to editorial suggestions and provocations. The publisher's three anonymous referees were unfailingly generous and constructive in their comments. We also acknowledge with warmest thanks the help of Patrizia Bassini in the organization of the original meeting of the group and of Humaira Erfan-Ahmed in the production of the final text.

Peregrine Horden
Elisabeth Hsu

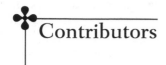# Contributors

Guy Attewell, formerly of the Wellcome Trust Centre for the History of Medicine at University College London, has since 2010 been a researcher in the Department of Social Sciences of the French Institute of Pondicherry. His publications include *Refiguring Unani Tibb: Plural Healing in Late Colonial India* (Hyderabad: Orient Blackswan, 2007).

Patrizia Bassini obtained a doctorate from the Institute of Social and Cultural Anthropology, University of Oxford, for a study of home-based medicine on the Sino-Tibetan frontier. She held an OUP John Fell Fund post-doctoral fellowship before returning to live in Amdo-Tibet, where she currently works with NGOs.

Barbara Duden held a chair in the Institute for Sociology and Social Psychology in the Leibniz University Hannover where she taught from 1997 until her retirement. Among her numerous publications is *The Woman beneath the Skin: A Doctor's Patients in Eighteenth-Century Germany* (Cambridge, MA: Harvard University Press, 1991).

Peregrine Horden is Professor of Medieval History at Royal Holloway, University of London, and an Extraordinary Research Fellow of All Souls College, Oxford. He is co-author, with Nicholas Purcell, of *The Corrupting Sea* (Malden, MA: Blackwell, 2000), and is at work on its sequel. He also writes on the history of charity and medicine. His recent publications include *Hospitals and Healing from Antiquity to the Later Middle Ages* (Aldershot: Ashgate, 2008), and he is preparing a general book on early hospitals for Yale University Press.

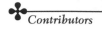

Elisabeth Hsu is Professor of Anthropology at the Institute of Social and Cultural Anthropology of the University of Oxford, and Fellow of Green Templeton College. Recent co-edited volumes include: *Wind, Life, Health* (Oxford: Blackwell, 2008), with Chris Low, and *Plants, Health and Healing* (New York: Berghahn, 2010), with Stephen Harris. Her most recent authored book is *Pulse Diagnosis in Early Chinese Medicine: The Telling Touch* (Cambridge: Cambridge University Press, 2010).

Peter Murray Jones is Fellow and Librarian of King's College, Cambridge. He has published extensively on medieval medicine and science, image-making in medicine, medical books and the circulation of medical information. His books include *Medieval Medicine in Illuminated Manuscripts* (London: The British Library, 1998).

Helen King is Professor of Classical Studies in the Faculty of Arts of the Open University and Visiting Professor at the Peninsula Medical and Dental School. She has written extensively on the history of ancient and early modern medicine. Her books include *The Disease of Virgins: Green-Sickness, Chlorosis and the Problems of Puberty* (London: Routledge, 2003), and *Midwifery, Obstetrics and the Rise of Gynaecology* (Aldershot: Ashgate, 2007).

Shigehisa Kuriyama is Reischauer Institute Professor of Cultural History at Harvard University, where he a faculty member in the departments of East Asian Languages and Civilizations and of the History of Science. His prize-winning monograph is *The Expressiveness of the Body and the Divergence of Greek and Chinese Medicine*, pbk edn (New York: Zone Books, 2002).

Ellen Messer is Visiting Associate Professor in the Friedman School of Nutrition Science and Policy, Tufts University. She has written extensively on cross-cultural perspectives on the human right to food; biocultural determinants of food and nutrition intake; sustainable food systems (with special emphasis on the roles of NGOs); the impacts of agrobiotechnology on hunger; and the cultural history of nutrition, agriculture, and food science.

David Parkin is Professor Emeritus of Social Anthropology in the University of Oxford. His many books include the monograph *The Sacred Void: Spatial Images of Work and Ritual among the Giriama of Kenya* (Cambridge: Cambridge University Press, 1991), and *Holistic Anthropology: Convergences and Emergences* (Oxford: Berghahn, 2007), co-edited with Stanley Ulijaszek.

Emilie Savage-Smith recently retired as Professor of the History of Islamic Science at the University of Oxford and is an authority on the history of medieval Islamic medicine, magic, scientific instruments and cartography. Her recent books include *A New Catalogue of Arabic Manuscripts in the Bodleian Library, University of Oxford*, vol. 1: *Medicine* (Oxford: Oxford University Press, 2011), and *Medieval Views of the Cosmos*, co-authored with Evelyn Edson (Oxford: Bodleian Library, 2004).

Francis Zimmermann is Professor of South Asian anthropology at the École des Hautes Études en Sciences Sociales, Paris. He has published widely on Ayurveda. His books include *The Jungle and the Aroma of Meats: An Ecological Theme in Hindu Medicine* (Berkeley: University of California Press, 1987), *Le Discours des remèdes au pays des épices* (Paris: Payot, 1989), and *Généalogie des médecines douces. De l'Inde à l'Occident* (Paris: PUF, 1995).

Introduction

Peregrine Horden

The human body contains blood, phlegm, yellow bile and
black bile. These are the things that make up its constitution
and cause its pains and health. Health is primarily that state
in which these constituent substances are in the correct
proportion to each other [Greek *metrios*, 'moderately, in due
measure'], both in strength and quantity, and are well mixed.

—Hippocratic treatise, *The Nature of Man*[1]

In the ethnographic literature on New Guinea and elsewhere,
we see that a number of common patterns appear ... First,
there is a set of ideas about the most significant substances
in the human body, of which we can cite blood, grease, and
water in particular as examples. Second, there is a concern
with the flow and management of these and other substances,
in terms of ideas of balance between hot and cold and wet
and dry conditions. It is this concern that justifies our calling
these thought-worlds examples of humoral systems of ideas.

—Pamela Stewart and Andrew Strathern, *Humors and Substances*

The local model of health and illness [in a Turkish Black Sea
village] does not include a general idea of the possibility of
infection ... [T]he basis of health is explained as a balance
within the system of the body and soul ... The social context
of the individual is also considered to be important for health,
since social imbalances can bring about *nazar* (the 'evil eye').

—S. Wing Önder, *We Have No Microbes Here*

This collection of studies offers a path through the world's major systems of thought about the nature of health and the causes of disease.[2] They are systems that have flourished across the globe at various times during roughly the last two millennia. We believe that studying them through historical evidence and modern ethnography can promote illuminating comparisons. Such study may also suggest the urgent need to reformulate the categories through which the global story of medicine and healing should be told.[3]

The systems we shall look at can be characterized in a preliminary way by their explanation of health and illness in terms of the balance or imbalance of some fundamental properties or constituents of the body. The body here is the human body, but often to be understood in terms of the larger 'body' of its social and natural environment. Two major questions suggest themselves, which the chapters that follow collectively address. The questions bear on the relationship between theory and practice. First, what is the nature of the balancing required? That is, how is balance defined or conceptualized, by whom, and in what circumstances? What exactly is to be balanced or rebalanced, and by what means? Second, how far, and in what ways, are these fundamental properties or constituents, and this process of balancing them, important – whether in word or deed – in actual encounters between sufferer and healer? How far, if at all, does practice reflect theory?

Following the path through world medicine beaten by seeking answers to those questions might seem a relatively straightforward task. Our subtitle refers to humoral medicines. The first epigraph above, from the Ancient Greek 'Hippocratic corpus', apparently gives a brief paradigmatic statement of humoral pathology. Humoralism is a type of medical theory that postulates the proper relationship between fundamental substances in the body as the determinant of health and the disturbance of that relationship as the cause of disease (Nutton 1993). Here are the 'standard' four *chumoi* or humours, blood, phlegm, yellow bile and black bile. Each person and each part of each person has his or her individual mixture of humours, which is subject to a range of influences external to the body from diet to season and climate. It is a clear, attractive, logical system. And it is easy to find seeming analogues to it, so that the path across world medicine is easy to trace. 'The health concepts and practices of most people in the world today continue traditions that evolved during antiquity ... Folk curers throughout the world practice humoral medicine' (Leslie 1976: 1). And not only 'folk' curers, such as those implied by the second epigraph above. The ancient medicines of Asia, whether Indian (Ayurveda) or Chinese (so-called traditional Chinese medicine) have been identified as similar enough to the ancient Greek paradigm for their fundamental constituents to be given in English as 'humours' (e.g., Wujastyk 2003).

Our chapters could have been grouped into three clusters to reflect that particular approach. The first and largest would embrace the supposedly paradigmatic medicine of Graeco-Roman antiquity (King) and some of its main offshoots or descendants. These are the Hippocratic-Galenic tradition in medieval Islam (Savage-Smith), in medieval Europe (Jones) and in eighteenth-century Europe (Duden), just before the humoral paradigm in European medicine began to atrophy.[4] We should also include here the 'Greek medicine', Yunani *tibb*, of the modern Indian sub-continent (Attewell). Another less cohesive cluster would be formed by the learned Asian medical traditions: the varieties of 'traditional' Chinese medicine (Hsu), Ayurveda (Zimmermann) and medicine in Japan (Kuriyama) and Tibet (Bassini); Yunani *tibb* might of course be listed here too. The third and smallest cluster in the volume would represent sub-Saharan Africa (Parkin) and the hot/cold classification systems of Latin America (Messer).

Yet grouping and classifying therapeutic cultures on a global scale in this way is fraught with difficulty. We have 'humoral medicine' in our subtitle, but only for brevity. We cannot readily define humoral medical systems and isolate them from the rest. Heavily emphasized inverted commas must be understood as surrounding 'humoral'. As we shall see, the whole notion of humour is too problematic. The definition and number of the humours changes even within a few canonical texts of the Hippocratic corpus. In the long tradition of premodern Western European medicine, the underlying ideas prove remarkably enduring, but this was precisely because of their vagueness and adaptability. The Hippocratic humours, literally fluids in classical Greek, are not quite those of Galen in the Roman Imperial period; nor are they quite those of medieval scholastics; far less are they those of Duden's 'Baroque ladies'.

If that degree of variety is evident within one supposedly single tradition – derived from the Hippocratics – how much more is it true when we come to compare different traditions. The Graeco-Roman humours and their wider theoretical context cannot be mapped onto the three *dosha*s of Ayurveda (wind, bile and phlegm), the seven constituents of the body, and its waste products. Although it has often been mentioned in the same breath as Hippocratic or Ayurvedic medicine, ancient Chinese medicine is still less to be described as humoral. Its 'five agents' or 'phases' – the *wu xing* of wood, fire, earth, metal and water – correspond to neither elements nor humours elsewhere.

Thus, traditions that have sometimes too casually been aligned as humoral are significantly different from one another. In each, it is tempting to say, the body is differently, incommensurably, conceived (Kuriyama 1999). Even within a single tradition, medical ideas and practices that are held to derive from the same canonical texts vary not only over time but from one locality to another in the same period. On the other hand, few if any of these traditions have ever existed in pure form. Each has at different times been influenced by one or more of the others. This is most obvious in the case of the reception of Islamic medicine in the European Middle Ages; in that of Tibetan medicine with its signs of Greek, Ayurvedic and Chinese elements (Bassini); and of Yunani *tibb* over the last century or so as it has encountered Western medicine (Attewell). It is most controversial in the cases of the hot/cold classification of Latin America (indigenous, or imported from Europe?) or of the 'overarching' medical ideas of sub-Saharan Africa (did Islamic influence reinforce or modify earlier conceptions?). Such movements of medical ideas also make comparison difficult because they affect the heuristic value of any cross-cultural similarities uncovered (Alter 2005).

Not surprisingly, humoralism as a broad category of medical systems has often been abandoned in favour of a variety of attempts to divide up medical cultures in a more abstract way. Leslie (1976) adapted Redfield's notion of the Great and Little Traditions, but this made the duality no less contentious. Literacy – more precisely a style of medical thinking founded on an acquaintance with a canonical body of texts – has obviously been a significant aspect of some of the major medical traditions. The Hippocratics were different in their time (around 500 BC onwards) from their competitors in the eastern Mediterranean, not just in their theories of disease and consequent treatments but in the way their message was conveyed: in texts that may originally have transcribed public lectures or polemics, but that exercised an obviously much wider and longer-lasting influence in their written form. As texts of this sort accumulated, culminating for example in the massive oeuvre of Galen and the scarcely less imposing *Canon* of Ibn Sina (Avicenna as he was known in Latin Europe), so great learning came to be required of medical adepts. No practice without extensive reading. Hence Bates's (1995) suggested replacement of Great Tradition' with 'scholarly tradition' as a broad heading under which to align Hippocratic, Ayurvedic and 'traditional' Chinese medicines – even while acknowledging significant differences in epistemology between them.

If literacy has clearly been important in the transmission of some strands of medical expertise, on a global scale it can of course hardly have been decisive. Oral medical cultures have been shown to depend on precisely those sophisticated taxonomies and implicit theories often associated with the written word, while texts have very often depended on an orally transmitted 'tacit knowledge' for their proper understanding and clinical implementation. That is why Parkin has trenchantly criticized the notion that scriptural texts are essential to a Great Tradition' (Parkin 1990: 195; and this volume).

Such an approach of course broadens the discussion well beyond the literate medicines of Eurasia. It invites classification of healing systems on a genuinely global scale – ideally, to include for example the New Guinea 'humours' of sweat and grease mentioned in the second epigraph. Perhaps the most widely cited of these grand classifications has been that of Foster (1976). Foster distinguished the 'personalistic' from the 'naturalistic' in disease aetiologies. But that distinction at once collapses when a divine being is seen as the ultimate cause of 'natural' diseases and when the activity of demons or witches is thought to wreak havoc with the body's internal makeup (Janzen and Green 2003: 10–11).

In the same year as Foster's publication, Young (1976) instead proposed classifying explanations of illness according to whether they are 'internalizing' or 'externalizing'. Internalizing explanations rest above all on physiology. With them, 'probably the most widely used image is expressed in the idea that sickness is the consequence of a disturbed natural equilibrium which curers must try to restore' (Young 1976: 148).

5

The point of surveying this bewildering proliferation of taxonomies is not to choose between them, and to alight upon one term that seems to embrace those cultures and systems discussed below. None of these classifications is adequate to the diversity of substances, properties and relationships in question when we track medicines of 'humours' through history and across the globe. The point, rather, is to take up and explore Young's suggestion of the importance of balance or equilibrium. Our aim is to follow that concept as if it were a thread running through world medicine and to see where pulling on it leads us. We shall find that balance is not necessarily associated with an equilibrium or a symmetry or the maintenance of homeostasis, notions that reflect a modern biomedical understanding of the body. Balance varies enormously over time and space and may reside in the patient's own emotional life, or developing illness narrative, or in the wider body politic, or in collective moral-aesthetic ideals. It may be related to the regulation of social relations as much as to that of substances (as in the third epigraph). Moreover, how all this has translated into therapeutic practice is yet more diverse. Even the humours of properly humoral medicine turn out to have been less important at the bedside than was once thought. In short, each key term in our title – 'balance' and 'humoral' above all, but also of course 'body' and 'medicine' – is a useful introductory shorthand that must now be put to the question by history and ethnography.

Rather than arrange our chapters simply by continent or chronology, we have adopted what we hope is a provocative thematic layout. This will allow the chapters to prompt novel and suggestive long-range comparisons. The chapters in any one section of the volume are not, however, solely focused on the theme announced in its title, and a number of different arrangements would have been equally fruitful, some of which are hinted at in the preliminary account of each contribution that follows.

We begin in the ancient Mediterranean world of Greece and Rome, especially Greece. It was after all the literate Hippocratic-Galenic tradition that produced, eventually, the 'classic' system of four humours. Its durability and dominance in Europe – in scholarship as much as in medicine – ensured the projection of 'humours' onto other medical currents such as Ayurveda.

It would have of course been open to us to begin further east so as to counteract that projection. It would also have been possible to begin elsewhere, and earlier, in the eastern Mediterranean and Middle East. The belief for example implied in some Egyptian medical writings, that disease was caused by corrupt residues in the body, bears some resemblance to Hippocratic physiology. So does the emphasis in Babylonian medicine on fluids as a determinant of health (Nutton 2004: 42). In neither medical culture was anything resembling a humour articulated into a full disease aetiology.[5] On the other hand, underlying conceptions of ill health as caused by disruption of the natural order have been detected in ancient Mesopotamian culture (Robson 2008: 465). And, strikingly, *maat* (balance, order, justice), a concept with its eponymous goddess, seems to have been central to Egyptian medicine (Zucconi 2007: 27–8). Health depended on the 'balanced' flow of substances along the twenty-two *mtw* or vessels, as described in the Ebers papyrus, irrigating it by their passage as the Nile's waters irrigated the land.

How far the Greeks knew about, and were receptive to, these other medicines is a matter of continuing scholarly argument. In any case, what marks off the development of Greek medicine in the ancient world is its huge 'hinterland' of philosophical speculation. The world in which the authors later (somewhat artificially) gathered into the Hippocratic corpus began to write was one of very open debate and indeed polemic (Lloyd 1979). The boundaries between philosophical and medical ideas are hard to draw. The earliest surviving fragment of Greek philosophy gives us Anaximander's vision of the universe: opposing factors create 'injustice' that must be 'recompensed'. As with Empedocles' 'physics', in which four elements have to be kept in their proper relations, some notion of cosmic balance is apparently being invoked (Lloyd 1966: 16, 212). From the pre-Socratic philosophers to Plato, a variety of terms are deployed to characterize the proper state: *kosmos*, embracing notions of order and beauty; *dike* (justice); *taxis* (regularity, order); *summetria* (symmetry). At whatever level we look, from the entire universe down to the individual body, there is no single term that captures the ideal condition. For the philosopher Alcmaeon, of the sixth or fifth century BC, for instance, health is *isonomia* of the constituents of the body, almost an equality of rights, and ill health is *monarchia*, the dominance of one of them (fragment 4, with Lloyd 1966: 20; Nutton 2004: 47).

It is against this variegated philosophical background that we need to approach Helen King's chapter. The Greek words for humours – *ikmas* and *chumos* – she notes, mean 'fluid' or 'moisture' and derive from plant life. They are what enables flourishing. But among the Hippocratics, there was no single system of humours, no clear dominance of the classic quadripartite model that could later be integrated into a wider framework of seasons, ages of mankind, zodiacal signs and the like. That macrocosmic system was essentially a retrospective imposition on the Hippocratics by the great physician of Imperial Rome, Galen. Instead, in the Hippocratic originals we find a surprising range in the number of humours brought into play by medical authors; we find fluids that are not humours, and also the paired qualities of hot/cold and wet/dry. Even where the humours are held to be in balance in the healthy individual, it is a dynamic balance, changing with the seasons. But the Hippocratics do not even agree on whether humours are causes of disease or appear only as its by-products. Moreover, in the far more systematic Galen we encounter (not for the last time in this collection) the blockage of channels along which fluids move as a cause of ill health.

This notion of flows that are free or blocked seems to apply especially to Hippocratic women. In gynaecology, bile, pus and mucus seem to be the 'humours' most in question; but overall the Hippocratic female body is a body of blood, collected and, ideally, poured out. That is women's 'balance'. In the female case history from one of the books of *Epidemics* (here meaning prevalent ailments, or possibly 'clinical' encounters) with which King concludes, some humours are implied in the background. Yet there is sweat and urine but no bile or phlegm. To the extent that the patient's own view of her body is recoverable from the text, she speaks of 'heaviness', 'gathering' and 'clenching'. It is not what flows that matters, but whether there is flow at all.

This opening chapter radically unsettles everything that textbooks have taken as fundamental to humoral medicine. It could have been followed up in a number of ways – with alternative ancient traditions to that of Hippocrates and Galen, such as Methodism (which focused on the flow of corpuscles through the body's pores; Tecusan 2004), with Roman views of women's bodies (Flemming 2000) or the late antique to medieval gynaecological tradition (Green 2009). Further on in the collection we shall move through the Middle Ages. For the moment, though, we jump to the eighteenth century, the last century of that humoralism in European medicine that looked back, for its axioms and its canonical texts, to the ancient authors discussed by King. We thus bracket the entire 'humoral tradition' in the West.

We also stay with women patients. In 1987 Barbara Duden brought to the attention of medical historians the eight-volume collection of over 1,800 case histories of female patients that was compiled for his junior colleagues by a small-town German physician, Dr Johannes Pelargius Storch of Eisenach (Duden 1991, the English translation). In her chapter here, Duden revisits and refines the vision of female illness she proposed in her monograph. Like King's, her humours are oriented flows, and she sees continuity stretching back across the centuries between Storch's case books, in which she finds women's voices audible, and those of the Hippocratic *Epidemics*. To bring out the particularity of the female experiences she is uncovering, Duden deploys an unusual vocabulary. What matters is the 'autoception', which is not exactly perception of the self, but of the fleshy body, the *soma* – perceived 'haptically', through touch.[6] Humoralism in Duden's chapter is this sense of the body as constructed of liquids in their proper proportions, in 'order' when the body is healthy but always liable to fluxes or to being altered by stagnation. The patient's narration of these flows and blockages is literally a biology, a 'story of life'. As in the Hippocratic case history, Storch's women speak of flows of blood, of discharges of sweat and vomit, of unclean menses, of 'vicarious' menses, and flows from other orifices, as well as of 'clumps' in their innards. We shall meet comparable flows, blockages and entanglements in other chapters.

Duden wants to see the 'haptic autoceptions' reported to Storch as characteristic not just of the Baroque, but of the whole of the premodern. Some women in earlier periods seem to have sensed their bodies in comparable terms, complaining of fluxes (Rankin 2008: 129, 134); but then so too did men. Relying on seventeenth-century Italian and seventeenth-to-eighteenth-century German evidence respectively, Pomata (1998: 129–31) and Stolberg (2011: 89, 127) have both seen talk of fluxes as characteristic of early modern patients of both sexes. It remains to be seen whether this reflects the durability of a Hippocratic conception of the body (as a body of flows) and its 'lay' uses by patients, as against a Galenic conception of the body (as one of solid organs) (Pomata 1998: 135).

Meanwhile, the final contribution to the opening section keeps us in the early modern period, while also looking forward to other chapters on Asia. Shigehisa Kuriyama's unusual and distinctive view of Japan in the Edo period further disturbs any preconceived notions of what humours have been, and how they may be used to explain illness. There is no such thing as Japanese medicine, although *Kanpo* has some claim to be the main alternative medical system to biomedicine in contemporary Japan, distinct from 'traditional' Chinese medicine, the dominant premodern influence in the country (Ohnuki-Tierney 1984: 91–99; Jong-Chol 1995). The form in which *Kanpo* is taught today goes back to the sixteenth or seventeenth century. That is roughly the period of Kuriyama's chapter.

Could money ever be a humour, he asks, but not in any loose metaphorical sense? In Japan of the Edo period it actually was a humour – and could be again. (Contemporary political resonance is not lacking.) The expansive commercial activity of the period, in which money may to some have become more precious than life, has been seen as witnessing not an industrial but an 'industrious' revolution.[7] Families intensified their production for the market and could thus purchase a wider range of consumer goods. Those pursuing wealth to (as we would say) a pathological extent developed, Kuriyama argues, a quite specific symptom. It echoes the descriptions of other chapters here: 'accumulations knotted in their abdomen'. The underlying cause (as in 'classic' *Kanpo*) was a 'faltering in the flow of blood and breath'. This had to be diagnosed by palpations of the abdomen and dispelled by a massage to knead away the knots. The cause was a culture-wide phobia of idleness, of any slowing of money-making activity. Bullion must circulate, and must itself be made to work by being lent out. This psychology of industriousness and indebtedness is what, for Kuriyama, explains money's almost literal incorporation as a humour.

This first section of the volume brings out the diversity of humours and other liquids flowing – or not – in the sick body. It brackets not just the time span of the humoral tradition in the West but also, by moving from German to Japan, the Eurasian landmass. The next section, which emphasizes practice, resumes a chronological arrangement. We have already seen how limited the deployment of the 'standard' four humours in both Ancient Greece and Baroque Germany may have been. We now fill in some of the long history of Graeco-Roman medical learning and its cultural descendants. King stressed the huge extent to which that medical learning was moulded by Galen. He retrospectively remade Hippocrates in his own image, fixing the theory of humours and largely defining human anatomy and physiology for over a millennium and a half. Indeed the bequest of antiquity to the Middle Ages is Galenism: the dominance of virtually every field of medical endeavour (gynaecology apart) by the writings of one man, writings so vast in scale that, to make them manageable, they often had to be abbreviated and repackaged.

Galenism came to the Islamic world through the translation movement that began in Baghdad in the later eighth to ninth centuries. Its pre-eminence as medical theory seemed unassailable. As Emilie Savage-Smith notes at the start of her chapter, perhaps the clearest sign of the dominance of Galenic humoralism as the major explanatory model in the world of Islamic learning is its adoption by the later developing Medicine of the Prophet. The advantage of the four-humours theory was, as noted above, that on to it could be attached a cosmology – elements, seasons, ages of man, astrological signs. And yet this much-vaunted 'modularity' seems not to have determined actual therapy to anything like the extent we might have expected. What come to the fore in Savage-Smith's account are not the four humours, but the paired qualities of hot/cold and wet/dry, and the temperaments predicable on their various combinations, with respect to parts of the body as well as the whole. Even where humours do seem to have been involved, as with purging or bleeding, there could be no simple restoration of equilibrium since in the process all humours were evacuated simultaneously. Moreover, a person's natural temperament, in health, might be one in which a particular humour or quality predominated. There was no normal equilibrium. Balance does appear in Savage-Smith's analysis, but it is as likely to involve the ingredients of drugs or the comparison of the qualities of the illness with those of its proposed remedy. She offers a radical reappraisal of Islamic medicine – and by implication of humoralism elsewhere.

In Latin translations from the Arabic, this is the sort of medicine that created the scholastic medical culture of medieval Europe. That is where we move next with Peter Jones's chapter. Until the availability of these translations, and the development of first medical schools and then university medical faculties, early medieval medicine in Western Europe was only very loosely or residually humoral. The medicine of this early period – up to around AD 1100

– contrasts (so it is usually held) with the far more systematic and coherent learning of the later Middle Ages, a learning underpinned by Aristotelian philosophy. On the theoretical front it may have been so, although the extent of the contrast should not be overestimated (Horden 2011). But in clinical practice, humours tended to remain in the background throughout the Middle Ages, as Jones shows. Temperament or complexion once again mattered much more. Meanwhile, at the other pole from humoral – or complexional – theory stood the *experimentum*, experimental in a sense far removed from that of modern science. The *experimentum* worked, but no one knew why. It was relatively simple treatment, and might seem untypical; but such records of *experimenta* as we have could, as Jones argues, be a reliable guide to the generality of practice.

His findings echo those of other scholars, Savage-Smith included, who detect a separation between the elaborate procedures recommended by theoretical treatises and the far simpler treatments actually offered (see also Álvarez-Millán 2000). Through King's chapter, we see that this separation may go right back to the beginnings of literate medicine in antiquity. From Jones's contribution we learn that, especially in the wake of bubonic plague, the ultimate challenge to humoral medicine, practice seems only to have been weakly determined by humoralism. *Experimenta* trumped complexion. The 'occult sciences' such as alchemy and astrology also enjoyed new favour as a remedy was sought for this terrifying pandemic. Plague was poison, of the heart or the whole body. In other chapters we encounter pathological blockages of a healthy 'flux'. Here we see a desperate search for ways of obstructing the spread of a toxin. To poison there is the counterbalancing purity of the quintessence, of elixirs, of potable gold – or, in a homeopathic form, of the equipollent impurity of 'magical' medicine derived from excrement. In short, variety once more, as at the beginning, with the Hippocratics: variety where we might have expected the highest degree of unity provided by the consistent intellectual and institutional framework of scholastic medicine.

In the following chapter, by Guy Attewell, we turn eastwards to examine the long-term influence of Islamic medicine. This is the medical current of Yunani *tibb*, Greek medicine, but spread in its essentials to the Indian sub-continent with Islam. Claiming descent from Ibn Sina (d. 1037) and beyond him from Hippocrates and Galen, it is, nonetheless, as a developed medical system, an invention of the nineteenth century, not earlier. Humours, along with temperaments and concepts of excess, corruption and depletion are, Attewell notes, 'but one domain of a matrix of the so-called "foundational principles"'. Yet they dominate all descriptions of the history and practice of this medicine, and this is because of their perceived utility in defining and defending it. Just as humoral theory, fortified by Aristotelian philosophy, validated the status claimed by learned medieval Islamic and European physicians, so the humours of *tibb* could be deployed for broadly political purposes. The practice here is thus, in part, political. For Attewell, the key period is the turn of the twentieth century. Some practitioners of *tibb* (*hakims*) were criticizing these fundamentals just when others were leaning on them to establish themselves institutionally.[8] Practitioners debated not only among themselves, however. Through the later part of the twentieth century they engaged on one side with biomedicine, and with 'indigenous' practices such as Ayurveda on the other. In all this, humoral theory was not the immutable given that its proponents asserted, but a flexible construction, variously invoked in debate and polemic.

It had a history as such a construction. In the later nineteenth century, ideals of balance of equipoise chimed with an elite morality of moderation in comportment. (We shall see something similar in Hsu's chapter on ancient China.) That ideal came under pressure in the wake of the third pandemic of bubonic plague (that of the fourteenth century and later, brought into the reckoning by Jones, being the second). But the overall ideal of health was not necessarily framed in humoral terms, qualities proving just as significant; and the *hakims'* 'clinical' practice does not always seem to have reflected the so-called foundational principles. Indeed, in the case study presented by Attewell (Hakim Tabatabai of Lucknow) there is, once more, an 'experimental' emphasis on remedies that simply worked.

This second section of the collection closes with Ellen Messer's chapter. We are now at the other 'end' of the world. But her study of Mesoamerica can stand for a range of cultures not only in Latin America but in North Africa too. These are cultures in which the binary relation of hot and cold is the major element in diagnosis, therapy and everyday diet, and in which the continued adjustment of 'temperatures' has been seen as central. The hot/cold paradigm is typically considered a reduction of a more complex humoral system.

13

Yet we have seen from several chapters how variable and unsystematic the use of humours in medical discourse can be, and how qualities including hot and cold are in many cultures more important. So the degree and nature of the reduction is ripe for re-examination. Indeed, as Messer shows, consensus about many basic features of Mesoamerican 'hot/cold' systems is a long way off. How important is hot/cold in practice, as against, for instance, wet and dry or sweet and bitter? How far are classifications in particular domains such as eating or healing seen as fitting together into an overarching 'dual cosmovision'? What is the desired state of balance: neutral or on the hot or the cold side? Is this system indigenous, with a long history, or a Spanish colonial import?

Here we should note resonances with other chapters: engagement with biomedicine (as in Attewell), such that for example Alka Seltzer is 'hot'; the implications of a morality of moderation in ideas and practices of therapy (Attewell, Zimmermann, Hsu); magical or divine causation (Attewell, too, is at pains to stress that there is no inevitable secularizing tendency in the use of humoral or complexional theory); the aetiological role of emotions (here fright, leading to 'soul loss'; compare Hsu on anger), and finally hints of disjunction between 'reasoned knowledge' and practical 'action' (seen in the chapters by Savage-Smith, Jones, Bassini).

One aspect of Messer's chapter forms a particularly helpful link with its successor, by David Parkin: the indigenous as against the colonial. Parkin's chapter opens the next section, 'A Balance of What?', and shows how one particular tradition emanating from the north, the 'humoral' medicine of Islam, can fit into a pre-existing set of ideas about social and individual health and disease. Parkin's scope is nothing less than sub-Saharan Africa. He presents it not in simple terms of cultural unity or fragmentation but as an area of overlapping, interconnected traditions, a 'tangled skein'. In this entanglement 'many and perhaps most healing methods ... are premised on an idea of relational balance'. Healers of misfortune, which includes but is of course not restricted to sickness, have to decide, when diagnosing, whether an elemental imbalance is involved (humoral, or hot/cold), whether deviant social behaviour such as witchcraft has brought about an imbalance of a different kind, or whether congenital physical disorders have produced a 'natural imbalance'. In Parkin's chapter, importantly, we are mostly looking at therapeutic cultures which do not routinely depend on canonical texts, or indeed on literacy at all. The possible explanatory paradigms of social ills remain multiple, as do the forms of redress for them. Overall, in the tangled skein, body and cosmos need to be in, or to be restored to, harmony. Another telling image, by now familiar from earlier discussions, is that of blockage or entanglement, interruptions to crucial flows – to be countered by cooling, cleansing or the restoration of social inequality. Again, though, epidemic disaster may be seen as testing paradigms of explanation to their limits. In previous chapters it was bubonic plague; here it is AIDS.

For the remaining chapters in this section we return to Asia, and we start with anger. Anger has been mentioned in several chapters, along with other emotions that upset some type of appropriate relation between fundamentals and need to be treated as part of the treatment of bodily infirmities. And anger is the focus of Elisabeth Hsu's chapter on 'traditional' Chinese medicine, based on her own ethnography as well as the close reading of very early texts. Challenging the view that Asian medicine did not recognize emotions as direct causes of ill health, she tracks between the ancient and the modern, drawing inspiration en route from Elias's concept of the 'civilizing process' (Elias 1979, 1982). She posits in ancient China, first, a moralizing of anger – that is, the cultivation by elites of a 'morally appropriate emotionality' in which excess was socially unacceptable and recognized as pathogenic – and second, a medicalizing of anger, so that, in the canonical medical texts emotion came to be an integral part of hot/cold ethno-physiologies. The rebalancing sought after transgression/sickness was a balanced social interaction that had both medical and moral dimensions.

In Graeco-Roman medicine some of this would not be surprising. The Hippocratics did not medicalize the emotions in this way, but Galen did, so that when Galenism emerged carefully reshaped in Islamic translation, pathological emotions such as fear and beneficial emotions such as cheerfulness were fully registered as determinants of health (the misleadingly labelled 'non-naturals' referred to by Savage-Smith, Jones, and Attewell). 'For is not anger a sickness of the soul?' Galen had written, 'Or do you deny the sense of the ancients, who gave the name of "affections of the soul" to these five: grief, rage, anger, desire, and fear?'[9]

15

Next, we turn to Ayurveda. Here is indisputably one of the Great Traditions, a learned text-based medicine with fundamental constituents of the body in its theoretical armoury that have sometimes, unthinkingly, been translated as 'humours' (they are wind, bile and phlegm). How are these fundamentals related in health and sickness? Francis Zimmermann argues for the importance of interpreting the transactions between fundamentals in two distinct ways: on the one hand, there is proportionality of qualities and degrees, which is what is implied by classic humoral theory of the Hippocratic kind; on the other hand, the 'congruence' of opposed natures and qualities, the adequacy of their therapeutic fit with one another. This second interpretation is the one that comes to the fore in Zimmermann's discussion of his work with a learned healer in Kerala in the 1980s, a healer who was diagnosing and treating diseases due to wind (rheumatic disease, arthritis).

A generously synoptic view of this practice is essential. The land and its long-distance trade are held between them to generate medicines that display, to the initiated, a pre-established harmony with the illnesses they are used to treat. Once again there is a continuum from plants to humanity involved (as in the medicines surveyed by King and Messer). The whole person is treated: mind and speech as well as body. The body is full of imperceptible fluids – fluids in flux (hardly for the first time in the collection). Their state is inferred from the harmoniousness – or lack thereof – in the patient's gesture and discourse. Ill health is manifested in the signs of 'breaks, gaps, abrupt reversals' – not far, conceptually, from Duden's blocked German women or Parkin's entangled African sufferers. Hot and dry, cold and wet also come into play, condensed – but not reduced – into the polarity of bile and phlegm. Like Dr Storch, Zimmermann's Keralan teacher did not touch his patients; he listened to their narratives. His prescriptions aimed not at restoring an equilibrium so much as a congruence – between fundamental quasi-humours perhaps, but also between fundamental and medicament, and between individual and environment. The 'humours' of which he spoke are images, concepts or categories in a taxonomy of qualities and processes. In daily practice, Zimmermann concludes, the terms are 'devoid of any ontological implications'. They constitute simply a terminology.

It is worth bearing that conclusion in mind as we move finally, with Patrizia Bassini, to Tibet. Bassini frames her discussion with a tripartite

16

distinction. This is between: first, the textual paradigm of learned medicine, in this case the scholarly tradition that began in Tibet in the seventh century AD as a blend of medical currents from, largely, India and China; second, the narrative mode for representing suffering, which has already been encountered in several other chapters; and third, the practice of healing. Bassini reveals the imbalance of the learned Tibetan medicine practised in monasteries as a disorder in relations with the world of the divine. The narrative mode, by contrast, offers the hearer a story of perpetual unease, an emotional imbalance. The practice is one of endless rituals to ward off harms from evil forces in a capricious landscape. With all three modes, a connection is indeed discernible between individual, social order and environment. As in Ayurveda, health for the learned practitioner depends on the proper movement of such bodily constituents, as well as on the 'congruence' (to recall Zimmermann's term) of three 'humours'. But these three are also to be identified with the three fundamental Buddhist defilements of desire, anger and ignorance. When patients tell stories they link illness, especially 'heart distress', to their feelings about collective or personal events such as sedentarization or bereavement. And in Bassini's fieldwork they also find the cause of their ailments in offences committed with respect to the divine beings in the landscape. These offences have disrupted order and hierarchy (a balance of a kind) which has to be re-established through propitiatory rituals. We are a long way from canonical texts, which provide only one thread in a 'tangled' set of ideas.

In medieval Tibetan historiography, King Songtsen Gampo is said to have summoned physicians from across Asia to his court. One of them was called Galenos and he came from 'Byzantine lands'. The legend reflects the influence of Graeco-Islamic medical ideas on those of Tibet from the seventh century onwards (Meyer 1995: 110; Akasoy, Burnett and Yoeli-Tlalim 2010). We are also brought back to the nearly contemporaneous medicine of the late antique Mediterranean. To that extent, by closing in Tibet the collection comes full circle.

Fluids, even within the body, and certainly coming out of it, ought to be highly visible and intelligible – far more so than a physiology of organs. Claims have occasionally been made for the empirical basis of the classic humours such as phlegm. And yet it has become clear that there are no simple explanations in humoral history. The contributors examine a wide range of liquids in flux, only some of them properly called humours. Before the advent of the biomedical laboratory none of these could be measured at all exactly with respect to the classic ingredients of balance such as volume, weight or potency. The proportions could be inferred only from the imbalance which was the defining feature of ill health. Balance must therefore be an abstraction, partially detectible only in its opposite. And the balances we discuss are far more various than those bound up in 'humoral pathology'. In this volume, we question both the 'lumping' together of humoral medicines (Hippocratic, Ayurvedic and others) and the 'splitting' of oral and literate traditions. We question the role of even the classical humours in so-called humoral practice. And we find a range of balances, equivalences, congruences and proportional relationships to be in play across the history and ethnography of world medicine – emotional, physical, social, environmental – involving gods and witches as well as blood or wind, medicines and healers as well as patients. 'Humoral medicine in practice' *is* 'the body in balance'. There is no tighter way of defining it. But the body in balance depends on factors much more diverse than those encompassed by humoral medicine. What is balanced, and what balance means, admit no simple answer; rather, they are, like Parkin's sub-Saharan 'tangled skein', a novel way of comparing and classifying forms, ideas and methods of healing from right across the globe.[10]

Notes

Acknowledgements: for advice and references I am grateful to three anonymous referees, to Nicole Archambeau, William Crooke and Vivian Nutton, and not least to my co-editor, Elisabeth Hsu.

1. This passage comes from *The Nature of Man* 4, trans. Lloyd (1978: 262). In her chapter below, Helen King quotes a slightly different, more literal translation.
2. For 'medical systems', see Leslie (1976).
3. See Hsu's closing discussion, 'What Next?' (this volume).
4. Not coincidentally, this is the point at which, as Savage-Smith (this volume) notes, the term 'humoral pathology' was invented.
5. For Babylon, see Robson (2008) and Geller (2010). For Egypt, see King (this volume), n. 4.
6. Note that Stolberg (2011: 2, 127) takes a different view of the evidence and is less inclined to think that women's experiences are directly represented here.

7. For the controversial application of the term further west, see de Vries (2008).
8. Compare Jones's report of the critique of scholastic medicine launched by one of its *alumni*, Nicholas of Poland (Jones, this volume).
9. From Galen's treatise *On the Passions and Errors of the Soul* (Galen 1997: 110–11, with details of editions on xliii). For context see Harris (2001).
10. This could of course be extended in a number of directions. For example, the 'balances' involved in astrological medicine (e.g., Akasoy, Burnett and Yoeli-Tlalim 2008), or those in ritual practices of cultures not covered here, such as that of the Navaho (Milne and Howard 2000: 555, 565).

References

Akasoy, A., C. Burnett and R. Yoeli-Tlalim (eds). 2008. *Astro-Medicine: Astrology and Medicine, East and West*. Florence: SISMEL-Edizioni del Galluzzo.

——— (eds). 2010. *Islam and Tibet: Interactions along the Musk Routes*. Aldershot: Ashgate.

Alter, J. (ed.). 2005. *Asian Medicines and Globalization*. Philadelphia: University of Pennsylvania Press.

Álvarez-Millán, C. 2000. 'Practice versus Theory: Tenth-century Case Histories from the Islamic Middle East', in P. Horden and E. Savage-Smith (eds), *The Year 1000: Medical Practice at the End of the First Millennium* [*Social History of Medicine*, 13 (2000)]. Oxford: Oxford University Press, pp.293–306.

Bates, D. (ed.). 1995. *Knowledge and the Scholarly Medical Traditions*. Cambridge: Cambridge University Press.

de Vries, J. 2008. *The Industrious Revolution: Consumer Behaviour and Household Economy, 1650 to the Present*. Cambridge: Cambridge University Press.

Duden, B. 1991[1987]. *The Woman beneath the Skin: A Doctor's Patients in Eighteenth-century Germany*. Cambridge, MA: Harvard University Press.

Elias, N. 1979[1939]. *The Civilizing Process*, Vol. 1: *The History of Manners*. Oxford: Blackwell.

——— 1982[1939]. *The Civilizing Process*, Vol. 2: *State Formation and Civilization*. Oxford: Blackwell.

Flemming, R. 2000. *Medicine and the Making of Roman Women*. Oxford: Oxford University Press.

Foster, G. 1976. 'Disease Etiologies in Non-Western Medical Systems', *American Anthropologist* 78: 773–82.

Galen. 1997. *Selected Works*, ed. and trans. P.N. Singer. Oxford: Oxford University Press.

Geller, M.J. 2010. *Ancient Babylonian Medicine: Theory and Practice*. Oxford: Wiley-Blackwell.

Green, M.H. 2009. *Making Women's Medicine Masculine: The Rise of Male Authority in Pre-modern Gynaecology*. Oxford: Oxford University Press.

Harris, W.V. 2001. *Restraining Rage: The Ideology of Anger Control in Classical Antiquity*. Cambridge, MA: Harvard University Press.

Horden, P. 2011. 'What's Wrong with Early Medieval Medicine?' *Social History of Medicine* 24: 5–25.

Janzen, J.M., and E.C. Green. 2003. 'Continuity, Change and Challenge in African Medicine', in H. Selim (ed.), *Medicine Across Cultures*. Dordrecht: Kluwer, pp.1–26.

Jong-Chol, C. 1995. 'Kanpo: Japanese Herbal Medicine', in J. Van Alphen and A. Aris (eds), *Oriental Medicine*. Boston: Shambhala, pp.247–52.

Kuriyama, S. 1999. *The Expressiveness of the Body and the Divergence of Greek and Chinese Medicine*. New York: Zone Books.

Leslie, C. (ed.). 1976. *Asian Medical Systems: A Comparative Study*. Berkeley: University of California Press.

Lloyd, G.E.R. 1966. *Polarity and Analogy: Two Types of Argumentation in Early Greek Thought*. Cambridge: Cambridge University Press.

——— 1979. *Magic, Reason and Experience: Studies in the Origins and Development of Greek Science*. Cambridge: Cambridge University Press.

——— (ed.). 1978. *Hippocratic Writings*. Harmondsworth: Penguin.

Meyer, F. 1995. 'Theory and Practice of Tibetan Medicine', in J. Van Alphen and A. Aris (eds), *Oriental Medicine*. Boston: Shambhala, pp.109–42.

Milne, D., and W. Howard. 2000. 'Rethinking the Role of Diagnosis in Navajo Religious Healing', *Medical Anthropology Quarterly* 14(4): 543–70.

Nutton, V. 1993. 'Humoralism', in W.F. Bynum and R. Porter (eds), *Companion Encyclopedia of the History of Medicine*. London: Routledge, pp.281–91.

——— 2004. *Ancient Medicine*. London: Routledge.

Ohnuki-Tierney, E. 1984. *Illness and Culture in Contemporary Japan: An Anthropological View*. Cambridge: Cambridge University Press.

Önder, S.W. 2007. *We Have No Microbes Here: Healing Practices in a Turkish Black Sea Village*. Durham, NC: Carolina Academic Press.

Parkin, D. 1990. 'Eastern Africa: The View from the Office and the Voice from the Field', in R. Fardon (ed.), *Localizing Strategies: Regional Traditions of Ethnographic Writing*. Washington, DC: Smithsonian Institution Press, pp.182–203.

Pomata, G. 1998. *Contracting a Cure: Patients, Healers, and the Law in Early Modern Bologna*. Baltimore, MD: Johns Hopkins University Press.

Rankin, A. 2008. 'Duchess, Heal Thyself: Elisabeth of Rochlitz and the Patient's Perspective in Early Modern Germany,' *Bulletin of the History of Medicine* 82: 109–44.

Robson, E. 2008. 'Mesopotamian Medicine and Religion: Current Debates, New Perspectives', *Religion Compass* 2(4): 455–83.

Stewart, P.J., and A. Strathern (eds). 2001. *Humors and Substances: Ideas of the Body in New Guinea*. Westport, CT: Bergin and Garvey.

Stolberg, M. 2011[2003]. *Experiencing Illness and the Sick Body in Early Modern Europe*, trans. L. Unglaub and L. Kennedy. Basingstoke: Palgrave Macmillan.

Tecusan, M. 2004. *The Fragments of the Methodists*, Vol. 1. Leiden: Brill.

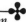

Wujastyk, D. (ed. and trans.). 2003. *The Roots of Ayurveda: Selections from Sanskrit Medical Writings*. London: Penguin.

Young, A. 1976. 'Internalizing and Externalizing Medical Belief Systems: An Ethiopian Example', *Social Science and Medicine* 10: 147–56.

Zucconi, L.M. 2007. 'Medicine and Religion in Ancient Egypt', *Religion Compass* 1(1): 26–37.

A Body of What?

Chapter 1

Female Fluids in the Hippocratic Corpus

How Solid was the Humoral Body?

Helen King

In this chapter I want to begin by setting out the current position in scholarship regarding humours in the Hippocratic corpus, although I will also refer to the later Graeco-Roman medicine that developed their use. I will concentrate on the classical world in the fifth and fourth centuries BC, demonstrating that, rather than a single humoral system being dominant, many different ideas about the body were in existence.[1] These often involved notions of hot and cold, wet and dry, and of health essentially as a matter of balance, with the fluids that left the body being used as a guide to events inside it; medical writers also reported patients' sensations of 'heaviness' or of 'gathering' within the body. However, explanations of disease and suggestions for treatment did not necessarily include humours, whether in the broader sense of 'fluids' or in the more specific sense of the 'four humours'. The Greek *ikmas*, humour, simply means moisture, and is something plants need to sprout; it is not, in origin, a medical term but instead relates to a widespread analogy between the human body and the world of plants, as does the other main word for a humour, the Greek *chumos*.[2] The second part of the chapter will examine the specific issues raised by the female body, looking at some case histories from Book 7 of the Hippocratic *Epidemics* in order to reflect on whether female patients would necessarily have shared male doctors' interpretations of the inside of their bodies.

Revisiting the 'Four Humours'

For the history of premodern European medicine more broadly, the established view that it was dominated by a humoral understanding of disease is increasingly being challenged. For example, Michael Stolberg (2011) has argued that, for early modern Europe, the humours formed only one aspect of the model of disease causation, and by no means the most important one. Although in this period patients would identify themselves by temperament – for example, as 'sanguine', dominated by blood – they did not always connect this to humours, regarding other factors such as their build, their strength, 'morbid matter' and bad air as equally important in causing disease.[3]

But what of the ancient world? While it is still widely assumed by those outside the field that the humours, and specifically, the 'four humours' – blood, phlegm, yellow bile and black bile – characterize 'the' Hippocratic model of the body, and thus represented the foundation of fifth- and fourth-century BC medicine, there is growing agreement amongst classical scholars themselves that the theory of the humours was a relatively late addition to ancient medicine. Vivian Nutton summarized the situation as follows: 'There was a variety of competing humoral theories, and competing humoral interpretations, not only in the fifth century B.C. but also for a considerable time to come in the Hellenistic and Roman worlds' (Nutton 2005: 19).

The four-humour model owes its power to its promotion by the great physician Galen, but, as Daniel Le Clerc realized even at the beginning of the eighteenth century, 'the rigidity of the four-humor system as Galen uses it is not characteristic of Hippocrates'.[4] It was when Galen made the deliberate choice to foreground the four humours, possibly basing this on what he was taught by some of his own teachers, but focusing on a single Hippocratic treatise in which they feature – *On the Nature of Man* – that this became more than one theory among many.[5] I will return to the Galenic reinforcement of a four-humour system later in this chapter.

While some Hippocratic medical treatises do mention blood, phlegm, yellow bile and black bile, many treatises ignore them and instead feature other fluids and other ways of accounting for disease and health. A casual reader of the modern literature on ancient medicine would not, however, realize that this variety existed.

For example, Antoine Thivel, noting 'the almost total absence of references to the humours in the most ancient authors', suggested that humoral theory came into existence only in the late fifth century BC (Thivel 1990: 281–82).[6] While he went on to condemn as 'lamentable' the still widespread idea that Hippocratic medicine consisted simply of *On the Nature of Man*'s four-humour theory, at the same time he continued to insist that 'Greek medicine is a humoral form of medicine; it is there that its originality lies' (Thivel 1990: 282–83). In his monumental work *Hippocrates*, Jacques Jouanna similarly noted, 'The one domain of Hippocratic physiology where the imagination of certain physicians succeeded in creating a system of perfect clarity, in order to account for an entirely obscure world, is that of the humors' (Jouanna 1999: 314).

These statements about humoral medicine, I think, remain too optimistic, despite their caveats; it appears that the power of Galen's insistence that Hippocratic medicine is based on the humours remains such that it is very difficult for modern scholars to abandon altogether humoral medicine as the dominant model. Nutton (2005: 117) has suggested that *On the Nature of Man* may be more properly seen as 'aberrant' in its humoralism, observing that the comments of Wesley Smith about how Galen 'looked for a Hippocrates in his own image' (Smith 1979: 50) have yet to be taken fully on board by scholars.[7]

Jouanna's reference to a 'system' raises the question of how frequently the humours appear as a 'system' in Hippocratic physiology; indeed, how far can we even think of a single 'Hippocratic physiology'? Even if we look at those Hippocratic treatises, such as *Epidemics* 1 and 3, that used to be linked directly to the 'Father of Medicine' in the days when it was still fashionable to try to identify the 'genuine works of Hippocrates' (Langholf 2004: 249; Mattern 2008: 29), humours are not found at the centre of the picture. Caterina Licciardi has noted that, in these two treatises, the humours feature in descriptions of patients' symptoms, with bilious or phlegmatic matter being present in discharges, but nevertheless 'the humours ... never played the role of causative agents' (Licciardi 1990: 328). In *Epidemics* 2, 4 and 6, regarded traditionally either as the work of Hippocrates' son Thessalus or as notes by the great man himself, phlegm and bile do appear as causes of disease, but blood does not, while in Books 5 and 7 of this collection, which appear to be the last to have been compiled and for whose Hippocratic authorship nobody has argued, bile (both yellow and black) features as a cause, but only in the first part of Book 5 (Licciardi 1990: 331–32, 334–35). These texts concentrate on describing the symptoms rather than speculating on causes.

In ancient Graeco-Roman medicine, the 'obscure world' of the body's interior, to which Jouanna refers, became known to the physician through observation of what came out of the body, leading to the belief that, inside as well as outside, fluids streamed through the channels, met occasional blockages, and were attracted to 'structures' (*schemata*).[8] These 'structures' are seen as largely secondary to fluids. The author of another Hippocratic treatise, *On Ancient Medicine*, puts it like this: some structures are hollow, 'some solid and round, some flat and suspended, some are stretched out, some large, some thick, some are porous and sponge-like'.[9] Those structures that are wide at one end and narrow at the other – such as the bladder, the skull and the womb – are best able 'to attract and absorb moisture from the rest of the body', 'and are always filled with fluid'. Other structures, 'such as the spleen, lungs and female breasts', are described in the same chapter as being 'spongy and of loose texture'; when these attract fluid, they become hard and, unlike the womb, are unable to discharge the excess gradually. To understand the body it is thus necessary to appreciate the nature of its fluids and of the structures which collect them. The Hippocratic treatise *On Humours* – which, despite its title, does not use the canonical four humours and gives a far wider range of explanations for disease – suggests that different fluids have 'preferred routes' out of the body: some are best removed downwards, some upwards; some should be washed out, others dried up.[10]

But just which fluids counted as 'humours' for an ancient Greek medical writer? Jacques Bos recently defined humoralism as 'the view that the human body is composed of a limited number of elementary fluids' (Bos 2009: 30). Certainly, reference is made to the body's fluids, and sometimes to there being four, in a number of treatises. But writers disagreed as to whether such fluids are naturally present in the body, only becoming dangerous if there is too much or too little of them, or whether they are intrinsically harmful substances made from blood. Galen, for example, discussed Plato's *Timaeus* in relation to the Hippocratic corpus in order to show that 'Hippocrates' scientific method was directly approved by Plato' (Lloyd 1991b: 407). While enlisting Plato in support of what he represents as the Hippocratic theory that humours are responsible for most diseases, Galen commented that Plato was wrong about the humours in that, unlike Hippocrates, he did not demonstrate that they are natural to the body.[11] This question of whether humours are natural parts of the healthy body, or only produced in disease, is addressed differently by the various treatises of the Hippocratic corpus. For example, *Places in Man* has been characterized by its most recent editor, Elizabeth Craik, as showing 'humoral theory ... at its most inchoate'. It shows most interest in moisture (linked to phlegm), with bile apparently arising 'from diseases, rather than diseases from bile (which would then always be present to some degree, at least in some people)' (Craik 1998: 14).

Writers also disagreed on how many humours there were. Some Hippocratic treatises ignore humours in favour of elements, or have humours but not four of them. So the treatise *Regimen* operates with two elements, fire and water, with the human body in flux between the two, while in *Affections, Diseases* 1, and *Airs, Waters, Places,* fluids are the constituent parts, but only two fluids are named: bile and phlegm. The lost works of other writers of the Hippocratic period, which did not find their way into the Hippocratic corpus, are only known to us from summaries in the papyrus known as *Anonymus Londinensis*, dating from the second century AD but discovered only at the end of the nineteenth century and thought to derive from the work of a pupil of Aristotle.[12] Four-humour theories may owe their origin to an attempt to incorporate the four elements of the philosopher Empedocles (Thivel 1990: 283), but in this papyrus we can find further variations: the three-humour theory of Philolaus of Croton (blood, bile and phlegm) and another three-humour theory linked with Thrasymachus of Sardis (bile, phlegm and pus) (Nutton 2004: 80). Philolaus regarded the three humours not as constituent parts of the body but as the result of changes within it.[13] The fourth-century BC physician Diocles of Carystus named four humours (blood, phlegm, bile and black bile) which came from the food consumed and were then affected by heat to make the different substances (van der Eijk 2001, fr. 27, 40). In the Hippocratic *On Generation/On the Nature of the Child* and the related *Diseases* 4, an alternative four-humour theory is found, with each of the four being linked to an organ: blood (heart), phlegm (head), water (spleen) and bile (a receptacle on the liver).[14] According to Galen in *On the Natural Faculties* 2.9 (Loeb 216–18), Praxagoras had a ten- or, as he did not include blood in his list of ten, even eleven-humour theory (Steckerl 1958, fr. 21; Smith 1979: 188; Nutton 2005: 118). Finally, there are also fluids other than humours which play a very important role in ancient medicine, including urine, sweat, mucus, milk, tears and semen.

But it is in only one of the sixty or so 'Hippocratic' texts – *On the Nature of Man*, thought to date to the late fifth century BC – that the specific 'canonical' four of blood, phlegm, black bile and yellow bile are named, and here they are seen as intrinsic to the body rather than as the products of disease. In anthropological terms, the colours could be seen as significant, Berlin and Kay (1969) having argued in a controversial book that if the colour field is divided into four then these four will be black, white, red and either green or yellow. *On the Nature of Man* states that:

> The body of man has in itself blood, phlegm, yellow bile and black bile; these make up the nature of his body, and through these he feels pain or enjoys health. Now he enjoys the most perfect health when these elements are duly proportioned to one another in respect of compounding, power and bulk, and when they are perfectly mingled. Pain is felt when one of these elements is in defect or excess, or is isolated in the body without being compounded with all the others. (*Nature of Man* 4, trans. Loeb 4.11–13)

Actually, a better translation of the Greek of the first sentence would be, 'The human body has in itself blood and phlegm and bile, yellow and black'; this more literal translation makes the point that, even here, this is not entirely a four-humour theory but more like a three-humour theory with a later subdivision added on. But the writer of this treatise (or of this section of it, as it was recognized even before Galen as being a composite work) then goes on to link the humours to ever more 'fours': the four seasons, four elements and four qualities, so that in winter it is the cold and wet phlegm that dominates the body, while in spring it is the hot and wet blood, and so on (*Nature of Man* 7, Loeb 4.18–22).[15] In winter, it is diseases in which phlegm plays a crucial role that are most common; in spring, it is the blood-based conditions such as nosebleeds and dysentery. In the treatise *On Humours* a similar seasonality appears, but there are different causative factors: 'Droughts accompany both south winds and north winds. Winds cause differences – and this too is important – in all other respects also. For humours vary in strength according to season and district; summer, for instance, produces bile; spring, blood, and so on in each case' (*On Humours* 14, Loeb 4.89).

In *On the Nature of Man*, the humours are all present in every body, all year round: 'so long as a man lives he manifestly has all these elements always in him; then he is born out of a human being [*anthrôpos*] having all these elements, and is nursed in a human being having them all' (*Nature of Man* 5, Loeb 4.15). However, 'as the year goes round they become now greater and now less, each in turn and according to its nature' (*Nature of Man* 7, Loeb 4.21–22). Here, the humours are intrinsic to the body, but health is not a simple balance; the levels depend on the seasons of the year, so that what is a normal amount of blood in the spring would be regarded as an excess of blood in the winter. Furthermore, in terms of the practical medical application of the humours, 'if you give the same person to drink the same drug four times in the year, you will find that he vomits the most phlegmatic matter in the winter, the moistest in the spring, the most bilious in the summer and the blackest in the autumn' (*Nature of Man* 7, Loeb 4.22). This seems to envisage a multipurpose purge: one drug, four results. Interestingly, here there is not a simple match between humours and qualities – it is the most phlegmatic/most bilious, but then the most moist (rather than the most bloody) in the spring and the blackest (rather than the most 'black-bilious') in the autumn. But it is only in this one treatise, out of sixty or so, that this fairly developed picture of the familiar four humours occurs.

If we look outside the medical texts of the Hippocratic corpus we can find further evidence for multiple models of the humours in fifth-century BC Greece. The famous account by the historian Thucydides of the plague of Athens, which affected Greece in 431/430 BC, provides a complementary lay view. In his extensive list of the symptoms that were experienced in all parts of the body, Thucydides mentions the production of 'every kind of bile named by the doctors' – not of 'both kinds of bile', which would perhaps suggest the four-humour model with its two 'biles' – but 'every kind', suggesting perhaps that the historian was most familiar with a multi-bile model, or alternatively that he was aware that different medical practitioners functioned with different lists of the bilious options (*Peloponnesian War* 2.49.3). For example, the treatise *Regimen in Acute Diseases* distinguishes between 'black bile' and 'bitter bile': 'the sharpness obtained from vinegar is more beneficial to those with bitter bile than those with black bile because it dissolves bitter substances, turns them into phlegm and fetches them up. Black bile is lightened, brought up and diluted, for vinegar brings up black bile' (*Regimen in Acute Diseases* 61, Loeb 2.116).[16]

Here, it is worth noting, bile can be transformed into phlegm; the humours are not represented as fixed entities, but as mutable. In *Timaeus*, Plato also refers to 'all sorts of bile and serum and phlegm' in the body, and argues that 'some physician perhaps, or rather some philosopher, who had the power of seeing in many dissimilar things one nature deserving of a name', was responsible for applying the label 'bile' to several different substances (*Timaeus* 85c). He suggests that different kinds of bile are 'distinguished by their colours', mentioning black, greenish and reddish 'biles' to which certain physicians have given the common name of *cholê* (*Timaeus* 83c1–2). For Plato, Harold Miller argued, 'As humors originating *para physin* [against nature], phlegm and bile have no natural function in the structures and processes of the body' (Miller 1962: 185). The different kinds of bile are all present in blood only as the result of corruption in the body reversing the process of the formation of flesh; in *Timaeus* 83e, Plato describes all the types of bile, serum and phlegm as 'agents' (*organa*) of disease (Miller 1962: 181).

The origins of the terms for the canonical four humours have been the subject of much scholarly debate. As Jouanna has pointed out, the Greek *phlegma* originally meant not a cold wet substance but its reverse: fire, with the verb *phlegein* meaning 'to blaze'. In Philolaus, for example, according to the writer of *Anonymus Londinensis* (18.41–44; Jones 1947: 72–74), phlegm is 'hot'. In *On the Natural Faculties*, Galen says something similar about Prodicus, who used the term phlegm for a burned and roasted humour, and called the white substance which others named 'phlegm' instead *blenna* (2.9, Loeb 200–202). Jouanna suggests that the word *phlegma* was originally used in medical contexts for inflammation, and then shifted to become 'a humor resulting from inflammation', although the original sense can also be found in some Hippocratic treatises (Jouanna 1999: 315; see also Craik 1998: 16; Nutton 2004: 79). In common with writers throughout antiquity, Plato regarded bile, not phlegm, as the source of 'burning' diseases; it was commonly believed that black bile, thrown on the earth, would produce fermentation. Moreover, it has been noted by scholars that black bile appears to be the new kid on the block; it does not appear as a separate humour in earlier medical texts. Indeed, although *On the Nature of Man* offers us a four-humour model, the first three chapters of the treatise only talk about blood, phlegm and 'bile'. As we have already seen, in *On the Nature of Man* 4, the two types of 'bile, yellow and black' appear as subdivisions of this 'bile'. In one later reference in the same treatise, we even find 'the *so-called* black bile' (*Nature of Man* 7, Loeb 4.22). Nutton has argued that black bile was originally seen as a degenerate form of a single, simple 'bile', which turned black in certain medical conditions.[17] Galen, who towards the end of his life wrote an entire treatise *On Black Bile*, preserves in his *On the Natural Faculties* fragments of Diocles of Carystus, who drew an analogy with the process of wine fermentation, suggesting that yellow bile was like the lighter residue of this process, black bile like the heavier; but he also suggested that black bile had both a natural state and a corrosive state in which it was 'sharp like vinegar'.[18] In *On the Nature of Man*, the constituents of the human body are always the same 'according to both convention and nature' (*nomos* and *physis*), but the names of the constituents are 'separated, according to convention' (*Nature of Man* 5, Loeb 4.12). While their names are 'conventional', their forms are different in terms of their nature (*physis*), their colour, and their 'feel to the hand'. There is a real difference, but what we call them is simply a convention.

The value of the four-humour model in the form in which it appears in *On the Nature of Man* is that it is a very powerful image, linking microcosm and macrocosm, as the seasons affect the relative amounts of the fluids in the human body. The author of the first part of *On the Nature of Man* was not writing in a vacuum but explicitly arguing against another theory found in ancient Greek philosophical writers, that of monism, in which everything in the body is made from a single element such as air, earth, fire or water (associated for example with Anaximenes), or a single fluid; he opens the treatise with the polemical statement, 'I do not say at all that a man is air, or fire, or water, or earth, or anything else that is not an obvious constituent of a man' (*Nature of Man* 1, Loeb 4.2), and later he states his opposition to 'those who assert that man is composed of *a single* element' (*Nature of Man* 6, Loeb 4.14). He notes that among medical writers – as opposed to philosophers, who also discuss this topic – 'some say that a man is blood, others that he is bile, a few that he is phlegm' (*Nature of Man* 2, Loeb 4.4). Such people – like the writer himself, actually – base their theories on observation. 'They see those who drink drugs and die through excess purgings, vomiting in some cases bile, in others phlegm; then they think that the man is composed of that one thing from the purging of which they saw him die' (*Nature of Man* 6, Loeb 4.16). Geoffrey Lloyd (1995: 33–34) has argued that the author of *On the Nature of Man* wants to play up strongly the differences between the fluids of the body, in their names, their colours, their tangible qualities and their forms, specifically in order to make clear his opposition to monism (see *Nature of Man* 5, Loeb 4.12–14).

The reason why the four humours became so powerful in Western medicine was, as noted already, that Galen, writing towards the end of his long career (about AD 189), chose to elevate the section on humours in *On the Nature of Man* to the status of a 'genuine work of Hippocrates' when writing his commentary on it. For Galen, the first part of *On the Nature of Man* 'contains, as it were, the foundation of the whole Hippocratic science'.[19] Volker Langholf has pointed out that Galen wrote a treatise – now lost – concerning the claim 'that Hippocrates holds in all his other treatises the same doctrine as that in *De natura hominis*' (Langholf 2004: 245). Galen not only used, but also developed in far more detail, this four-humour model, and his version of the four humours was then taken up by Arabic medicine.[20] However, there is no reason to argue that *On the Nature of Man* is any closer to the historical Hippocrates than is any other part of the Hippocratic corpus. The treatise as a whole clearly combines three previously separate texts, and in the second part (Chapters 9 to 15) we find a passage on the channels through which blood moves (*Nature of Man* 11, Loeb 4.30–32). This passage was attributed by Aristotle to Polybus, Hippocrates' son-in-law, but he is the only person of that period who thought this.[21] Galen, in contrast, attributed not the second but the third part (on regimen, Chapters 16 to 23, a section in which only phlegm and an undifferentiated 'bile' feature) to Polybus. For Galen, the central section – with which he disagreed completely – was written by a late writer who padded out an earlier work in order to sell it to a library for a higher price.[22] But the first part (Chapters 1 to 8), a speech where the four humours appear, Galen ties to Hippocrates himself. This is a perfect example of how much earlier writers tried to link these anonymous texts to named individuals.

It was only in Galenism, the version of Galen's many theories that developed after his death, that the four humours were tied tightly not just to the four seasons, four elements, four qualities and four types of fevers, but also to the four temperaments, four points of the compass, four ages of man and, by the Middle Ages, even the four evangelists. Important here was Galen's treatise *On Black Bile*, which – like Plato in the *Timaeus* – gives 'biles' of other colours and describes many non-humoral fluids in addition to variations on the canonical four.[23] For example, yellow bile is described as 'not always yellow' but sometimes cream, sometimes the colour of egg yolk. There are also leek-green fluid and 'woad-like' fluid (*On Black Bile* 5, CMG V 4,1,1,79–82). Like the author of the pseudo-Aristotelian *Problems* (probably third-century BC), Galen also argues for two kinds of 'black bile' – a good type and a bad type; the bad type involves seething and fermentation (*On the Natural Faculties* 2.9, Loeb 212). The *Problems* noted that that the temperature of the bile changed its effects on the body. If there was too much of it, but it was neither too hot nor too cold, then the individual would 'tend to excel in education, art and politics' (*Problems* 30.1, 954a11–b3, Loeb 2.160–62; Bos 2009: 35). Even in Galen, then, there is far more going on in terms of the fluids of the body than simply four humours.

What Does Four-humour Theory Mean for Therapy?

In *On the Nature of Man*, as we have already seen, it is assumed that each humour must be present in the body – 'he enjoys the most perfect health when these elements are duly proportioned to one another in respect of compounding, power and bulk, and when they are perfectly mingled' – but that the relative proportions at any one time depend on other factors, most notably the seasons. Furthermore, as well as making the point about one drug producing four results according to the time of year when the drug is administered, the writer states that any of the four humours can be 'evacuated' by giving a single relevant remedy, the remedy for blood being not a drug but an incision:

> If you were to give a man a medicine which withdraws phlegm, he will vomit you phlegm; if you give him one which withdraws [yellow] bile, he will vomit you [yellow] bile. Similarly too black bile is purged away if you give a medicine which withdraws black bile. And if you wound a man's body so as to cause a wound, blood will flow from him. (*Nature of Man* 5, Loeb 4.14)

But, the writer says in the following chapter, it is actually more complicated than this. If you give someone a drug to withdraw phlegm, then he will start by vomiting phlegm but then go on to vomit yellow bile, then black bile, and finally blood (at which stage he will die). This is because the drug, as it enters into the body, will start by working on the fluid closest to its own *physis* ('nature'), but will then work on the other fluids. This is, therefore, a complicated picture, with some drugs targeting just one humour and others evacuating whatever is seasonally dominant, but it also contains the belief that the fluids are sufficiently related that one drug can move through all four of them. In *Places in Man*, with its interest only in bile and phlegm, therapy is used to moisten the body by producing more phlegm, or drying it by expelling fluid (Craik 1998: 17).

Therapy by drugs was recognized by ancient medicine as being difficult to achieve; hence the greater interest in dietary manipulation to control the production of fluids in the body.[24] In the Hippocratic treatise *Affections*, drug handbooks are mentioned in passing, apparently arranged by type of action, so that 'warming drugs' and 'cooling drugs' would have their own sections.[25] A theme running through medical discussions of drugs to stimulate sexual performance, in particular, is their danger. Chris Faraone has argued that love potions carried two different risks for men: while the increase in desire could lessen a man's self-control, the plants that could arouse this desire were also believed to cause permanent impotence if given at the wrong dosage (Faraone 1992: 100–1). Lay people were as familiar as doctors with the risks inherent in the variable effects of the substances they applied to the body, depending on dosage; for example, the Hippocratic writer of *Places in Man* was well aware that *mandragoras* – used in love potions – is antispasmodic in a small dose, cures insomnia in a moderate dose, but leads to delirium in a larger dose, and also that the line between small and large is not easy to recognize (e.g. *Places in Man* 39, Loeb 8.78). Faraone cites the mistress of Philoneus' error, described in Antiphon 1, *Against the Stepmother* (19; Loeb *Minor Attic Orators* 1.8): she gave her man a love potion but put in a little more of the drug in order to make him love her more, thus inadvertently killing the object of her desire.[26] Nor were love potions the only area in which drugs should be treated with caution. In a Hippocratic case history, Scamandros of Larissa took two doses of a purgative; his story ends: 'Having drunk the saturated drug again at evening, he died at sunrise. It seemed that he would have survived longer if not for the strength of the medicine' (*Epidemics* 5.15, Loeb 7.166). The writer of *Epidemics* 7.38 (Loeb 7.340) appears to be blaming a drug for producing the tetanus which killed a patient and, in a section of *Epidemics* 5, cases in which patients take a purgative and then die are grouped together.[27]

As I have already noted, humours were by no means the only fluids within the ancient body mentioned by Hippocratic writers, and treatment would be aimed at moving these as well. Sweat, for example, features in the appendix to *On Regimen in Acute Diseases* which states that 'all diseases are resolved through either the mouth, the cavity or the bladder; sweating is a form of resolution common to them all' (Appendix, 39, Loeb 6.303). Mucus (*myxa*) is another important fluid, and the term is applied to the fluids in the joints in *Places in Man* 9 (Craik 1998: 127–30; 2002).

A further fluid identified as having considerable medical importance was semen, and it is instructive to look at how far medicine delivered therapy for sexual disorders by means of controlling the production of sexual or other fluids. The line between 'food' and 'drug' is impossible to draw in ancient texts; in some circumstances one could argue that what separates them is the intention behind their use, but in the case of sexual prescriptions doctors simply used what was already believed about different foods, although sometimes delivering the substance by means other than the diet (King 1995: 355–56). In addition to charms and spells being used to affect potency, a number of foodstuffs were believed to have an effect on sexual desire, the fluids of the foodstuffs clearly being significant in choosing which to use. A Lydian gourmet sauce called *kandaulos* was described in a fragment of Menander as *hypobinetionta bromata*, literally 'food that makes one somewhat desirous of a screw' (Harvey 1995: 277). Certain foods were believed to increase desire in a man, including bulbs and particular herbs; some were equally thought to have effects on women.[28] Aphrodisiac and antaphrodisiac were very close and could even be found in the same plant; thus the *orchis* was thought to have two roots, one large and aphrodisiac, the other small and having the reverse effect.[29] Athenaeus, citing Heracleides of Tarentum, states that bulbs, snails and eggs 'produce semen, not because they are filling, but because their very nature in the first instance has powers related in kind to semen' (Athenaeus, *Sophists at Dinner* 2.64a–b), presumably a reference to the sticky fluids they contain or can produce.

However, not all ancient medical intervention into sexual disorders or reproductive medicine took the form of altering the fluids in the body. Simple mechanical procedures were also common. Objects shaped like a penis, such as worms, cucumbers (of the squirting kind) and horns are commonly used in ancient treatments for women. For example, in a treatment for a woman who has lost her ability to conceive, given in a section of *On Barren Women* (222, Littré 8.430–32), the dry gourd used after a series of injections into the womb is explicitly 'just a little smaller than the male organ' (*andros aidoion*) and the woman 'sits herself on the glans [*balanos*, literally 'acorn'] of the gourd'.[30] Here, something other than humours lies behind the recommendations, and this use of mechanical methods is widespread in Hippocratic medicine.

Remedies to assist conception raise the question of whether women have humours in the same way that men do. *On the Nature of Man*, the origin of the four-humour theory, would suggest an affirmative answer, although there is no explicit reference to women in this treatise, only the comment that any individual 'is born out of a human being [*anthrôpos*] having all these elements, and is nursed in a human being having them all' (*Nature of Man* 5). In another part of the Hippocratic corpus, the *Diseases of Women* treatises, to which I will now turn, the female body is presented as wet and spongy, dominated by blood, and it is rare that other humoral fluids are even mentioned; this is indeed a 'body of fluids' rather than a 'body of organs', and it is even a 'body of blood' (King 1998). The collections of case histories known as the *Epidemics* appear to share much the same model (Hanson 1989). For women of childbearing age, the ideal is to bleed every month, and to lose a considerable amount of blood; only in this way can a woman's health be preserved. Women are naturally in flux, with blood being produced, collected and poured out. The production of blood is also seen as essential if a woman is to be able to manufacture a child, as it forms the raw material for this production. In these treatises, in contrast to other ancient medical texts, it is unusual that blood-letting is practised, perhaps because the aim is to restore women's natural menstrual bleeding, but also because a reduction in blood production, by control of the patient's regimen, may be seen as sufficient.

Menstrual blood, while being 'blood' (that is, normal blood rather than some malign variant), could contain other humours.[31] Part of the final chapter of *Places in Man*, in which women are considered separately, notes that normal menstrual flow starts off as 'full of blood', but 'when it comes less heavily it contains pus-like substance. In younger women the flow is more full of blood, whereas older women have more mucus-like menstrual flow, as it is called' (*Places in Man* 47, Loeb 7. 100; trans. Craik 1998: 89). Here, pus and mucus are not actually present, but the substances in the blood resemble them. In addition to these normal variations, for which no treatment is necessary, a patient can have an unhealthy amount of another fluid in her menstrual blood. In one instance in *Diseases of Women*, the physician is instructed to see which humoral fluids can be extracted from the menstrual rags. In *Diseases of Women* 1.11 (Littré 8.44–6) a patient is described as having 'phlegmatic' menses, and is treated with a drying diet, exercise, vapour baths, emetics and purgative pessaries. This appears to suggest that the concept of phlegm as 'wet' is accepted here; the answer is to use up the wetness and make sure no more is produced. Women patients in the *Epidemics* collections of case histories produce bile in gynaecological contexts – as in the case of a stout woman who took a purgative in order to conceive (apparently deciding on her own initiative, or on that of a midwife, that she was not conceiving because she was 'too wet'), then had 'twisting in the intestines and swelled up', and survived after passing 'much bile below' (*Epidemics* 5.42, Loeb 7.184). So, rather than phlegm, she produced bile, perhaps because her self-diagnosis was wrong, and she had identified the wrong humour as the excessive one, or perhaps suggesting that the writer of this section believes that humours can transform into each other. A female slave treated in *Epidemics* 5.35 (Loeb 7.182) was purged and produced a little bile 'up' and a lot 'down'. Like the stout woman in 5.42, she had taken a purgative drink, a *katapoton*, but here the purpose is not stated.

According to the beliefs common to *Diseases of Women* and *Epidemics*, then, women are dominated by blood, but also contain bile and phlegm, and substances that resemble pus and mucus. This is a body of fluids, but not precisely a body of humours.

Treating the Wife of Theodoros

In this final section I want to develop these comments on women, humours and Hippocratic medical practice by turning to a single case history of a female patient with fever from the *Epidemics* (7.25), and asking how helpful humoral theory is in understanding it. In the process of analysing this case I will raise a number of questions concerning our reading of the Hippocratic corpus; for example, while at some points I shall be using other case histories from the same treatise to develop my analysis, I shall also look to other treatises, thus assuming that we can use one treatise to illuminate our understanding of another. But I am also aware that this procedure can be a dangerous one, perhaps assuming a continuity that is not there. Is it possible to hear the voices of patients, and to discover whether their views of their bodies differed from the theories put forward by doctors? Is there any evidence for patients functioning with a non-humoral model of their bodies?

The most recent editor of *Epidemics* 6, Wesley Smith, characterized the *Epidemics* collections as 'technical prose from the time when prose was coming into being and authors were realizing its potential; unique jottings by medical people in the process of creating the science of medicine' (Smith 1994: 2). While some books of the seven that make up *Epidemics* have brief case histories, sometimes arranged entirely by the days of the illness, books 5 and 7 are unusual in the high level of detail they give. This makes them, superficially, more accessible to the modern reader, but they are not as easy to read as generations of eager physicians, anxious to flex their diagnostic powers, have thought. Sometimes the symptoms make no apparent sense either in our system or in theirs – for example, when a man in Abdera passes 'things like lizards' (*Epidemics* 4.56, Loeb 4.148), or an account of how, when the womb moves to touch the hip joints, there are 'something like spheres/balls' in the stomach (*Places in Man* 47, Loeb 8.96). In such cases, it is difficult to know whether we are getting a patient's view of the symptoms or whether we simply do not understand the text (which of course may be corrupt).

In the case the wife of Theodoros from *Epidemics* 7.25 (Loeb 7.326–30), we have an exceptionally vivid account that appears to include patient input, and which ends with her death. The *Epidemics* 7 deathbed is a place of 'much wet, gushing, foul-smelling excrement' (7.88) and pus, also characterized by an 'overwhelming smell' (7.5).[32] But, although there may be little he can do to help, it is still the domain of the Hippocratic physician, whose presence can sometimes be detected from his incidental remarks: 'there was redness in the cheek as he was approaching the end' (*Epidemics* 7.5, Loeb 7.306), 'Sweat about the feet and legs as she was dying' (*Epidemics* 7.41, Loeb 7.344), 'Very alert looks, until the final moments' (*Epidemics* 7.7, Loeb 7.310), or 'His feet grew cold, there was heat more at the temples and the head as the end was imminent ... All signs were bad. He said he wanted something under him, stared fixedly, resisted a brief time, and died' (*Epidemics* 7.10, Loeb 7.314). The end of one case history suggests that the doctor does not just sit and watch: 'In the last period the patient could hardly perceive a touch on his feet' (*Epidemics* 7.5, Loeb 7.306).

Over the course of her last seven days, we have a sense of how the final symptoms of the wife of Theodoros were perceived by those witnessing her death. When she is delirious, she sometimes conducts herself rationally (*emphronôs*) but often does not. Delirium is disturbing to those witnessing it, and in other passages of the *Epidemics* it can be described as *kosmôs*, translated by Wesley Smith as 'in a decorous way' or 'inoffensively'.[33] Her fever followed a haemorrhage; there is nothing to indicate whether this was *post partum*, but it is more likely to refer to naturally occurring blood loss than to blood-letting, simply because blood-letting on female patients is very unusual in the Hippocratic texts (although later strongly recommended by Galen; see King 2002).

Is there anything humoral in this account? The writer notes at the outset that the case occurred in winter, so a humorally minded reader would assume that this means the cold wet humour of phlegm is dominant. Fevers, according to *On the Nature of Man* 15 (Loeb 4.38), mostly come from (yellow) bile. If we take these two texts

together, thus privileging *On the Nature of Man* in the same way
as Galen did, we could see this as a woman with fever in winter,
thus dominated by the hot and the dry, in a season when the cold
and the wet prevail; this could be seen as making this a particularly
dramatic and worrying fever. After the fever leaves, she has a new
symptom, 'heaviness of the right side, as from the womb'; it is not
immediately clear whether this is her gloss or that of the writer, noted
as a provisional diagnosis. But we are then told it was 'the first time
it had happened', which I take to mean that the interpretation of a
uterine origin is made by the doctor. If the woman patient has never
had the feeling before, how would she know it was 'from the womb'?
A further possibility is that she is describing the (new) sensation in
her right side in terms of the (familiar) sensations she already knows
in her womb.

Chest symptoms then become the focus; the pain there is 'terrible'
(*deinê*). She is treated with fomentations – applications direct to the
affected part – but there is no further treatment mentioned until a
suppository on the third day. Although largely in chronological order
over the seven days of the illness, the account sometimes jumps
around; delirious talking on the fifth day towards night is mentioned
twice. Her own voice comes through in the wording 'it seemed to her'
(*edokei autêi*) that the fire or fever was less, but this is contrasted
with the healer's own interpretation based on observing the blood
vessels at her temples, her rapid breathing and her delirious talking.[34]
In general, while she is relying on her feelings, at least until she
falls into a coma, the physician appears to be reading her condition
from hearing (her trachea whistled; her talking), vision (white
tongue; yellow whites of the eyes), what comes out (expectoration,
excrement, much sweat; bloody urine, urine like semen), taste
(astringent urine 'like fig juice'), and touch (hands like ice; swelling
of the right hypochondrium; soft belly).[35] In contrast to many case
histories in the *Epidemics*, we are given a sense of the patient's social
context within the rest of the household; she 'threatened her child
irrationally',[36] and she 'sat up and rebuked' those present.[37]

Jouanna, in his analysis of this very full (and thus, as I have
already noted, atypical) case history, has linked it to another
Hippocratic text, *Prognostics*, noting that the case history mentions
several features listed as 'bad' in the latter treatise; for example, that
the patient lies on her back and has difficulty turning over, that she

sleeps with her eyes open, and that her sweat is cold (Jouanna 1999: 305–7). He thus suggests that the case history assumes knowledge of the principles outlined in *Prognostics*; anyone familiar with these principles would see how the physician has identified the signs of a fatal outcome from an early stage. However, it is far from clear how far one should read one Hippocratic text in the light of another, especially since dating is so uncertain.

I would argue that humoral theory does little to help us understand this case from either the doctor's or the patient's point of view. There are certainly fluids in the story – a great deal of sweat, and also several kinds of urine – but no mention of blood beyond the initial haemorrhage, and no bile or phlegm at all. Hot and cold feature far more prominently, as there is burning heat as well as icy sweat. There is heaviness on the second day, and then 'greater heaviness' on the sixth day. Whereas the fluids and the temperature are accessible to both doctor and patient, the heaviness seems to be something felt by the patient and articulated to the doctor. However, even this cannot be certain, as on the sixth day the patient was delirious and therefore may not have been able to communicate her sensations to the doctor. It is noteworthy how little treatment there is in this whole case history; this could be due either to the literary genre of the Hippocratic case history, which rarely gives detailed remedies, or to an early decision by the doctor that this patient was going to die, and so remedies would have no value and may even lead to him being accused of causing her death.

But this particular case history raises a further question. The comment 'it seemed to her' (*edokei autêi*) inserted into the doctor's narrative makes the reader wonder how far the women patients of Hippocratic doctors shared their models of the female body with those treating them. In *Epidemics* 7.25, of course, the woman patient's view is contradicted by the doctor; she feels that the burning is less, but in fact it is not. In the scholarship on ancient gynaecology, Paola Manuli (1980, 1983) most famously described Hippocratic theories about women's bodies as 'hygienic terrorism', while Aline Rousselle (1980) suggested that the material in the gynaecological texts was essentially women's lore, taken over by male physicians. Where it is a woman's *kyrios*, her father or husband, who summons and pays the physician, it is above all he who needs to feel that the explanation offered for her condition makes sense: but, if she is to be healed by the encounter, then she too needs to believe what is said. The remedies offered by all healers, whether female or male, equally relied on theories intended to account for women's symptoms, such as the theory that the womb was too dry and had risen up the body in search of moisture. If the patient did not believe in the theory, she would have no encouragement to follow the regimen offered as a cure. Rather than seeing theories of the nature of woman and remedies to treat their diseases as either women's or men's knowledge, a third option is thus probably nearer the truth; namely, that the image of women presented in these texts was one that both men and women would recognize and accept, while both sexes had knowledge of, and access to, the plant substances used to treat sexual diseases. As Lesley Dean-Jones put it, the Hippocratic treatment of women 'must have been acceptable to them and have squared with their view of their own physiology' (Dean-Jones 1994: 27).

Readers familiar with Barbara Duden's work on the patients of Johann Storch in eighteenth-century Germany (Duden 1991, this volume) may wonder if *Epidemics* 7.25 is a text that provides access to women who were aware of the movement of humours within their bodies, and who were encouraged by their physicians to describe this to them. However, Michael Stolberg (2011: 2) has pointed out that even sources as apparently promising as these are mediated through the physician: Storch may only be telling us what women felt if it made sense within his own terms of understanding. This relates to a wider issue in the history of medicine: To what extent is it possible to discuss 'patients' from the past? In a valuable article, Flurin Condrau analysed the move in the social history of medicine to 'the patient's point of view' and examined the argument that case histories show us the doctor's construction rather than that of the patient (Condrau 2007: 529). He suggested that it may in fact only be in sources other than case histories that we can hear the patient's voice. It is relevant here to consider Alisha Rankin's recent study of another, this time identifiable, female patient, the sixteenth-century noblewoman Elisabeth of Rochlitz. In her case, the doctor appears to have thought in humours, while the patient spoke about 'fluxes'. Based not on a case history but on Elisabeth's letters, account books and recipe collection, Rankin argues that Elisabeth had 'a very fine-tuned conceptualization of illness and its expressed symptoms, and a very different set of concerns than the practitioner'; moreover,

Elisabeth was a 'proactive' patient (Rankin 2008: 110, 112). On one occasion Elisabeth mentions a flux she felt in her chest which 'made her feel she was choking' (Rankin 2008: 130). Early modern European women do appear to have been aware of a sensation of a flux, or flow, within their bodies.[38]

Is the 'heaviness' felt by the wife of Theodoros an example of such female sensations for an earlier historical period? In *Epidemics* 7 there are two other cases in which a woman's own feelings or beliefs about her condition are flagged up, and these may help to answer this question. In 7.28 (Loeb 7.334), the female patient, the wife of Polemarchos, 'said she felt as though there was a gathering about her heart [*kardiê*]'. In 7.11 (Loeb 7.314), the female patient, the wife of Hermoptolemos, sick with a fever in the winter, 'said that her heart had been damaged'. How should we understand these words from the female patients in the *Epidemics*? It is not that the author or compiler of this book has a particular interest in the heart – it is mentioned on only two other occasions in book 7. I have already raised the question of whether it is legitimate to read one Hippocratic treatise by means of another, and in this context it is worth noting that the heart does feature in the *Diseases of Women* treatises; it is a site to which the womb can move, causing suffocation and anxiety, and vomiting bile will relieve the symptoms (*Diseases of Women* 2.124; Littré 8.266–8), while elsewhere we read that the womb can also press on the heart (*Diseases of Women* 2.200; Littré 8.382). The heart also plays a key role in *Disease of Virgins* (Loeb 9.360), in which the author's explanation for the deranged behaviour of young unmarried girls is that their menstrual blood has been retained in the area of the heart. The verb in *Epidemics* 7.28 (Loeb 7.334) is *sunagô*, which is used on four other occasions in *Epidemics* 7. It is the verb used twice for bringing the upper and lower jaw together (*Epidemics* 7.8, Loeb 7.310; *Epidemics* 7.37, Loeb 7.340) and also for closing the eyes (*Epidemics* 7.25, Loeb 7.330) and for 'drawing the whole body together' (*Epidemics* 7.11, Loeb 7.318). Perhaps we could translate it as a 'clenching' of the heart?

These references to women mentioning their hearts show that they felt aware of this organ, and of 'gathering' there. Either they saw this as important enough to mention, or the doctor who observed them considered it significant. Is it blood that gathers, or is it the womb itself? When the womb moves to the heart it causes difficulty in breathing; in *Diseases of Women* 2.201 (Littré 8.386) we are told, 'If the heart is suffocated by the womb, it is compressed, and respiration is difficult and frequent' – precisely the symptom experienced by the wife of Polemarchos. In *Diseases of Women* the verb for suffocation is *pnigein*, and in *Epidemics* 7.28 (Loeb 7.334) the wife of Polemarchos feels *pnigmos* in her pharynx.

There are many overlaps between the fifth and seventh books of *Epidemics*, and the case of the wife of Polemarchos is one of those that are duplicated between them. The second version of the story appears in *Epidemics* 5.63 (Loeb 7.196), and in both cases she has not only *pnigmos*, which is relieved by blood-letting, but also a persistent fever and pain and swelling in the right knee. In *Epidemics* 5, the phrase 'she said she had gathering around the heart' uses the verb *sullegô*, which has a similar sense of 'collecting'. It is commonly used for blood 'collecting' in one place (such as in *Nature of Man* 11, Littré 6.58) but I have not found any text in which a Hippocratic writer talks about anything specifically 'collecting' around the heart.

What is happening here? Are these two women, with their insistence that something is 'collecting' or 'gathering' at the heart, speaking up for a belief not recognized by the Hippocratic writer? In a section of the Hippocratic corpus in which humours do not feature significantly, are they telling us that, for them, sensations of anonymous fluids moving within their bodies are normal, and any blockage in this movement is worth reporting to the doctor? The notion of 'gathering', 'clenching' and 'collecting' recalls Barbara Duden's comment that it was 'hardening' or 'lumping' that was seen by Storch's female patients as dangerous, because it was interpreted as stopping the normal movement of fluids (Duden, this volume). These comments may in turn recall the passage of *Places in Man* already mentioned, when there are 'something like balls' in the stomach; as Elizabeth Craik has noted, this treatise generally suggests that 'flux which coagulates is bad' (Craik 1998: 232). She argues that it draws on sources also used by the gynaecological treatises and notes that, in two of the latter, we find references to 'a hard thing like a ball' in the area of the ribs, and here the absence of menses is a symptom (Craik 1998: 26). Is this again a 'gathering' thought to be retained blood?[39]

For the Hippocratic case history, the problem, as ever, is that we cannot always reconstruct the principles by which the writer decides what is significant and what need not be noted down. In essence, if he mentions it, he must think it worth mentioning. This suggests that the Hippocratic doctor does respect the subjective sensations reported to him by his patient, whether male or female. This may be because they actually fit perfectly well into his construction of the patient's body: a woman who feels her heart clenching under the accumulation of blood is one who interprets her body according to Hippocratic views of blood and its movement within the female body that it dominates. Alternatively, the fact that we learn of this from a reported sensation of the patient may reflect a greater interest among women in fluids and in the dangers believed to arise if they 'gather'.

Within the parameters of the body of fluids, there is no one model of what these fluids are, and little agreement on how to treat the disorders they can cause. While *Epidemics* 7.25 is an unusually full case history, neither its disregard for four-humour theory nor its suggestion of a flux theory existing alongside it are unique. The 'four humours' are a rarity in the Hippocratic corpus, only as influential as they were in later thinking because Galen chose to understand *On the Nature of Man* as an example of the work of the great Hippocrates himself. Even in the broader sense of 'fluids', humours represent only one aspect of disease in the Hippocratic corpus. Hot and cold, wet and dry, climate and season, air and the behaviour of the individual play roles in causing disease; adjustment of the diet and the patient's way of life can be used to cure it. The humoral 'body in balance' is just one of the models used by the doctor, while the sensations described by the women patients examined here are not about balance so much as 'hardening' or 'gathering'. The concept of flow remains at the heart of many of these passages, but it is not what flows that matters so much as whether flow takes place at all.

Notes

1   Many of the ancient sources used here – such as Plato, and Thucydides – can be readily found by the non-specialist in English translations. For the Hippocratic treatises, where an English translation exists in the Loeb Classical Library series, I shall be using that, in the interests of ease of access for non-specialists. That series will also go online in 2013; meanwhile, a list of open access versions of many volumes is maintained at http://www.edonnelly.com/loebs.html. Where a translation does not yet exist in Loeb, I shall use the edition of Littré (1839–61). Other ancient medical texts are

cited in the *Corpus Medicorum Graecorum* edition (*CMG*) where possible; these are available online at http://cmg.bbaw.de/online-publications.

2. On *ikmas*, see, e.g., Thomas (2000: 50–52). *Ikmas* is used, for example, in the Hippocratic *Diseases* 4.2–3 (Loeb 10.102–4), where an explicit analogy between plants and human bodies is used. *Chumos* too is used for plant juices, for example in *Epidemics* 6.6.3 (Loeb 7.262) but also in the sense of 'humour'. Another use of the human–plant analogy would be the Hippocratic treatise *On Generation/Nature of the Child*, where the development of limbs in the embryo is likened to a tree branching. See Lonie (1981).

3. The contributors to Horstmanshoff, King and Zittel (2012) seek to re-examine the non-humoral fluids and their place in the physiology of the body in ancient, medieval and early modern medicine.

4. The phrasing of Wesley D. Smith (1979: 22), citing Le Clerc (1729: 15).

5. On Galen's teachers, see Smith (1979: 64–72). For a recent summary of Galen's education, see Johnston and Horsley (2011: xiv–xviii).

6. Thivel also argues that the Indian version of the humours was very different from that in Greek medicine, and points out that the ancient Egyptians operated with 'breaths' rather than 'humours' (Thivel 1990: 281–82).

7. This point is also made by Thivel: 'this system is unique in the Hippocratic corpus' (Thivel 1990: 283).

8. On the uses of *schema* in the Hippocratic surgical treatises, see Jouanna (2002).

9. *On Ancient Medicine* 22 (Loeb 1.56–60). On this passage, see Schiefsky (2005: 320–23).

10. *On Humours* 1 (Loeb 4.64).

11. See Lloyd (1991b: 408); Galen, *On the Doctrines of Hippocrates and Plato*, *CMG* V 4.1.2, 510.8–12. and 512.4–12.

12. See Jones (1947). Classical scholars increasingly challenge the label 'Hippocratic corpus'; they emphasize that there were many medical treatises of the period not included in this group. The Thirteenth *Colloque Hippocratique*, held in Texas in 2008, had as its theme 'What's Hippocratic about the Hippocratics?' Philip van der Eijk addressed 'to what extent the Hippocratic writings are bound together by any sort of intrinsic characteristic that distinguishes them *as a group* from other medical literature and thought of the same period. This is an important question, for if the answer is negative, the justification for treating the Hippocratic writings as a *corpus* or *collection* collapses' (van der Eijk 2008, conference abstract).

13. *Anonymus Londiniensis* (18.30–35, Jones 1947:72), Lloyd (1991a: 62–63), Langholf (1990: 41–42).

14. *On Generation/On the Nature of the Child* 3 (Loeb 10.10) and the related *Diseases* 4.1 (Loeb 10.100). As Thivel (1990: 285) points out, the writer bases his conclusions about anatomical structures on his assumptions about physiology.

15. Smith (1979: 220) discusses *Nature of Man* as a 'composite work'.

16. I am here giving the translation of Lloyd 1978: 202–3. For 'bitter bile' see also *Regimen in Acute Diseases* 61 (Loeb 2.116).
17. At some points in *Nature of Man* it is specifically yellow (*xanthês*) bile; see also Nutton (2004: 83–84). Langholf (1990: 47) argues that the author of *Nature of Man* had worked in an area where he observed the black urine of malaria sufferers, and created the concept of black bile to account for this.
18. *On the Natural Faculties* (2.8–9), see van der Eijk (2001, i: 50–53). *On Black Bile* was written around twenty years after *On the Natural Faculties*, a dating supported by its references to Galen's commentary on *Nature of Man*, itself written in about AD 190 (5; *CMG* V 4,1,1,79–82).
19. *CMG* 5.9.1, cited in Smith (1979: 170).
20. E.g., Ibn Hindū (2010: 60–61), discussed by Savage-Smith (this volume).
21. Aristotle, *History of Animals* (512b12–513a7), Jouanna (1999: 56–57).
22. See Smith (1979: 114); Smith (1979: 169–70) cites the relevant passage from Galen. The *Anonymus Londinensis* papyrus also attributes the section on the four humours to Polybus; Jouanna (1999: 62, 400). See Langholf (2004: 238–47), who sums up scholarly approaches to *Nature of Man* as either a composite or a unitary work; he suggests that the first part, with its use of the first person, is a personal discovery and that the third part is based on earlier, traditional material which is being used to try out this discovery.
23. *Timaeus* (83c1–2); see also note 18 (above).
24. This section reuses some material already published in King (2011: 116–18).
25. E.g., *Affections* 9, Loeb 5.16: 'give the remedy recorded in the *Remedy Book* for pain in the side'; *Affections* 15, Loeb 5.28: 'give the drugs written in the *Remedy Book* as stopping pain', and so on.
26. Faraone (1999: 114–15). See also [Aristotle] *Magna Moralia* (1188b30–38).
27. *Epidemics* (5.34–37; Loeb 7.182). In two cases this is squirting cucumber.
28. E.g., Theophrastus, *History of Plants* (9.18.9); cf. Pliny, *Natural History* (26.99).
29. Theophrastus, *History of Plants* (9.18.3).
30. Totelin (2007: 532). As Skoda (1988: 161–63) and Totelin (2007: 535) show, *balanos* was used for the glans of the penis both by the writers of comedy and by Aristotle (e.g., *History of Animals* 1.13).
31. On early modern discussions of whether menstrual blood was indeed 'blood', see King (2007: 54–56).
32. *Epidemics* (7.88, Loeb 7.334; 7.5, Loeb 7.306).
33. Smith translates 'in a decorous way' (*Epidemics* 4.17, Loeb 7.104–05); 'inoffensively' (*Epidemics* 4.55, 7.148).
34. This symptom is associated with imminent death; compare 'rapid breathing, as of dying people' (*Epidemics* 5.55, Loeb 7.192 = *Epidemics* 7.77, Loeb 7.374).
35. See Nutton (1993) on the five senses in Hippocratic medicine and in Galen.
36. The Greek word *pais* can also mean 'slave'.

37. 'Those present' (*hoi pareousoi*) also feature in *Epidemics* 5.2 (Loeb 7.152), where Timocrates of Elis fell asleep and seemed to those present 'not to be breathing, but to have died'; these household members and other visitors are listed as features of the 'economy' (*oikonomie*) of the sick person in *Epidemics* 6.2.24 (Loeb 7.234), to be taken into account by the doctor.
38. See also Pomata (1998: 35–42).
39. Craik (1998: 224) discusses 'the use of common sources' for *Places in Man* and the gynaecological works; see *Places in Man* 47 (Loeb 7.94–100), *Nature of Woman* 38 (Littré 7.380–82), *Diseases of Women* 2.129 (Littré 8.276–78).

References

Berlin, B., and P. Kay. 1969. *Basic Color Terms: Their Universality and Evolution*. Berkeley: University of California Press.

Bos, J. 2009. 'The Rise and Decline of Character: Humoral Psychology in Ancient and Early Modern Medical Theory', *History of the Human Sciences* 22: 29–50.

Condrau, F. 2007. 'The Patient's View Meets the Clinical Gaze', *Social History of Medicine* 20: 525–40.

Craik, E. 1998. *Hippocrates* Places in Man. Oxford: Clarendon Press.

——— 2002. 'Phlegmone, Normal and Abnormal', in A. Thivel and A. Zucker (eds), *Le Normal et le pathologique dans la Collection hippocratique*. Nice: Publications de la Faculté des Lettres, Arts et Sciences Humaines de Nice-Sophia Antipolis, pp.285–301.

Dean-Jones, L.A. 1994. *Women's Bodies in Classical Greek Science*. Oxford: Clarendon Press.

Duden, B. 1991. *The Woman Beneath the Skin*, trans. T. Dunlap. Cambridge, MA: Harvard University Press.

Faraone, C. 1992. 'Sex and Power: Male-targeting Aphrodisiacs in the Greek Magical Tradition', *Helios* 19: 92–103.

——— 1999. *Ancient Greek Love Magic*. Cambridge MA: Harvard University Press.

Hanson, A.Ellis. 1989. 'Diseases of Women in the *Epidemics*', in G. Baader and R. Winau (eds), *Die Hippokratischen Epidemien*. Stuttgart: Franz Steiner, pp.38–51.

Harvey, D. 1995. 'Lydian Specialities, Croesus' Golden Baking-woman, and Dogs' Dinners', in J. Wilkins, D. Harvey and M. Dobson (eds), *Food in Antiquity*. Exeter: Exeter University Press, pp.273–85.

Horstmanshoff, M., H. King and C. Zittel (eds). 2012. *Blood, Sweat and Tears: The Changing Concepts of Physiology from Antiquity into Early Modern Europe*. Leiden: Brill.

Johnston, I. and G.H.R. Horsley (eds and trans.). 2011. 'Introduction' in *Galen, Method of Medicine* Vol. 1 (Loeb Classical Library). Cambridge, MA: Harvard University Press.

Jones, W.H.S. 1947. *The Medical Writings of Anonymus Londinensis*. Cambridge: Cambridge University Press.

Jouanna, J. 1999. *Hippocrates*, trans. M.B. DeBevoise. Baltimore, MD: Johns Hopkins University Press.

—— 2002. 'ΣXHMA dans la littérature chirurgicale hippocratique', in A. Thivel and A. Zucker (eds), *Le Normal et le pathologique dans la Collection hippocratique*. Nice: Publications de la Faculté des Lettres, Arts et Sciences Humaines de Nice-Sophia Antipolis, pp.445–65.

King, H. 1995. 'Food and Blood in Hippokratic Gynaecology', in J. Wilkins, D. Harvey and M. Dobson (eds), *Food in Antiquity*. Exeter: Exeter University Press, pp.351–58.

—— 1998. *Hippocrates' Woman: Reading the Female Body in Ancient Greece*. London: Routledge.

—— 2002. 'The Limits of Normality in Hippocratic Gynaecology', in A. Thivel and A. Zucker (eds), *Le Normal et le pathologique dans la Collection hippocratique*. Nice: Publications de le Faculté des Lettres, Arts et Sciences Humaines de Nice, pp.563–74.

—— 2007. *Midwifery, Obstetrics and the Rise of Gynaecology: The Uses of a Sixteenth-century Compendium*. Aldershot: Ashgate.

—— 2011. 'Medicine and Disease', in P. Toohey and M. Golden (eds), *Sexuality in the Classical World (500 BC–350 AD)*. Oxford: Berghahn, pp.107–24.

Langholf, V. 1990. *Medical Theories in Hippocrates*. Berlin: Walter de Gruyter.

—— 2004. 'Structure and Genesis of Some Hippocratic Treatises', in H.F.J. Horstmanshoff and M. Stol (eds), *Magic and Rationality in Ancient Near Eastern and Graeco-Roman Medicine*. Leiden: Brill, pp.219–75.

Le Clerc, D. 1729. *Histoire de la médecine ou l'on voit l'origine & le progrès de cet art*. The Hague: Isaac van der Kloot.

Licciardi, C. 1990. 'Les causes des maladies dans les sept livres des *Epidémies*', in P. Potter, G. Maloney and J. Desautels (eds), *La Maladie et les maladies dans la Collection hippocratique*. Québec: Éditions du Sphinx, pp.323–37.

Littré, E. (ed. and trans.). 1839–61, *Oeuvres complètes d'Hippocrate*, 10 vols, Paris: Baillière (reprinted Amsterdam: Hakkert, 1961–62).

Lloyd, G.E.R. (ed.). 1978. *Hippocratic Writings*. Harmondsworth: Penguin.

—— 1991a. 'Who is Attacked in *On Ancient Medicine*?' in G.E.R. Lloyd, *Methods and Problems in Greek Science*. Cambridge: Cambridge University Press, pp.49–69.

—— 1991b. 'Galen on Hellenistics and Hippocrateans: Contemporary Battles and Past Authorities', in G.E.R. Lloyd, *Methods and Problems in Greek Science*. Cambridge: Cambridge University Press, pp.398–416.

—— 1995. 'Epistemological Arguments in Early Greek Medicine in Comparativist Perspective', in D. Bates (ed.), *Knowledge and the Scholarly Medical Traditions*. Cambridge: Cambridge University Press, pp.25–40.

Lonie, I.M. 1981. *The Hippocratic Treatises 'On Generation', 'On the Nature of the Child', 'Diseases IV'*. Berlin: De Gruyter.

Manuli, P. 1980. 'Fisiologia e patologia del femminile negli scritti ippocratici dell'antica ginecologia greca', in M. Grmek (ed.), *Hippocratica*. Paris: CNRS, pp.393–408.

———— 1983. 'Donne masculine, femmine sterili, vergini perpetue: La ginecologia greca tra Ippocrate e Sorano', in S. Campese, P. Manuli and G. Sissa (eds), *Madre materia: Sociologia e biologia della donna greca*. Turin: Boringhieri, pp.109–236.

Mattern, S.P. 2008. *Galen and the Rhetoric of Healing*. Baltimore, MD: Johns Hopkins University Press.

Miller, H.W. 1962. 'The Aetiology of Disease in Plato's Timaeus', *Transactions and Proceedings of the American Philological Association* 93: 175–87.

Nutton, V. 1993. 'Galen at the Bedside: The Methods of a Medical Detective', in W. Bynum and R. Porter (eds), *Medicine and the Five Senses*. Cambridge: Cambridge University Press, pp.7–16.

———— 2004. *Ancient Medicine*. London: Routledge.

———— 2005. 'Galen: The Fatal Embrace', *Science in Context* 18: 111–21.

Pomata, G. 1998. *Contracting a Cure: Patients, Healers, and the Law in Early Modern Bologna*. Baltimore, MD: Johns Hopkins University Press.

Rankin, A. 2008. 'Duchess, Heal Thyself: Elisabeth of Rochlitz and the Patient's Perspective in Early Modern Germany,' *Bulletin of the History of Medicine* 82: 109–44.

Rousselle, A. 1980. 'Observation féminine et idéologie masculine: Le corps de la femme d'après les médecins grecs', *Annales* 35: 1089–115.

Schiefsky, M.J. 2005. *Hippocrates* On Ancient Medicine. Leiden: Brill.

Skoda, F. 1988. *Médecine ancienne et métaphore: Le vocabulaire de l'anatomie et de la pathologie en grec ancien*. Paris: Peeters/Selaf.

Smith, W.D. 1979. *The Hippocratic Tradition*. Ithaca, NY: Cornell University Press.

———— 1994. 'Introduction' in *Hippocrates* Volume 7 (Loeb Classical Library). Cambridge, MA: Harvard University Press.

Steckerl, F. 1958. *The Fragments of Praxagoras of Cos and his School*. Leiden: Brill.

Stolberg, M. 2011[2003]. *Experiencing Illness and the Sick Body in Early Modern Europe*, trans. L. Unglaub and L. Kennedy. Basingstoke: Palgrave Macmillan.

Thivel, A. 1990. 'Flux d'humeurs et cycle de l'eau chez les présocratiques et Hippocrate', in P. Potter, G. Maloney, J. Desautels (eds), *La Maladie et les maladies dans la Collection hippocratique. Actes du Ve Colloque international hippocratique*. Québec: Editions du Sphinx, pp.279–302.

Thomas, R. 2000. *Herodotus in Context: Ethnography, Science, and the Art of Persuasion*. Cambridge: Cambridge University Press.

Totelin, L. 2007. 'Sex and Vegetables in the Hippocratic Gynaecological Treatises', *Studies in History and Philosophy of Biological and Medical Sciences* 38: 531–40.

van der Eijk, P. 2001. *Diocles of Carystus: A Collection of the Fragments with Translation and Commentary*, 2 vols. Leiden: Brill.

Chapter 2
Fluxes and Stagnations
A Physician's Perception and Treatment of Humours in Baroque Ladies

Barbara Duden

The opportunity to explore notions of imbalance in a medical practice embedded within humoralism is a precious one. It allows me to review a theme I started to explore many years ago and have gone back to again and again. Here I put forth a thesis, which began as an intuition, developed into a hypothesis, and by now is a conviction that orientates my reflections about experienced and lived 'bodies' in the West prior to the end of the eighteenth century. It is an insight gained from the perspective of the historian of the experienced and lived body. My aim is to make it plausible that the substance of the traditional medical encounter was the patient's 'felt *soma*' that he or she revealed to the physician in the form of a narration. I will argue that the subject of this story – the oral narration of a time, place and status-specific feel of the flesh brought to the physician by the patient – was the haptic experience of oriented flows, of humours. In spite of great differences in times and cultures, a set of characteristics of this experienced humoral flesh, irrespective of linguistic, cultural, epochal changes in *etyma* (the literal sense or root of a word) and style, remained constant over many centuries, and this is the percept and concept of *soma*, of flesh, based on variations of intensity and fluidity of oriented flows. These modulate a variety of distinct, epochal expressions of the history of the body.[1]

Humorality then, since antiquity and well into the eighteenth century, does not primarily refer us to medical theories that were based on a humoral framework but to somatic autoception, to the feel of one's flesh as proportionate liquids, admixture of humours, interior fluid movements, vivid fluxes and ominous stagnations. I fear that categories like humoral pathology or humoral theory when applied to the body in a period prior to the eighteenth century inadvertently and retroactively medicalize the past. A focus on the history of successive medical paradigms of humoral pathology or the 'theory' of four humours may turn out to be an impediment for an understanding of the physician's practice, its social significance and its traditional effectiveness. Instead, we should begin the analysis by taking seriously the humours as experience, as autoception.

Let me turn to the Baroque ladies and their physician. I will again draw on the medical cases of the small-town physician of Eisenach in Germany, which I have already used to study the practice of Johann Storch. In the years between 1719 and 1741 this physician wrote down in daily protocols what his female patients complained about. He published his cases in yearbooks, and at the end of his life he assembled his notes as individual case histories and published them in volumes arranged according to the bodily states of women. Eight volumes, dealing with girls in menarche, with women pregnant, miscarrying, in labour, lactating and lying in, and women's diseases in general (Duden 1991). In addition, the author, a Halle-trained physician, continuously draws and comments on similar cases from the medical literature between the sixteenth century and his time. The physician took his notes in the vernacular German and not in Latin. The arrangement of his cases fits into the flourishing epistemic genre of *Observationes*, which originated in the second half of the sixteenth century and had become a primary form of medical writing by the early eighteenth century, its key feature being an unprecedented emphasis on practice and thus a strong focus on detailed description of what the physician had heard, touched and observed in conversation with his patients.[2]

Medical case histories in the vernacular, such as those of Johann Storch, do not foreclose the possibility that the historian might reconstitute what has been said or felt by the sick in front of their physician. I will comment on typical aspects of humoral self-perception as I find them voiced by the women patients in this early eighteenth-century practice, and I will stress the analogous perception of the physician regarding the balance (*Ordnung der Natur*) and imbalance (*Unordnung der Natur*) of inner fluid movements in each case: its narrative nature, its habitual aspect incarnate in the humours, the polymorphous nature of fluids, orientation and disorientation, obstruction and stagnation. These aspects I have found typical for the humoral flesh of early eighteenth-century Protestant Germany.

From the very beginning of my research I had to tackle a phenomenon that I found extremely difficult to understand. These women speak about their flesh in terms of something exquisitely liquid. They speak about their *Geblüt*, 'fluxes' (for example, *Steckfluss*, *Goldaderfluss*, *flussartige Materie*, *Flussfieber*, *weißer Fluss*), inner fluid motions (*Flussregungen*) and imbalances of their juices. Unquestionably at the centre of this physician's practice stood something that is foreign, both to the modern clinic, and to the register of symptoms or syndromes usually attended to in the history of nosology: a somatic stirring, a swelling and ebbing of liquids, an inner hardening and lumping that the women perceived as stagnation (*Verstockung*), and deep anxiety when their *Geblüt* 'stopped', when their fluxes would not flow.

When first confronted with these phenomena I was lost. Clearly, the subject of the encounters between single women and their physician was a flesh spoken about in terms of flows, fluid movements and stagnations; on the other hand, to apply classical paradigms as a pattern of explanation seemed anachronistic. Quite obviously these women, literate court ladies and illiterate charwomen, educated wives of Protestant ministers and poor servant girls who probably had never touched a scholarly book of medicine, could not bring a disease to their physician that would match the doctrine of Hippocratic or Galenic, iatrochemical, iatromechanical or vitalist humoral theory. Nonetheless, what emerged in hundreds of cases was an acute, intense awareness of inner movements of fluids, an anxiety about stagnations of the *Geblüt* and a reported relief with the onset of some discharge – as vomiting, sweating, oozing from an ulcer or menses.

It dawned on me that I had to rethink the historical nature of the humours. What the physician and his women patients were about was not some remnants of a worn-down and by now threadbare doctrine of the four humours; the substance of the exchange that

I strained to understand was, without exception, always a story. The less I tried to understand these encounters in terms of medical history paradigms, the more I realized that they were – in the full sense of the word – biology: *logos*, or talk about, *bios*, which in Greek means lived life. And this *bios* was voiced in the nature of quivering liquidity. Even if the physician regularly, yet incidentally, refers to the woman mentioned above as 'choleric' or to another as 'sanguine-choleric', in doing so he does not intend to refer to objectifiable humours. Dr Storch recorded, so I learnt through close reading, evidence of autoception in lived times: of an intuitive self-reference, of a fit between *autos*, i.e. ego, and the haptic perception of some dis-ease, dis-order, im-balance in interior liquid movement.[3]

The subject of the encounters in the practice of this physician was not a diseased, isolable body as a physical entity but the patient's 'felt self' in terms of the interior movement of fluids. I had to inquire into the historical nature of 'fluids' to grasp the stuff of experience which was then called the flesh: 'fluxes' and 'fluids' not as concepts in medical nosology but as names for experiences in lay people's explanations of their own flesh.

The Flow of One's Own Story, Narration and Experienced History

A pathology of solids, an imagined pathology in a localizable organ or a pain in a distinct spot in the body, today will inevitably be targeted by the physician's question: 'Where do you have pain?' If the tests are made in the laboratory, additional talk by the patient can be dispensed with. Self-perception in terms of fluids by the person calling on a physician or the percept of a sickness in terms of haemorrhages by its very nature demand that a story be told. It will not do just to point to a bodily spot. Fluids are moving matter. Fluids always have a time dimension, a past, a present, and a direction into the future. The flow of times, the experience of inner liquid movements and the flow of the life story run together. A narration has to set in if a *Fluss* (flux) is at stake.

What then is the object of this Baroque physician's attention? The answer seems obvious. Of course – one will say – a patient. But how does the physician come to know a patient? Certainly not by observation, that is, through visual inspection. Storch rarely touched a patient, and his eye-sight was an instrument of minor importance compared to his ears. Storch and his contemporaries acquired their knowledge through close attention to the revelation of the patient. 'The patient revealed to me', 'the patient confided to me', 'the patient disclosed to me' (*eröffnete, vertrauete an, ließ wissen, entdeckte mir, erzählte*) are common turns in hundreds of *casus*. And, what the women reveal to the healer is something to which they, and they alone, are privy. It is the story of the autoception of their juices, their *Geblüt*.

In hundreds of single cases recorded as stories by the physician we find the meandering thread of the *Geblüt* in these women's lives. Let me give just some examples to illustrate the minute, concrete, situational details which were reported to the physician and inserted into his protocol of the *casus*. A woman who was breastfeeding took part in a baptismal banquet and there experienced how two neighbours quarrelled over their seating – immediately the lying-in flow of the new mother dried up (Storch 1752: 56); a noble lady ran to the fountain in her undershirt when she 'suffered a fit of apoplexy' (*Steckfluss*) during the night, as 'the sergeants who were coming to report to her husband surprised her along the way', so that she could 'pass only with the greatest embarrassment' (Storch 1752: 56).

A twenty-two-year-old noblewoman kept getting fatter. The physician was called in 1720 'to advise her on her violent headaches'. He notes:

> However, when I discovered that she had had sickly attacks on numerous earlier occasions, I made it my concern to further investigate the circumstances, and was informed of the following: several years before, during spring in another village, she had tired herself out very much by dancing. Not only had she cooled herself off at an open window, but at night she also went along on the hunt for mountain cocks. From that time on she had been burdened with intensely painful fluxes and occasionally with womb anxiousness, in fact, she also had an oozing flux in her side [*inguine*] between her fat belly and thick legs. (Storch 1752: 146)

In order to know what to administer – in this case a well-timed phlebotomy at the ankle – the physician must first understand the story as the story of her moving fluxes.

In 1718 a young married woman had herself bled at the arm at the time of her menses – an 'improper time' in Storch's view – and she 'noticed right away that the monthly flow stagnated'. Subsequently she had headaches and did not conceive 'stemming from the improper bleeding'. This incorrect bleeding was still remembered and subject of the conversation two decades later, in 1737. With this same woman, the physician reflected, 'one should not forget, after all, that she had been strongly inclined to anger since her youth, on account of which during recent years this had repeatedly caused pains and induced the blood flow to surge' (Storch 1752: 81).

When discomfort and dis-ease is perceived in the mould of interior fluid movement, the body cannot be split off from the story of the person. Flow by its nature is historical, originating in a past and streaming towards a future. In order to give sense to a present autoception of hardening or looseness, of aberrant flux or healing discharge, of ulcers, rashes and headache, the patient relates her past. It must be narrated, revealed to disclose the sense of the present imbalance. When Storch noted down and later printed all these seemingly trivial details, like the landlord grabbing the patient's arm in a fight, or details about other family members' ongoing menses as integral parts of this *casus*, he kept to the same logic. In order to assist the person restore her individual balance, the physician has to listen to her unravelling her 'biology' and maybe even that of her kin. Most of the *observationes clinicae* of this period are stuffed with personal details, smallest incidents, minute events, and it is because of this story-telling character that medical history had difficulties in their analysis, concentrating more on paradigmatic changes in medical theory than on an analysis of the somatic experience of those seeking to be cured. The revelation of past inner movements is a precondition for the physician to understand the actual tendency in these women's *Geblüt*, and to be able to help their nature.

Flow is Habitual: Imbalance Cannot but Be Personal

Flows as the stuff of self-perception not only involve the history of the ego, they also incarnate habits, periodic and often involuntary repetitions of an inclination, a tendency of the flesh. The Greek term for 'habit' is *hexis*, defined as the 'second nature' of a person. To illustrate this humoral nature of a person's *hexis* let me quote verbatim:

A fiftyish choleric woman, whose main task in life had been the expression of anger [*deren vornehmste Verrichtung in ihrem Leben die Ausübung des Zorns gewesen*], had a run-in with her landlord on January 28th, 1723. The man grabbed her arm and forcefully showed her the door. This so deeply offended the woman that since then her arms and legs tremble, her heart hurts [*cardialia*], and she has a strong cramp in her hands and legs. (Storch 1752: 440)

In a squabble with her landlord, this constitutionally angry woman had tried to spit out her swelling gall in a bitter flow of words. In vain, no one had listened to her, so the poison that could not exit clumped in her innards: 'Bad blood and bitterness had by now so hardened her, that ordinarily she would not have been affected by this outbreak of rage. But this time she had been ridiculed and had been refused a hearing, and, as a result, the poison, which she was wont to spit out, had got stuck inside' (Storch 1752: 440).

Storch's patient was unable to emit the poison that had accumulated in her by means of bitter words. And by this time she was drowning in her own gall. At this juncture, she sought help from the physician. He answered with a triple prescription: a tincture of rhubarb to clean the intestines, polichrest powder to soften the cramped 'mother', and *tartarum* (*Weinstein*). A day later the woman reports that her innards are getting unstuck, that she felt relief (*Besserung*). The bad blood that had turned in the wrong direction and got stuck had 'loosened up and re-oriented itself'.

When women of Eisenach disclose the habitual 'tendencies' (*Gewohnheit, anhaltende Regung*) of their *Geblüt*, the physician hears something that we should not confuse with the concept of 'constitution' according to humoral theory. This term, 'constitution' has an objective ring. It sounds like the quantifiable preponderance of some *Geblüt* – as if yellow gall or sanguine blood 'constitute' the person so endowed. The choleric *Geblüt* in casus 67 refers to something innate, born into one's fluids, that with time and practice has become an embodied habit, a tendency of this (some) body somatized in habitual practice. The 'choleric woman', by submitting to her inborn disposition, established habits, acquired a second nature, in which she kept her unpleasant character in a sort of balance by constant nagging. Then, 'gall' could be spitted out through nasty words, abuse poured out, insults showered upon someone. Or the bitter or vitriolic stuff might be discharged by

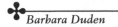

inducing vomiting or with the help of rhubarb. She could take a certain intensity or amount of poisonous blood and could endure more, the more her habitual nature had taken biographical shape. But dis-ease would set in and drive her to seek some rescue, if the poison got 'stuck', could not 'move' or 'flow' out. The physician tended to this habitual flesh, he recognized the danger involved in the humours' propensity to clumping, the *cessatio fluxus* which Galen had called a 'metastasis'.[4]

Metamorphosis: The Polymorphous, Changing Nature of Interior Fluids

In the history of medicine, early eighteenth-century physicians' reasoning was often categorized in the perspective of a theory of blood pathology when I began my inquiry into these sources. This classification resulted in two suppositions: an assumption that in medical practice the 'humour' could be identified with blood that might be broken down into chemical ingredients; secondly, the notion that the issue in question is 'pathology', a 'pathological' state of one or several of the humours. However, 'humours' in Storch's practice escape the effort of the historian to isolate something like 'normality' and to conceptually draw a line where the pathology of diseased humours sets in. The somatic living fluid voiced by Storch's patients is shapeless, smudgy, ambiguously iridescent, versicoloured. Not only does it unforeseeably change direction, it also transforms its nature.

Almost a century had passed since William Harvey's discovery of the measurable bulk of circulating blood; in 1673 Antony van Leeuwenhoek had posited 'small round globules' in the blood and reported this extraordinary finding to the Royal Society; half a century had passed since Robert Boyle had subjected blood *in vitro* to dry distillation in 1684, measured its chemical ingredients and physical properties, contradicting the millennial certainty that blood is an essence that can be interpreted only *in vitam*. In spite of these discoveries dis-embedding 'blood' as a scientific fact, the volatile liquids experienced by Storch's women patients escape an objectification into some substance that would lend itself to laboratory analysis. In Storch's practice, fluids, by their very nature, change composition – taste, colour and touch.

The wife of a princely footman, twenty years of age, lay sick after her first childbirth with 'cold sweat', 'heat' and a feverish rash. Over the course of several days she suffered repeatedly from loose bowels and complained about the 'drying up of milk'. She had frequent diarrhoea 'that looked whitish like milk'; later, the diarrhoea came out 'white, like curdled cheese' (Storch 1751a: 606). The physician in this case surmised that the discharge, 'white like curdled cheese', 'originated in the regurgitated milk'. To substantiate his diagnosis he listed a number of other authors who also had observed that women's milk could take irregular paths. Milk was thought to pass from the breasts to the stomach and from there to be excreted as white milk; it might also be excreted as spittle or urine, or in an incision opened on a swelling. The physician's reflection on the interior anatomy, on the ducts channelling the interior fluids, do not contradict the perception the woman brought to his practice. A young girl seeks help and has plasters placed on her swollen breasts, whereupon 'the menses broke out which in colour, smell and taste resembled milk' (Storch 1748: 225). Pungent food flavoured the fluids when a nursing woman took elderberry juice as a purgative, whereupon her child 'fell into a sweat, which in colour and taste was like the elderberry juice' (Storch 1751b: 132).

Thus the quality of fluids changed with one's comportment. It is evident that emotions also season the self's fluids, or, to be more correct, that fluids are tasted in the woman's emotional states: sweet blood by the sight of a beloved person, bitter blood after a quarrel with her husband, dark blood in sorrow and desolation after a child's death, salty blood from disappointment. The liquid's physical qualities cohere with the emotionally spiced perception of anger, lust, envy, jealousy or longing.

Orientation and Dis-orientation: Errant Flows

'Humours', fluid, 'flux' by its motile nature, always implies a direction; fluids are dynamic and oriented; they always suggest a rising and falling, a vivacity or slackness, a turbulent or sedentary quality, a flowing or stoppage. If we grasp this we are cautioned not to insert their historical nature into the same topology as 'organs' in an anatomical atlas. Fluids are incomparable to 'organs', at least to 'organs' drawn from the dissection of corpses, dis-embedded, situated and fixed in visualizations and then re-inserted into the interior of a living person.

One complaint in the Eisenach practice is particularly frequent and is at the same time difficult for a modern mind to understand: the women are particularly troubled or relieved by discharges taking the 'wrong direction', fluids gone stray, 'aberrant', even habitually 'aberrant' fluxes. The women disclose to the physician the habit of their flesh to seek unbefitting orientations and improper exits, and the physician provides the Latin names for this tendency of the *Geblüt* to seek *insolitae viae*, unbefitting exits. The physician diagnoses these misplaced discharges when they happen in women as *menses vicariae* (vicarious menses). They found their exit from the nose in a widow; from a festering wound in a sixteen-year-old maidservant; in a suppurating boil, several years running, which had formed on the forehead of a country girl; from a 'sore thigh' of a woman 'well into her thirties', who suffered this irregular discharge of her 'monthlies' for a long period; from a tonsillar abscess that was forming in the throat of a sixteen-year-old daughter of a chancery clerk when her menses were obstructed.

The medical literature of the sixteenth to the early eighteenth century – theoretical treatises as well as case histories – abounds with examples of *menses vicariae* and *insolitae viae*, of the blood swelling, pushing, urging towards an unbefitting exit.

As Gianna Pomata (1992) has shown, according to a surprising number of educated physicians' records, men too experienced these roaming fluxes, especially if their *haemorrhoids* had dried up, that part of the body where men might most properly and conveniently discharge an excess of blood. By turning to the men's side, Pomata helped us better understand the epoch-specific notion of *Geblüt* and physicians' practice. Men periodically bled through noses or haemorrhoids, the tip of the finger or even the penis. Routinely, this was not interpreted as 'pathological' but as necessary and therapeutic, a sign of the capacity of *soma* or nature to get rid of superfluous or peccant blood. Healthful bleeding from the golden vein in men and periodic bleeding of women was perceived as analogous, and men worried and also turned to a physician in case of a stoppage (obstruction) of their blood-flow. 'There is no doubt that the focus on monthly and cyclical aspects of different forms of bleeding in men in this period is related to a lively interest in physicians' discourses' (Pomata 1992: 59).

Pomata (1992: 67) quotes Thomas Bartholin's *Anatomia Reformata* (1651) on the vein or golden veins: 'These are around the anus and the intestines, visible also from the outside; in all men, at regular intervals, they spontaneously open and thus happens an evacuation of thick blood, which is good for their health'. The theoretical background for this interest in the menses and the golden vein, the *viae insolitae*, the erroneous ways of the blood, was the theory of plethora, superfluous blood, which periodically assembles in the flesh and must be emitted. Pomata argues that all these stories – medically interpreted as plethora or fermentation – reflect the deeper logic of the physicians' duty: to help 'nature' to find her way, and to be aware not to block or obstruct nature in her healthful expellant, balancing intentions or movements.

The 'disorientation' of fluids due to some blockage is an old theme in the Hippocratic and Galenic tradition: the Hippocratic texts counsel healthy purging through regular emitting of blood and acknowledge the body's effort to get rid of 'blocked menses' by discharges in other parts of the body. Galen interpreted throwing up blood as being related due to a suppression of the menses or haemorrhoidal flux (Pomata 1992: 67 n.53). Cyclical haemorrhoidal bleeding or periodic discharges through open veins were not only tolerated by patients but perceived as a normal state of their flesh, and physicians provided analogous therapies to prevent or counter-act disease. 'If sickness is provoked by the retention of blood in women, or in men by the blockage of their haemorrhoidal flux, it is useful to stimulate these parts and elicit the habitual excretion of blood' (Aretaeus, cited by Pomata 1992: 67). Misplaced discharges are not something 'pathological' within 'humoral theory' but signs of nature's effort to get rid of burdening matter.

Reading the Eisenach complaints as evidence of haptically perceived oriented flows, we have to admit a directionality in the lived flesh that is alien to later interpretations of self by lay people as well as in clinical anamnesis. I mentioned story telling and narrative, the habitual and the polymorphous aspects in the liquidity of lived *soma*; now we must grasp the fluid body's innate 'intentions'. In Storch's reports women interpret discharges, swellings and ulcers as wrongly-placed, yet healthy purges.

In a sudden fright, in the exasperation of receiving unexpected bad news, from the sight of a barn on fire, the blood rushes to

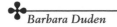

the heart burdening it by masses of liquids; in other instances the flux swells upwards, overwhelming the head, laming the tongue, obscuring vision, obstructing hearing. These turbulent 'accidents' – the vernacular German word used is *Sturm*, 'storm' – are violent reactions in a flesh that is disturbed, im-balanced. In other instances the *Geblüt* slackens and 'sits' in a part of the body, causing pain. Suppurating ulcers, oozing scabies, nosebleed and so on are interpreted by lay perception eventually as the healthy effort of the flesh to rid itself of these burdens and re-balance itself. The physician diagnoses bad matter, *materia peccans*, and with his prescriptions of unguents and plasters, *vesicatoria* or rhubarb assists the discharge. To purge oneself, to cleanse oneself, to loosen threatening stagnation by evacuation is paramount to both patient and physician. The haptic perception of oneself probably helped evacuations – periodic blood flows, artificially induced bloodletting, suppurating wounds, swellings or sweat – to be experienced as a relief. We can thus better understand why the women, according to the physician's records, seem to have felt improvement after purging, a feeling of being unburdened by evacuations.

The physician listens and scrutinizes his repertory to help the woman's nature, either getting rid of wrong matter, keeping a habitual yet unbefitting exit or bringing her back to the ordinary ways of proper discharge. Discharges of fluids might be disoriented, in need of re-orientation, but rarely interpreted as 'pathological'. Certainly not 'pathological' according to that definition of the word that in Europe became common in the later eighteenth century. Eisenach's women's grand-daughters would no longer experience itches or swellings as healthful efforts of their nature and thus endure living with suppurating skin. The encounter with medicine would by then echo back an iatrogenic body, that is, a medically restorable body that had no healing intentions of its own.

Obstruction, Stoppage and Stagnation

A 'delicate, choleric woman' came to Eisenach, consulting the physician Storch, and complained of 'persistent cold feet and legs, shortness of breath, and hot flushes'. On a later occasion 'she disclosed that she had had an oozing flux between her toes after confinement. She had cured it by sprinkling it with white lead powder, and she suspected that this flux had been driven back and was now manifesting itself inside. I agreed with her' (Storch 1751a: 749).

As the Eisenach women disclose to their physician the stories of their discomforts, one image is particularly prominent. We have seen how the appearance and re-appearance of discomforts is channelled by the movement of the 'flux' (*Fluss*) — from hip to toe, from throat to breast, from nose to womb. But dis-ease is acutely embodied in the slackening, thickening and temporary obstruction of their fluids. The head aches, the joints ache, the eye-sight is darkened, the mood is low, the spirits are depressed because of a congestion of *Geblüt*. A multitude of pains, aches, and dis-eases and a great variety of illnesses — from hydropsy to coughing, from paralysis to cramps in the womb, from pneumonia to 'stones' in the bladder — are ascribed to the obstructed movement of fluids. The loss of the soma's capacity to rid itself of superfluous or bad matter is a frequent lay cause of discomfort. The flesh gets blocked (*verstockt*) or closed (*verschlossen*), and an inner hardening (*Verhärtung*) or an amassing of stones (*Sammlung von Resten/Steinen*) sets in.

The physician tries to liquefy the *Geblüt*, to loosen the *stasis*, to quicken movement and to help the woman's nature to evacuate properly and thus bring her back to her proper balance with respect to the interior composition, quantity, intensity and orientation of her fluids. In his medication, the physician relied on the women's *physis* to re-establish the disturbed imbalance by prescribing a proper diet, herb, pills, unguents or bloodletting at the right spot, to support the proper, and that is always the personal, habitual *modus* and *tonus* of her fluxes.

These sensations of inner fluid movements, reported by the women, involve simultaneously several aspects: firstly, they perceive themselves kinaesthetically (experienced kinesis, movement) as quick, lively, dull, sluggish, obdurate, hardened, blocked, clogged-up; secondly, what they perceive is grasped by a haptic apperception of something which swells, presses, pinches, oppresses them, lies heavily on them; thirdly, they stress syn-aesthetics; that is, taste and smell, gall and comfort coalesce, as do hot fits and cold shudders. Many phrases evoke this synaesthetic blending, like black, bitter and stagnant gall or sweet and lively blood; fourthly, these aspects of somatic apperception are oriented; that is, the flux swells up or down, goes to the right or the left, to the head, to the shoulder or to the feet, moves inwardly or towards the outside. The fluid 'body' is perceived as oriented stuff or fluxes which are haptically grasped in the confluence of one's interior senses.

Conclusion

So far I have kept close to one physician's records. I wanted to convey their – the women's – perception, autoception of their *Geblüt*, because I am convinced that Dr Storch administered to their 'bio-logies' – that is, to their felt, oriented autoception. Obviously, the stuff which is the fundamental reference for both the patient's complaint and the physician's reflection and intervention is an oriented, polymorphous experience of flows that were taken for granted. Since I first tried to understand the dynamic, dialogical sense of the encounters in this practice, new research has unearthed very similar testimonies. In his book on '*homo patiens*', the experience of disease and the 'body' in the seventeenth century, Michael Stolberg has collected autobiographical and medical sources that tell of the same awareness of the balances of one's fluid movements and of the attention people paid to interior 'fluxes' (Stolberg 2011).

By the end of the eighteenth century, however, the notion of the therapeutic function of menses, as well as the theory of critical evacuations in general, is gone. The erroneous but healthful inner fluid movements (*menses vicariae*) are no longer perceived as a sign of provident nature but are classified as the patient's pathology, while the *menses in marium*, the menses in men, were now classified as abnormal and a symptom for a pathological disease entity. The primordial form of the physicians' therapeutic interventions that had been modelled by analogy to, as an imitation of, woman's periodic stirrings of fluxes and of the aim of her nature to restore her balance of humours, will be conceived in theory as *contra naturam*. This reversal in the medical paradigm – from attention to fluid somatic stirrings to 'solidar pathology' – opened a hiatus between two heterogeneous 'bodies' – the perceived haptic inner *soma* and 'the body' in the diagnosis of the physician.

Notes

1. In her extraordinary research, the classicist Ruth Padel (1992) collected and analysed testimonies for fluid apperceptions, be they from medical or poetical texts, in Greek antiquity. She revealed, to my knowledge for the first time, fluidity as a constituent of Greek somatics and emotions. See also King (this volume).
2. Gianna Pomata (2010) has analysed the emergence of this new genre of medical writing since the sixteenth century, thereby stressing its characteristic: the way the case narrative moved into the foreground of attention and detailed observations from the physician's daily practice were minutely recorded.
3. Ulinka Rublack (2001) found ample and vivid testimonies of similar sensory perceptions in sixteenth- and seventeenth-century personal records. Rublack stressed that bodily fluids and 'juices' and their movements or blockages are crucial if we want to understand early modern somatic apperceptions.
4. Pomata (1998) found in seventeenth-century Bologna medical records a similar 'dis-ease' of the blockage of inner fluids (*mal d'oppilazione*).

References

Duden, B. 1991. *The Woman beneath the Skin: A Doctor's Patients in Eighteenth-century Germany*. Cambridge, MA: Harvard University Press.

Padel, R. 1992. *In and Out of the Mind*. Princeton, NJ: Princeton University Press.

Pomata, G. 1992. 'Uomini mestruanti: somiglianza e differenza fra i sessi in Europa in età moderna', *Quaderni storici* 79: 51–103.

——— 1998. *Contracting a Cure: Patients, Healers, and the Law in Early Modern Bologna*. Baltimore, MD: Johns Hopkins University Press.

——— 2010. 'Sharing Cases: The *Observationes* in Early Modern Medicine', *Early Science and Medicine* 15: 193–236.

Rublack, U. 2001. 'Erzählungen vom Geblüt und Herzen: zu einer historischen Anthropologie des frühneuzeitlichen Körpers', *Historische Anthropologie* 9: 214–32.

Stolberg, M. 2011[2003]. *Experiencing Illness and the Sick Body in Early Modern Europe*, trans. L. Unglaub and L. Kennedy. Basingstoke: Palgrave Macmillan.

Storch, J. 1748. *Von Kranckheiten der Weiber*, Vol. 3: *Darinnen vornehmlich solche Casus, welche die Schwangerschaft betreffen*. Gotha.

——— 1751a. *Von Weiberkranckheiten*, Vol. 6: *In welchem vornehmlich solche Zufälle, so die Wöchnerinnen und Kindbetterin betreffen*. Gotha.

——— 1751b. *Von Weiberkranckheiten*, Vol. 7: *In welchem solche Zufälle, so die stillenden Weiber und Säugammen betreffen, auf theoretische und practische Art abgehandelt*. Gotha.

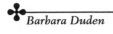
Barbara Duden

———— 1752. *Von Weiberkranckheiten, Vol. 8: Worinnen vornehmlich solche Zufälle, Kranckheiten und Gebrechen, so man der weiblichen Mutter zuschreibt, und den Weibern außer dem Schwangergehen begegnen, abgehandelt werden.* Gotha.

Chapter 3
When Money Became a Humour

Shigehisa Kuriyama

Can Money be a Humour? The notion may seem bizarre. Humours are part of the human body, and we commonly conceive the body and money as distinct and unrelated sorts of things. We identify human beings with warm blood and feeling flesh, and perhaps a soul, whereas we associate money with cold, dumb coins and inanimate bills. We suppose inquiry into money to be as useless for mastering physiology as the study of physiology is, presumably, for comprehending finance. We imagine doctors and economists as experts of utterly separate worlds.

Many in the past, however, have seen the two realms as more closely entwined. As Nicholas Oresme wrote in the fourteenth century, just as 'the body is disordered when the humours flow too freely into one member of it, so that the member is often thus inflamed and overgrown' (cited in Johnson 1966: 119), so a kingdom cannot survive when excessive riches flow to the prince. Money should be named 'the second blood', Bernado Davanzati declared in the late sixteenth century. Just as 'blood is the sap and the nutritive substance in the natural body', so money is the sap of the world which, 'in flowing from the large purses into small ones, brings into each new blood, which is spent and flows continually into the things which we use in life ... In this fashion, in circulating, it maintains the body of the republic' (cited in Johnson 1966: 120). Each state thus needs a certain amount of circulating money, Davanzati concluded, just as each body needs a certain amount of irrigating blood. When money all accumulates the head, the state is apt to suffer from 'atrophy, dropsy, diabetes, consumption, and other maladies' (Johnson 1966: 120).

For these early Europeans, the flow of humours in the body could illuminate the role of money in the state. For the Japanese doctor Nakagami Kinkei (1744–1833), conversely, the power of money helped to explain the differing vitality of bodies. Human beings are not equally strong, Kinkei notes (Miyake 1917: 113). Some people can endure winds and bitter cold without harm, while others succumb to even the slightest chill or draft. Why? Think of it this way, he says: people of superabundant vitality are like the fabulously rich merchant houses of the Mitsui or Kônoike, while others, with weaker constitutions, resemble the street vendors who scrape by on a few copper coins. Wind and cold and other causes of disease are like thieves that steal from a person's storehouse of life. In the case of the grand House of Mitsui, the thieves may abscond with a pile of gold, and the House will still be vigorous: 'The blood and breath of its business will continue to circulate smoothly, just as before', Kinkei remarks (Miyake 1917: 113). By contrast, feebler bodies are like the poor, who must expel the thieves right away, for even a small loss will exhaust their capital. In short, money is like blood, and blood like money.

Of course, such passages – and it would be easy to cite many more – suggest only that the two share some similarities; they prove nothing, and indeed, make no claims, about real identity. We read them as mere analogies and metaphors, just ways of talking. To say that money *is like* a humour is not at all the same as asserting that money *is* a humour. Yet it is precisely this latter possibility that I want to probe. In what follows, I propose to explore the idea that in certain contexts the figurative and the real may converge, and money can actually become a humour.

My plan is simple: I shall argue for latent potential by spotlighting an actual instance. That is, I shall try to show how money can become a humour, by portraying how it actually became a humour in a particular place and time – specifically, in Japan of the Edo period (1603 to 1868). I thus hope to elaborate, in one historical instance, the alchemy of money's transformation into flesh. Let me be clear: I shall not argue – and indeed, do not believe – that money is always, and necessarily, and universally, a humour. On the other hand, I do suspect that the case of Edo Japan is not unique and that research into other contexts could reveal other forms of money's incarnation.

For the key to its incarnation in Japan, I shall argue, was an intuition that can also be found elsewhere. I mean the intuition of money as a living power, a force that can wax and wane, and even die. To appreciate money's alchemical potential, I suggest we must ponder the mystery of its life.

'Life is more precious than money!' we find moralists repeating in Edo Japan. And at first we pay scarce heed. Of course, we say. Money is just an instrument of exchange, which allows us to more conveniently trade for food, clothing and other goods; that is, it is only a means to an end, and that end is the sustenance and enjoyment of life. It is useless when we are dead. Obviously. And yet … If the matter were really so plain, there would be no need to say it. To insist. Life is more precious than money! If people needed to be reminded it was because they so often forgot, because money so easily became the heart's supreme obsession.

'Alas! I am going to die,' groans a miser in Ihara Saikaku's *Nihon eitaigura*, first published in 1688, 'and I can't bear to think of all this money belonging to someone else' (Ibara 1955: 131). In his last moments on earth, he voices no concern for the family that he is leaving or the afterlife to which he is headed. But he is utterly distraught about parting with his lovingly accumulated wealth.

> Clinging to his money, and shedding bitter tears, he looked very pale – as a hornless blue devil. With this ghastly look on his face he struggled up and walked about all over the house until he fell down exhausted, very near the end. Full of alarm, his servants gathered round and supported his body. But he rallied once more, and asked again and again, 'Is the money still there? What about the money?' (Ibara 1955: 131)

A major feature of late seventeenth and eighteenth century Japan was the emergence of what historians have termed an 'economic society' (*keizai shakai*) – a new social order shaped by the growth of a nationwide market, an unprecedented abundance of goods and diverse services, and above all the universal spread and almighty reign of money (Hayami and Miyamoto 1994). Saikaku was one of the shrewdest chroniclers of this transformation, detailing with cool lucidity the frenzy that it stirred.

He gazed unflinchingly, on the one hand, at the horrors inspired by the lust for gold and silver, noting how it could drive people to blackmail, to the theft of dogs, to the starving of babies, to harvesting

71

the hair of the drowned – 'acts so disgusting and inhuman that it would have been better for the person never to have been born' (Azuma 1998: 122). But alas, 'when a man is infected, he cannot see the evil in even the most evil deeds' (Azuma 1998: 122). Unlike Confucian moralists, however, who longed nostalgically for a purer, more virtuous agrarian past, Saikaku revelled in the commercial culture of his time, and saw nothing base or evil in money itself. Quite the contrary. Yes, miserliness was deplorable, but frugality was a prime virtue. Yes, life was undeniably more precious than money, but no one could deny money's desirability. 'I believe deep down', he affirms at the start of the same work in which he relates the tale of the ghoulish miser, 'that money can grant all wishes in this world – save that of altering our mortality. That is the sole exception. Surely there is no greater bearer of treasures!' (Azuma 1998: 15).

Forget the exception, and the madness of the miser no longer seemed mad. And it was so easy to forget. 'Nothing is more important in the world than life,' Santô Kyôden declares in *On-atsuraezome chôju gomon* (1802) – only to concede, 'yet money carries equal weight' (Yamaguchi 1926: 628). And often greater weight: those who have sacrificed health for wealth, Kyôden sighs, are beyond counting, victims all of that magnificent trick (*dai karakuri*) by which money somehow appears more precious than life.

It is almost impossible for us, now, to appreciate the full jarring shock of the new economic society, to re-experience the sense of seismic upheaval. When historians tell us that Edo Japan was transformed by radical commodification, and write of the supreme sway of the market, we nod casually and read on. For today we take the hegemony of capital for granted, as the ordinary, almost natural, order of things; we have but the dimmest memory of a pre-monetized past. And so it requires the most strenuous effort of the imagination to hear the depths of wonder, and bewilderment, and outrage voiced by Saikaku's contemporaries when gold and silver, abruptly and everywhere, glittered more dazzlingly than life.

Yet our own time may offer an analogue. Like the spread of the money economy in early modern Japan, the recent spread of the internet has swept us with dizzying speed into a world that is at once exhilarating and confusing, exciting and troubling, full of promise and full of fears. And just as with the spread of the money economy, the sole certainty about the new communication technologies is that they are changing social relations, swiftly and ineluctably, into forms unrecognizably, worryingly different from what they were not so long ago. We have a queasy sense that all is not right. We fret about how people seem increasingly more focused on the machines that mediate communication than on the human beings with whom they communicate, and that they relate more often, and more readily, through electronic mediation than face to face, in the flesh. We are troubled by intimations of a diminished humanity.

The changes in feeling and behaviour that accompanied the surge of the new economic society in Japan felt even more disturbing, more wrong and pathological. Saikaku saw the dying fret about the fate of their gold, and the living set to murder for cash. Moralists intoned in vain that, 'life is more precious than money!' So we are not surprised to find Edo-era doctors, for their part, diagnosing the birth of a pervasive new disorder, though the disorder itself may puzzle us.

The problem they identified was not the blindness of greed, or other vague mental derangement, but an oddly specific physical symptom. 'Whether they be old or young, depleted or plethoric', observed Gotô Konzan near the end of the seventeenth century, 'most people today have accumulations [*shakki*] knotted in their abdomens' (Otsuka and Yakazu 1979: 155). 'Most people today'. People had not suffered in this way before. And yet it was an epidemic that transcended differences in age and physical constitution. In one form or other, in greater or lesser degrees, the problem of congealed knots in the belly now affected nearly everyone. The knots were a reflection of the time, a change in the body mirroring a changed world.

This was a change that ostensibly made medicine vastly simpler. Past teachings, Japanese doctors now urged – Chinese ideas about the interactions of the five phases and microcosmic–macrocosm correspondences, their dense maps of acupuncture points and conduits – were all unnecessarily complex and beside the point. To understand most suffering it was enough to grasp one principle: whether the pain appeared in the head or the feet, whether the patient felt feverish or chilled, all pathology stemmed from a faltering in the flow of blood and breath (気, *ki*, Chinese *qi*) around the body. 'The hundred diseases', Konzan asseverated, 'all arise from the stagnation (*ryûtai* 留滞) of vitality (*genki* 元気)' (Otsuka and Yakazu 1979: 155).[1]

Prevention and treatment were thus simple. To fend off sickness one had only to ensure constant, vigorous circulation. To cure a disease one just had to find and dissolve the knots and accumulations that had congealed because of sluggish flow. This fresh frame inspired Japanese doctors to devise a novel diagnostic technique: *fukushin* 腹 診, the examination (診) of the *hara* (腹), the abdomen.[2] While they continued to query the fleeting flickers of the pulse at the wrist, they now also palpated the chest and bellies of their patients with the more forceful touch of the masseur, seeking out solid masses of varying size and consistency. Over the course of the Edo era, they composed more than sixty treatises on the hermeneutics of abdominal signs, a corpus without parallel in world medical literature (Otsuka 1981).

Therapy, too, shifted to meet the challenge of stagnation. The turn of seventeenth and eighteenth centuries was marked by the appearance, for the first time in Japanese history, of the professional masseur (Katô 1974: 119–26, 397–400), and saw the publication of a flurry of treatises devoted to massage, all insisting on the usefulness, indeed the absolute indispensability, of massaging the belly. Since sickness was a matter of abdominal knots, it had to be cured by kneading the knots away.

Alternatively, the knots could be pulverized. Japanese acupuncturists crafted a unique method called *uchibari* 打鍼, or 'pounded needles', which casually abandoned the fourteen conduits and hundreds of points of Chinese acupuncture. Needling, in this radical recasting of tradition, no longer sought to coax subtle diversions of flow at precisely mapped points spread out around the body, but focused solely on finding and dispersing palpable nodules and masses in the abdomen. Whence the brute directness of *uchibari* technique: modified, thicker needles with blunter tips were struck with a small mallet, much as one might pound chisels to crack apart rocks.[3]

These are all procedures alien to modern Western medicine. Our doctors too occasionally palpate the abdomen, but their examinations are closely tied to local anatomy. They press below the hypochondrium, say, if they suspect a disease of the liver, or the right lower abdomen to confirm appendicitis. But few would think to palpate the belly when the patient complains of headaches or ringing in the ears, or suffers from rashes or sleeplessness. And none would dream of trying to cure such afflictions by kneading or pounding the belly.

It thus is tempting to dismiss practices such as *fukushin* as mere historical curiosities, quaint fantasies of interest only for what they reveal about the culture that conceived them. Yet abdominal palpation is still much prized today by many practitioners of traditional medicine in Japan. When a reprint series of Edo *fukushin* manuals appeared in 1994, the editors stressed how, by making available the lessons of old masters, they sought as much to advance contemporary clinical practice as to commemorate a cultural legacy (Matsumoto 1994: 26). These manuals, they asserted, had much to teach us about our own bodies here and now, not just about past beliefs. They had real medical as well as historical value.

In any case, this much is certain: the pathology of stagnation in Edo Japan was not just an abstract theory but an experience of objective, palpable presences. Whatever their origin or substance, whatever the insightfulness of the diagnoses that they inspired, whatever the efficacy of the therapies that tried to disperse them, knots and accumulations were unmistakably present, solid and graspable, there in the bellies of a great many people in early modern Japan.

It was not by chance that doctors focused where they did. *Hara*, the Japanese word that I am translating as belly or abdomen, had long evoked more than just the physical midsection of the body. Already in the mid tenth century, the author of the *Tale of Ise* described a lover so moved by a poem that he decided 'not to recite it out loud, but instead silently to savour it in his *hara*' (Fukui 1974: 171–72). Characters in the *Tale of Genji* (early eleventh century) typically experienced anger as an uprising in the *hara* (*hara ga tatsu*), a sensation still voiced today. Popular religion portrayed the *hara* as the abode of unruly worm-spirits (*mushi*), a lair of squirming cravings.

Hara, the focus of Edo medical interventions, was in other words not just the physical chest and abdomen but also the spiritual bosom, not just the centre of the body but also the core of the feeling person. It thus should not surprise us that stagnation, in early modern Japan, was an intimately felt discomfort as well as a palpable presence. The fleshy knots objectively confirmed from without, by the probing hands of doctors and masseurs, were subjectively experienced by patients, as recurring painful spasms (*shaku* 癪 and *senki* 疝気) and stubborn dull aches (*kenpeki* 肩癖). The chronic ache of accumulations was a widespread, constant complaint among the townspeople of Edo Japan, who sought relief not just in massage and acupuncture, but also in an endless array of commercial ointments and patent drugs.

So what was it about the new economic society that induced this epidemic of accumulations diagnosed by doctors, kneaded by masseurs, pounded by acupuncturists and suffered by patients? How should we understand the Edo epidemic of stagnation?

For the physician Kagawa Shûan, writing in the early eighteenth century, the tie between sickness and history was clear. The pathology of stagnation was produced by the commercial culture that followed upon stable Tokugawa rule; it could not have arisen in the turmoil of the preceding Warring States era. Peace had reigned now for over a hundred years. All was calm within the four seas, and people enjoyed rich abundance. They were frivolous and idle, overfed, overheated. Their bodies pursued relaxation and pleasure, while their minds laboured with worries. They worked themselves up over how much they could accumulate over their lifetime, they worried and schemed about the revenues that would sustain them through life. Add to these an inexhaustible thirst for wine and bottomless lust, and it is no wonder that people's vitality was weakened – life being treated so cavalierly. As the vital force declines, its flow cannot but become sluggish: this is how stagnation and knotting arises. And so all people suffered from knotting, or congelations, or colic (Otsuka and Yakazu 1982: 128–29).

The sickliness of the age, in sum, was engendered by Tokugawa peace and prosperity. Ease and abundance induced laziness, while money bred endless anxieties. A new social order had fostered a new pathology, but also new values. As hinted by Shûan's disapproving tone, the insistence on flow gave voice to an insistent spiritual imperative. Pleasure-seeking indolence was not only sickening but reprehensible. Accumulations were incarnations of moral failure, laziness made flesh.

The historian Hayami Akira has argued that economic growth in Edo Japan, in marked contrast to early modern England, was driven not by machines and technological innovation but rather by an intensification of labour (Hayami and Miyamoto 1994: 20–31). Whereas England underwent an industrial revolution, the transformation of Edo society turned on what Hayami dubbed an 'industrious revolution' (*kinben kakumei*) – a revolution marked not only by longer hours of more intense work but also by the elevation of industriousness into a cardinal virtue.[4] Idleness became a vice. It is especially this latter change that illuminates why, in Edo visions of health, the medical equation of vitality with brisk flow went hand in hand with ethical exhortations to work harder.

Kaibara Ekiken's *Yōjōkun* (1713), the single most popular health manual in Japanese history, perfectly reflects this spirit. Some people imagine, says Ekiken, that the art of cultivating vitality is exemplified by the retired old man passing his days in peaceful leisure, or, in the case of the young, by the hermit who lives far from the wearying cares of society (Kaibara 1981: 37). And so they suppose that the samurai who assiduously serves his lord and his parents, and strains hard to master the martial arts, or the farmers, craftsmen and traders who labour day and night at their calling and have scarce time to rest – that these people cannot properly care for their health. But Ekiken is adamant: those who believe this are wrong. Vigour is not nurtured by relaxed repose. On the contrary, it is labour (*rōdō*) that sustains life. Ceaseless work is vital. Idleness slows the flow of blood and breath, causing them to stagnate and congeal. Rest makes one sick.

The Edo obsession with stagnation was thus the obverse of a fierce compulsion to work. Which leads us to the question: what spurred this new compulsion? How should we understand the emergence of the ideal of industry? The crux of our topic lies here. Constant activity somehow came to feel like a physical and moral imperative, a visceral need. Somehow, rest felt wrong.

In his analysis of the industrious revolution, Hayami outlines how population growth and various shifts in the material conditions of agriculture made it both necessary and profitable for farmers to invest more time and energy in the cultivation of their fields. But his explanation sheds little light on Ekiken's exhortations, which were addressed more to the samurai, merchants and tradesmen of the cities. And it says nothing, more importantly, about industriousness as an internalized moral pressure, about idleness as a source of anxiety.

And yet it is especially this relentless pressure that needs interpreting – the restless inner compulsion. Edo manuals of regimen do not say, 'You can become healthier and wealthier by exerting yourself, and moving around', but rather, 'If you are not ceaselessly working and moving around, you will become sick'. Dawdle for even a moment, and the flow of life will slacken, blood and breath will start to congeal. Slowly but surely, small nodules will then form, and grow steadily, day by day, fed by countless brief spells of idleness, swelling imperceptibly from a nodule as miniscule as a grain of rice to become like a bean, then an egg, then a large ball. Only by perpetual busyness, by paring rest and sleep to a minimum, can one hold this grim accretion at bay. One must work tirelessly, without stop.

It is ultimately in this compulsiveness – the haunting worry that one was never working enough – that we must seek the key to the Edo fixation on sluggish flow. The real pathology of the time was less idleness than unease about idleness – a madness more subtle, yet more visceral, and ultimately more gripping than greed.

Why was repose so frightening? Suggestively, the same emphasis on work and movement in precepts about the life of the body recurs in Edo-era pronouncements on the life of money. 'If one constantly makes the body work', Kaibara Ekiken believed, 'then blood and breath will circulate, and digested food will not stagnate. This is the crux of the cultivation of life' (Kaibara 1981: 44). But precisely the same logic, Ekiken urged, governed the dynamics of wealth (Ekikenkai 1910: 452, 457). Merchants earn their living by making gold and silver go round, he says, and this circulation of money in society is no less vital than the circulation of blood and breath in the body. Stagnation and sluggish delay mean diminished profit, an erosion of money, and in the end, its death. 'You can have saved a hundred million pieces of gold and silver', the astronomer Nishikawa Joken cautions in *Chônin bukuro* (1719), his manual for merchants, 'but if you just let it accumulate in the vault, it becomes dead treasure: being put to no special use, the gold and silver become worthless to both yourself and to others. Gold and silver must circulate, and never stagnate in one place' (Nakamura 1975: 101).

Like the life of the body, the life of currency depends on flow. Secreted in storehouses – and here Joken echoes exactly the same words (*ryûtai* 留滞, 'stagnate', and *tsumoru* 積, 'accumulate') favoured by Konzan and other doctors – it becomes 'dead treasure' (*shihô* 死宝). Movement entails risks, to be sure; once the money flows out of your coffers, you may well incur losses. But such is the way of nature, Joken says; after wealth swells to an extreme, it must contract. And this is how it should be. For one's loss then enriches others. Gold and silver must go around. Just as the yin and yang must keep flowing, and never rest, just as their local accumulation creates imbalance and provokes disaster, so it is with money. 'It circulates among all the people, and should never stagnate in one place' (Nakamura 1975: 101).

As material objects, the gold and silver coins that pass from person to person are no different from the gold and silver hoarded in treasure vaults. But as money, the difference between them is the difference between life and death. Which is to say that money is not what it seems, and that its essence is separate from its material form. We must not confuse money with my 50 yen coin, say, or your 20 pound note. Just as clocks are only instruments for measuring time and not time itself, so stamped coins and printed currency are but convenient tools that allow us to count money. They are not money itself. Money can assume, and historically has taken, countless other guises, such as salt and rice, tobacco leaves, cowry shells and the teeth of dogs. Just think: most of your money now consists of mere numbers in bank computers, shifting arrays of electrons. Money exists, in other words, apart from tangible objects such as rice and shells, metal coins and paper bills, and persists even in their absence. It is the invisible soul that breathes life into lifeless things and transforms them into vital currencies.

Now the essence of this vital pecuniary soul may, in the end, be as unfathomable as the essence of the human soul. But we know this much: money lives not least because it is rooted in the desires and fears of living beings. 'Men are often criticised in that money is the chief object of their wishes and is preferred above all else', Arthur Schopenhauer observes,

> but it is natural, even unavoidable. For money is an inexhaustible Proteus, ever ready to change itself into the present object of our changeable wishes and manifold needs. Other goods can satisfy one wish and one need. Food is good only for the hungry, wine for the healthy, medicine for the sick ... They are all goods for a particular purpose, that is, only relatively good. Money alone is the absolute good: for it confronts not just one concrete need, but Need itself. (cited in Buchan 1997: 31)

The townsmen of Edo Japan would certainly have agreed. The explosion of new desires was the perhaps most striking manifestation of the new consumer society, as one after another, previously unimaginable luxuries came to feel like natural, implacable needs. Tokugawa rulers worried that the seemingly boundless escalation of extravagance and conspicuous consumption was eroding the social order, and tried, periodically, to brake it through sumptuary laws (Shively 1964). But all their efforts ended in failure: each time, the lure of more lavish, more dazzling and glamorous goods would not be denied.

And this actually was for the good, urged critics of government policy. Sumptuary restrictions, some argued, badly mistook the dynamics of a commercial world. Although restrictions on spending might appear, superficially, to conserve wealth, their real effect is to impoverish. It is precisely the hunger for luxuries, the passionate wanting, critics explained, which drives the circulation of currency and inspires the industry of merchants and craftsmen (Takizawa 1927: 37). Desire is vital. To repress it – to foster instead the accumulation of money in closed storage – is to drain an economic society of its animating force, to deprive it of its very life.

We catch glimmerings here, in the association of money with desire, of how it might be incarnated as a humour. Felt needs are unquestionably a physiological force, an energy that ebbs and flows in the body. But there is clearly more to the matter. For by itself, this association still leaves us in the dark about Kyôden's 'magnificent trick', the enigma of why people sometimes choose money over life. If the essence of money is felt want, there must be some want that reaches beyond the food and medicine, silk fabrics and precious stones, and the countless other goods that money can buy. For all these may gratify the living but they give no pleasure to the dead. There must be some other, special need that can make a person forget how 'life is more precious than money'.

Hoarded in vaults, Nishikawa Joken asserts, gold and silver will eventually die. To keep them alive, to nurture their growth and vigour, one must make them 'move and work' (*kore o ugokashite hatarakasete*). Money must not be allowed to play. Like the body, money must be made to work. But how does one do this? The answer is simple, and familiar to bankers everywhere: one makes money work by lending it out.

The simplicity of this answer is deceptive, however, because there is nothing at all simple about interest. It is the strangest, most magical property of money: circulating as loans, money bears children. The very words for interest in Japanese – *risoku* 利息 and *rishi* 利子, literally 'profit-breath' and 'profit-child' – express the intuition of money as something that breathes and breeds.[5] It is in this fecundity, I suggest, that we must seek the goad prodding restless industry. On the one hand, those who have money cannot afford not to lend it, to make it work: in a world of interest-bearing money, one is always and inevitably gaining or losing. There is no standing still. Each year, each month, each day that your gold sits inert in your money box, you are losing the interest that you should have earned. Time is money.[6] On the other hand, those who borrow this money cannot afford to rest. Money procreates day and night, without holidays, and idlers are quickly buried under its relentless accumulation. Nothing, warned Saikaku, is more fearsome than interest on a debt (Azuma 1998: 4).[7]

In the end, the life of money has more to do with borrowing than buying, more to do with debt than desire. 'Money of account', John Maynard Keynes declared, 'is the primary concept of a theory of money', and a money of account, he goes on, 'comes into existence along with debts, which are contracts for deferred payment' (Keynes 1971: 3). R.G. Hawtrey likewise observes:

> every piece of money is given a value or debt paying capacity in terms of the money of account. Thus the ideas of debt and money of account are more fundamental than that of money in the sense of legal tender currency. Debt cannot be defined in terms of money because money must be defined in terms of debts. (Hawtrey 1930: 545)

Other economists have of course promoted other views of money, but Keynes's and Hawtrey's accent on debt is particularly illuminating for our inquiry, for it suggests that the vital link between money and Edo restlessness may lie in the insistent pressure that indebtedness places on the soul.

Suppose that a friend, just scraping by, empties her savings to rescue us in a moment of desperate need. The monetary sum may be small but the resulting debt is enormous. For the cash that changes hands is merely the medium of a moral transaction. Although the transaction may be wrapped in warm sentiments of kindness and gratitude, both parties know the implacable obligation that has been incurred. The receiver of the favour owes the dispenser of the favour, and cannot rest easy until what is owed has been paid. An unreturned favour is now called an *oime* 負い目, but the same term applied, in Edo times, to outstanding loans.

A debt is a claim of the past upon the future, a promise to remember. A debtor who forgets, who neglects this duty to memory, risks dishonour and resentment, loss of friends. In those, moreover, committed to the imperatives of trust and friendship, prolonged delinquency can foster an unbearable sense of shame. Look in the plays of Saikaku's contemporary Chikamatsu Monzaemon and you constantly see characters who prefer to pay with their very lives rather than be thought remiss.

Previous generations, Kaibara Ekiken remarks, thought it shameful to borrow money; now, those who do not borrow are despised as stingy (Ekikenkai 1910: 465–66). This was a trend that he found disturbing. Borrowing is ill-advised, Ekiken says, because accumulating interest can ruin lives (Ekikenkai 1910: 463–64, 470). Borrowing is also reprehensible, because it is a symptom of extravagance, of people living beyond their means. But Ekiken's admonitions go further. He sternly cautions against borrowing anything from others. Bear the inconvenience of lack rather than assume the onus of debt. If you must borrow something, return it as quickly as possible. Check your home periodically for forgotten items borrowed from others and, if you find any, send them back right away. If you borrow a substantial tome, set aside all other books and concentrate on reading the one alone so that you can return it within two days (Ekikenkai 1910: 456–57).

Time is of the essence. It is a truth constantly confirmed by our own experience: the more days that elapse between a debt and its repayment, the more we feel we owe. Someone performs a kindness for us, or sends us a gift, and we ought to respond with some gesture of gratitude. If we reply immediately, a simple note may suffice. If we procrastinate for months, on the other hand, we feel obliged to write at greater length, with apologies and more profuse thanks – to discharge our debt, in short, with interest.

Curiously, economic theorists have largely overlooked this phenomenon. Eugen Böhn-Bawerk's magisterial *Capital and Interest* (1959) surveys the great variety of explanations for interest that have been proffered since antiquity, but the theories that he discusses concentrate on why lenders and investors can lay claim, justifiably or not, on money beyond what they lend or invest. The discourse of accumulation in Edo Japan, however, reminds us of the need to consider the psychology of the debtor as well as the privileges of the lender, and to reflect on how the sense of being beholden grows steadily heavier with time.

What is money? What is this mysterious force that has no fixed form and yet bears children? We spoke earlier of the puzzling absorption that it inspires: how it can make people forget their very mortality, how it must offer more than the purchase of earthly satisfactions. The psychology of indebtedness hints at what this something more might be. For if gratification is confined to mortal flesh, the demands of debt can be boundless and transcend life. Debts are akin to duties. (The word 'ought', recall, originates as the past participle of the verb 'to owe'.) They speak to the root values that ground life in meaning, social obligations that sometimes matter more than death.[8]

But debt and obligation are not necessarily felt with the same intensity, or for the same reasons, everywhere and at all times. A critical clue to the diverging local uses and perceptions of money – and the varying impact of money on the understanding and experience of the body – may lie precisely in such variations in the grammar and burden of indebtedness. In other places, at other times, money's abrupt transformation of social relations did not foster its incarnation as abdominal knots. To elucidate the specific inflections of money and the body in Japanese medicine, future studies will need to scrutinize the often seamless transitions, in Edo times, between the imperatives of *oime* and the strictures of *giri* – between the exponentially expanded and diversified circulation of debts created by the new economic society and the older compulsions of feudal duty.

Part of money's vitality may well derive from the flow of human desires. But to comprehend the knots that formed in Edo bellies, to appreciate money's incorporation as a congealing, accumulating humour, to grasp its palpable presence in a person's core of cores, we must also ponder the history of the sense of owing and the profoundly visceral experience of indebtedness.

Notes

1. Okubo Dôko (1709) similarly recognizes the focus on stagnation as a departure from traditional Chinese teachings, but explains that it reflects the pathological reality of Japan in his time. Eight or nine people out of ten, he suggests, suffer from blockages ensuing from sluggish flow.
2. The character 腹 is generally pronounced *hara* when it stands alone, and as *fuku* when combined with another character to form a compound.
3. Interestingly, because the first book to introduce acupuncture to Europe, Willem ten Rhijne's *De Acupunctura* (1683), drew on the author's observations of practice in Japan, the first Western picture of an acupuncture needle is accompanied by an *uchibari* wooden mallet.

4. For more on the ethic of labour in Edo Japan, see Yokota (1989).
5. The classical Greek term *tokos*, 'child', was also the standard term for monetary interest. Aristotle's criticism (*Politics* 1.10) of the unnaturalness of this breeding of money from money was long cited in European criticism of the practice of usury.
6. On the history of this phrase and its introduction to Japan, see Kuriyama (2002).
7. The problem of crushing debt, of course, also ultimately affected creditors as well as debtors. Over half the prosperous merchant families chronicled in Mitsui Takafusa's *Chônin kôken roku* (1727/28), for example, go bankrupt in the end, inexorably dragged down by the burden of money owed and never returned. See Crawcour (1961).
8. The most stimulating discussion of this association of money and debt remains Chapter XV, 'Filthy Lucre', of Brown (1985: 234–304).

References

Aristotle. 1962. *The Politics*, trans. T. A. Sinclair. Harmondsworth: Penguin.

Azuma, A. (ed.). 1998. *Nihon eitaigura* [The eternal storehouse of Japan]. Tokyo: Iwanami shoten.

Böhn-Bawerk, E. 1959. *Capital and Interest*. South Holland, IL: Libertarian Press.

Brown, N.O. 1985. *Life Against Death: The Psychoanalytic Meaning of History*, 2nd edn. Hanover, NH: Wesleyan University Press.

Buchan, J. 1997. *Frozen Desire: The Meaning of Money*. New York: Farrar Straus Giroux.

Crawcour, E.S. 1961, '"Some Observations on Merchants", a translation of Mitsui Takafusa's *Chônin kôken roku*', *Transactions of the Asiatic Society of Japan* 8: 1–139.

Ekikenkai (ed.). 1910. *Ekiken zenshû* [Ekiken, complete works], Vol. 3. Tokyo: Ekiken Zenshû Kankôbu.

Fukui T. (ed.). 1974. *Nihon koten bungaku zenshû* [The complete works of classical Japanese literature], Vol. 8. Tokyo: Shôgakkan.

Hawtrey, R. 1930. 'Credit', in E. Seligman (ed.), *The Encyclopaedia of the Social Sciences*, Vol. 3. New York: MacMillan, pp.545–50.

Hayami A., and M. Miyamoto (eds). 1994. *Keizai shakai no seiritsu, 17–18 seiki* [The establishment of an economic society, 17th–18th centuries]. Tokyo: Iwanami shoten.

Ibara S. 1955. *Nippon eitaigura: The Way to Wealth*, trans. S. Mizuno. Tokyo: Hokuseido Press.

Johnson, J. 1966, 'The Money=Blood Metaphor, 1300–1800', *Journal of Finance* 21: 119–22.

Kaibara, E. 1981. *Yôjôkun: Wazoku kun* [Precepts for nurturing life: precepts on education]. Tokyo: Iwanami shoten.

Katô Y. 1974. *Nihon môjin shakaishi kenkyû* [Studies on the social history of the blind in Japan]. Tokyo: Miraisha.

Keynes, J.M. 1971. *Collected Writings of John Maynard Keynes*, Vol. 5, ed. D. Moggridge. London: MacMillan.

Kuriyama, S. 2002. 'The Enigma of "Time is Money"', *Japan Review* 14: 217–30.

Matsumoto, K. (ed.). 1994. *Nihon kampô fukushin sôsho* [Collected works of Japanese works on abdominal palpation], Vol. 1. Osaka: Oriento shuppan.

Miyake, S. (ed.). 1917. *Nihon eisei bunko* [Library of Japanese health and hygiene], Vol. 5. Tokyo: Kyôiku shinchô kenkyûkai.

Nakamura, Y. (ed.). 1975. *Nihon shisō taikei* [Collection of works in Japanese thought], Vol. 59. Tokyo: Iwanami shoten.

Okubo D. 1709. *Kokon dôin kô* [Reflections on massage and exercise, past and present], unpaginated manuscript. Kyoto: Fujikawa Yû collection, Kyoto University.

Otsuka, K. 1981. 'Fukushin kô' and 'Fukushinsho no bunrui' [Reflections on abdominal palpation], in *Otsuka Keisetsu chosaku shû* [The classification of works on abdominal palpation], Vol. 65. Tokyo: Shunyôdô, pp.266–328.

Otsuka, K., and Yakazu, D. (eds). 1979. *Kinsei kampô igakusho shûsei* [Collected works of early modern Japanese medicine], Vol. 13. Tokyo: Meicho shuppan.

────── (eds). 1982. *Kinsei kampô igakusho shûsei* [Collected works of early modern Japanese medicine], Vol. 65. Tokyo: Meicho shuppan.

ten Rhijne, W. 1683. *De Acupunctura*. London: R. Chiswell.

Shively, D. 1964. 'Sumptuary Regulation and Status in Early Tokugawa Japan', *Harvard Journal of Asiatic Studies* 25: 123–64.

Takizawa, M. 1927. *The Penetration of the Money Economy in Japan and its Effects upon Social and Political Institutions*. New York: Columbia University Press.

Yamaguchi, T. (ed.). 1926. *Nihon meicho zenshû: kibyôshi nijûgoshû* [Collected Japanese classics: twenty-five picture-books], Vol. 11. Tokyo: Nihon meicho zenshû kankôkai.

Yokota, F. 1989. 'Hataraku koto no kinseishi' [The early modern history of work], *Kôbe Daigaku shigaku nenpô* 4: 63–79.

A Practice with What?

Chapter 4
Were the Four Humours Fundamental to Medieval Islamic Medical Practice?

Emilie Savage-Smith

The concept of four humours – what historians today call humoral pathology – is found not only throughout the Greek-based formal medicine of the medieval Islamic world (as exemplified by the *Qānūn* of Ibn Sīnā, known to Europeans as Avicenna), but also the pre-Islamic medicine attributed by Muslim scholars to the Prophet Muḥammad and his immediate followers (Pormann and Savage-Smith 2007: 43–45). The latter form of medicine was recorded by religious scholars in treatises known as 'prophetic medicine' (*al-ṭibb al-nabawī*/الطب النبوى). Treatises of this type were composed as early as the mid ninth century, but they became particularly popular in the fourteenth century, perhaps as a result of the occurrence of the Black Death in 1348 (Perho 1995).[1] The emphasis is on care and cure through food and simple medicines, proper conduct and invocations to God. Diagnosis and prognosis play little role in *al-ṭibb al-nabawī*, presumably because they suggest a notion of causality which might limit the omnipotence of God. There is a conscious avoidance of any claims of medicine to absoluteness. Yet, despite the qualms about the underlying notions of causality, the authors still accepted and utilized the humoral theory of disease. Thus, the notion that disease could be classified and explained in terms of the four humours appears to have been deeply ingrained in Islamic medicine in all its various forms.

89

Whatever its origins, the notion of four bodily humours was one of the unchallenged 'scientific' or medical ideas that were universally assimilated with little or no challenge throughout the Islamic world. Similar ideas that went unchallenged were the sphericity of the Earth, the Euclidean geometry of lines, angles, circles and cones, and the properties of numbers and principles of calculating with them (Savage-Smith forthcoming). As Dimitri Gutas has noted in his study of medical theory and scientific method in the age of Ibn Sīnā, 'the *theory* and principles of humoral pathology are to be accepted as given in natural science (Physics) and their investigation is declared off-limits to the physician' (Gutas 2003: 151, original emphasis). And so it was.

What I wish to consider here, however, is whether the four humours, and an attempt to balance them, played a primary – or even merely significant – role in therapeutics. In other words, did the imbalance of one of the four humours determine the course of treatment?

To test the common assumption that the four humours were at the centre of medical therapy in medieval Islam (and in the medieval world in general), I begin with a definition of humours given by an Arabic medical author named Abū al-Faraj ibn Hindū (d. 1029), an exact contemporary of Ibn Sīnā (d. 1037). Ibn Hindū was a Muslim philosopher, government official and physician, educated in medicine in Baghdad and employed by the Buyid court in Rayy, near modern Tehran. He was called Ibn Hindū because he was originally from Hindujan in Qum, a region of Iran that included Rayy (Mohaghegh 1999).[2]

In his treatise *The Key to Medicine and a Guide to Students*, Ibn Hindū provided the following definition:

> A discussion of humours [*akhlāṭ* اخلاط]: Humours are the foundations of the microcosm, which is the human being. Their equivalent in the macrocosm is the elements. This is because the body is composed of these humours just as all else in the world of creation and decay is made up of the elements.
>
> The humours are: blood, phlegm, yellow bile and black bile. Blood is hot and moist, the counterpart of air; yellow bile is hot and dry, the counterpart of fire; phlegm is cold and moist, the counterpart of water; and black bile is cold and dry, the counterpart of earth. These humours

are formed of the elements, which is why they resemble them and have related qualities.

It is for this reason that we say the human body is composed of the four elements. It originates from them – although through the intermediary of humours – and will return to them when decay sets in.

Know that the natures of the humours are as I described when they are normal and follow their natural course. However, some corruption or change might cause them to deviate from their normal state. Black bile, one of the basic constituents of the body, is naturally cold and dry. However, as a result of heat affecting the other humours, black bile may become dry and hot. Yellow bile [*al-ṣafrā* الصفراء] is also known as 'yellow bile' [*al-mirrah al-al-ṣafrā* المرة الصفراء], 'red bile' [*al-mirrah al-ḥamrā* المرة الحمراء] or 'yellow gall' [*al-mirār al-aṣfar* المرار الاصفر], and black bile [*al-sawdā* السوداء] known as 'black bile' [*al-mirrah al-sawdā* المرة السوداء] and 'black gall' [*al-mirār* المرار]. (Ibn Hindū 2010: 60–61)[3]

What I like about this definition is that it emphasizes the philosophical origins of the concept of four humours. The logical requirement of having four microcosmic substances equivalent or parallel to the four macrocosmic elements was the underlying motivation for the creation of the concept of four humours. Perhaps as a result of this cosmological origin, two of them (yellow bile and black bile) remained highly speculative with no clear counterpart in today's physiology. Yellow bile, often said to be red in colour despite its name, was generally considered a foam or scum produced during the formation of blood; after its production in the liver, half the yellow bile flowed with the venous blood while the other half was said to go to the gall bladder. Black bile was usually interpreted as a sedimentary dark matter also produced during blood formation, half of it remaining in the blood and the other half going to the spleen. That portion of the yellow bile that was siphoned off to the gall bladder can be compared to what we know today as bile: a golden-brown to greenish-yellow and bitter fluid secreted by the liver and poured into the small intestines via the bile ducts and concentrated in the gall bladder. The other portion of the yellow bile that was said to flow with the venous blood has no clear parallel in modern physiology. Similarly, black bile has no obvious equivalent in modern terms, though the darkest part of coagulated blood is black, and dark material is occasionally found in vomit, urine and excrement. In fact, one suspects that the postulation of these two biles only came about through the necessity for four fundamental substances in order to complete the symmetry of the system.

Case Histories

Let us now look at preserved case histories for evidence of the role of the humours in medical practice. There are over 900 case histories recorded by the students of Abū Bakr Muḥammad ibn Zakarīyā al-Rāzī (d. 925), working in Baghdad and Rayy. Most case notes simply record the symptoms. For example: 'headache, pain and cough', or 'continuous fever, red urine with pain', or 'headache and pain in right ear', or 'coughing for five months and vomiting a foamy blood for last three days' (Álvarez-Millán 2000: 295–96, 303; 2010; Harbī 2006). There are, however, a few instances in these case histories where humours are specified as the cause: 'Headache caused by a yellow bile vapour' or 'illness caused by an excess of bile that has crept to the head'.

While the cause of the illness may be explained in humoral terms as an imbalance of one humour, the therapy is never couched in humoral terms. Rather, therapy consists of the simple application of a medicament (or sometimes by bleeding or another form of evacuation) to suit the perceived symptoms. The justification for the use of one medicament over another is given in terms of the four qualities – warm, cold, dry, moist – associated with each medicinal substance, and not by an association with one of the four humours. In other words, there is no humoral justification given for the application of evacuation techniques or medicaments.

Throughout medieval Islamic medicine, individual medicinal substances (including foodstuffs) were classified by assigning to each a pair of primary qualities (dry or moist, warm or cool) and by grading their intensity on a scale from 1 (weakest) to 4 or 5 (strongest). Various methods of predicting the strength and effects of combined medicaments were proposed (Langermann 2003). In this way the notion of balance played a dominant role in therapy in the sense of balancing the primary qualities detectable in a temperament of a bodily part through employment of a mollifying or balancing medicine.

These case histories of al-Rāzī (and other similar ones), however, are very brief and terse, and consequently perhaps not the best guide to the role of humours in the therapeutics of the day.

Medical Manuals

In contrast to the abbreviated accounts preserved in case notes, the numerous manuals on therapeutics potentially provide a more detailed view of procedures. So let us look at an excerpt from a very influential therapeutic manual, *The Hundred Books on the Medical Art* by a Syrian Christian physician named Abū Sahl al-Masīḥī (d. 1010). There is persuasive evidence that he was the teacher of Ibn Sīnā (Sanagustin 2002: 304–8; Savage-Smith 2006). We know for certain that he was at the court in Khwārazm (south of the Aral Sea) at the same time as Ibn Sīnā, and when in 1010 a number of scholars at the court were summoned, rather abruptly, to the court of a rival ruler in Ghazna (now eastern Afghanistan), al-Masīḥī fled together with Ibn Sīnā in the opposite direction (westward). The two succeeded in fleeing as far as Māzandarān, a province to the south of the Caspian Sea, where they encountered a sudden sandstorm. Al-Masīḥī died in the sandstorm, but Ibn Sīnā continued travelling south-west into Iran. In Book 59 of his *Hundred Books*, which is titled 'On the Rules of Therapeutics', al-Masīḥī says the following:

> The procedures for treating diseases particular to one part of the body comprise four methods: (1) The first method is determined by the temperament [*mizāj* مزاج] of the ailing organ; (2) the second is derived from its physical form [*khalq* خلق]; (3) the third method is understood from its position [*waḍ'* وضع]; and (4) the fourth is determined by its strength [*quwwah* قوة].
>
> (1) As for the method derived from the temperament of the ailing organ, examples are those bodily parts in which heat dominates, such as flesh, or those in which coldness predominates, such as the nerves, or those parts balanced between the two, such as skin. If the natural temperament of any one of them should change, it is necessary that we restore it to its natural temperament by [using] things that deviate away from balance in the direction opposite to which it [the temperament] has inclined.
>
> (2) As for the procedure based upon the physical form [*khlaq* خلق] and shape [*hay'ah* هيئة] of the bodily part, we should observe [i.e., pay attention to] whether it is hollow or not. Those parts that possess a cavity either

have it only internally, as is the case with the stomach and the blood vessels in the hands and feet, or only externally, as is the case with nerves which are on the interior of the tunic [*ṣifāq*, probably peritoneum, possibly dura mater], or they have a cavity both internally and externally, as is the case with the lungs, which are surrounded externally by the chest cavity and internally have portions of the windpipe and pulsating vessels [arteries] dispersed and scattered in them.

Those bodily parts that are compact and not hollow are primary [*aṣl* اصل], such as the nerves that are in the hands and feet, and for that reason we begin, when necessary, by draining the parts and cleansing them of all the superfluities that have accumulated, which we judge by what is indicated for each one of them rather than by some other way [?]. That is because the parts which have no cavity either externally or internally require very powerful drugs for drainage of superfluities accumulated in them. The parts which have a concavity on either side [i.e., internally or externally], if they are compact and solid, require drugs which are in a middle category with regard to strength, but if the organs are light and porous, it is sufficient to use weak drugs. As for those bodily parts which have a concavity from one direction only, they require stronger drugs than the latter. Whenever a bodily part is light of substance and porous – such as the lung – it cannot withstand treatment with a strong drug, but when a body is compact and solid, such as the two kidneys, it withstands treatment with a strong drug. And when a bodily part is midway between the two – such as the liver and spleen – it requires a drug of medium strength.

(3) The method determined by the position of the part is one in which we look at the placement of the part and its relationship to what is adjacent. In treating a part with an abnormal temperament, one benefits from knowledge of the position of the part, because the closeness of the part allows for the drug to reach it and for the force of the drug to remain constant. We administer a drug whose potency will conform to what will cure the disease. If the position of a part is at some distance, the medication will not be able to reach it except by passing through another bodily part. We increase the dosage of a medicament by the amount that it is thought to loose from its potency during the passage which it follows before arriving at the [designated] part.

In the evacuation of disease matter [*māddah* مذة] from a bodily part, one also benefits from knowing the relationship of the part to what is nearby and adjacent. For example, when we wish to evacuate disease matter from the liver, we look at [i.e., consider] if the disease matter is on the concave side of the liver, in which case we would evacuate it with a laxative because the concave side of the liver is next to the intestine. But if the disease matter is on its convex side, then we evacuate with a drug that will induce urination, because the vaulted side of the liver is next to the kidneys ...

(4) As for the method based upon the strength of a bodily part, the physician is to determine whether the part is a principle and primary organ with a force [faculty, *quwwah* قوّة] linked to the rest of bodily parts – as is the case with the brain, the heart and the liver – and determine whether its function is a function of common usefulness to all the parts of the body – as is the case with the stomach and diaphragm – and determine whether it possesses acute sense perception, as does the eye. That is because when we need to apply a medicament to a bodily part which displays some or all of these characteristics, we should be cautious about using a drug whose potency would have a [detrimental] impact or would injure it.

But when it is not possible to do otherwise, we employ what we need of the drugs. When we need to administer a drug to the liver or stomach, it is by means of a dressing in which we have mixed the solvent drugs with other drugs that are astringent and fragrant in order that the strength of the organ remain the same. Similarly, when the stomach or liver in a person is weak, we protect it and refrain from sending to it during a fever a drink of very cold water, especially if the fever is very burning. In the same way, when we need to evacuate the body through the use of a laxative, we avoid – given a weak stomach or liver – drinking scammony [*saqmūniyā* سقمونيا] or euphorbia [*shubrum* شبرم]. If we administer the beverages, we mix it with something restorative so that it does not lessen the strength of the stomach or liver. (Masīḥī 2000, i: 528–30)[4]

Abū Sahl al-Masīḥī continues with further details regarding this fourth and final procedure making up the four methods of therapy. Throughout, however, there is no mention of either the assessment of the humours causing the complaint or the selection of a therapy designed to redress the imbalanced humour.

This treatise by al-Masīḥī had considerable later influence. Given that he was in all likelihood the teacher of Ibn Sīnā, and quite certainly a close colleague and friend, it is likely that it had an impact upon the most influential of all medieval medical manuals, Ibn Sīnā's *Qānūn*, or the *Canon of Medicine*. An example of al-Masīḥī's later influence is the fact that part of the section translated above is summarized (rather drastically) and cited by name by a late twelfth-century Muslim physician named 'Abd al-'Azīz al-Sulamī. He practised medicine in Damascus at the Nūrī hospital before moving to Cairo, around the year 1200, where he was appointed chief physician. In Cairo he dedicated to the vizier a diatribe (in question-and-answer format) against Damascene physicians which he entitled *Intelligent Examination of All Physicians*. Humours play such a small role in this tract that even in the chapter titled 'The Fundamentals of this Art', humours are not mentioned, except for a quotation from the ninth-century scholar Qusṭā ibn Lūqā stating that the art of medicine should include ten topics, one of which is 'the study of the humours and compositions on which the fundamentals of the human body are based' (Sulamī 2004: 114).

Humours in a Therapeutic Context

This is not to say that humours are never mentioned in therapeutic contexts. When they are, however, it is usually in a rather vague way. For example, Ibn Maymūn, known in Europe as Maimonides (d. 1204), stated in his book of aphorisms: 'If someone has putrid, thin humours in his body, it requires more nutrition, and if he has humours with the opposite quality, it indicates the opposite' (Maimonides 2007: 42). This sentiment, of course was extracted by Maimonides for his collection of medical aphorisms from Galen's treatise *De acutorum morborum victu et Galeni commentarius* (Maimonides 2007: 116 n.2), and it can be found throughout the Arabic literature in one form or another. In all such statements, there is no concern shown for restoring the balance of one particular humour vis-à-vis the others.

On the other hand, therapeutic instructions to remove an excess of humours are sometimes specified. In these instances, however, it is always (or nearly always) all the humours that are to be purged, and not a specific one. As an example, I offer three quotations from a treatise composed, probably in Baghdad or Samarrā' but possibly in Armenia, by Qusṭā ibn Lūqā (d. *c.* 912), a Christian physician of Greek origin from Baʿlbakk in Syria. It was written for a Muslim chief judge (*qāḍī al-quḍāh*/قاضي القضاة) who suffered from numbness in the foot. Bloodletting was, according to Qusṭā ibn Lūqā, the preferred method of treatment, but since his patron loathed and feared bloodletting, Qusṭā was compelled to devote most of the treatise to drug remedies that could be employed instead.

The notion of 'balance' figures prominently in Qusṭā's preface:

The preservation of every beloved one is desirable, and every living creature is preserved through a balanced mixture. It is thus necessary to desire the preservation of the judge and strive to keep his mixture balanced.

His bodily constitution gives evidence – by conclusions drawn from its colour and shape, stout or slender, and the extent of the blood vessels, wide or narrow, and the symmetrical form and healthy look of his face, and the state of the hair in quantity and quality; and from traces of the soul in his power of discrimination and the soundness of thoughts, and what the actions display of patience or pride – of a balanced mixture in his entire body, in each of its parts. (Qusṭā ibn Lūqā 2000: 3)

In a chapter on purgative drugs by which numbness is treated, Qusṭā states:

The purgative drugs by which numbness is treated are of two kinds: one of these extracts the humours that cause numbness from the body. The other heats the parts that have become cold, removes the chill and mixes with a cold humour if there is such in them.

As for the drugs that extract the humours from the body, the most efficient of them, and the one that cleans the body most completely, is the pill known as *qūqāqā* [قوقاقا]. It is a pill that Galen composed and he was of the opinion that it cleans the body of all humours. (Qusṭā ibn Lūqā 2000: 45)

Qusṭā says the following in a chapter titled 'On the Indications by which We Know which One of the Causes It Is that Has Made the Numbness Occur':

And the filled body is not filled by all humours proportionally; one of them exceeds its natural proportion in the body which is slightly cold ... for there is not pure blood in the vessels but all the blood in them contains all the humours – i.e., blood, phlegm, yellow bile and black bile – and the muscles are filled in proportion to their size in the body in its original constitution. [That a body is filled in this way] is indicated by dilated vessels, heaviness of the body and a feeling of tension in it and sluggish movements. (Qusṭā ibn Lūqā 2000: 25)

Qusṭā is here saying two things: first, numbness is due to the body being overfilled; it suffers from plethora (Greek *plēthos*, Arabic *imtilā'* امتلاء), and the muscles are consequently swollen and the nerves then suppressed. Secondly, all blood and all blood vessels contain all four humours in them. Evacuation is the main cure, through bleeding if possible. The cure, however, is not brought about by the restoration of balance amongst the four humours, which is in fact an impossibility given that there is no way of isolating just one humour in order to restore its proper proportion in the humoral mix.

This, in a nutshell, is the fundamental issue. When it comes to the humours playing a role in therapy, there was a problem: the blood vessels carried not only blood but also yellow bile and black bile and even (according to some interpretations) phlegm. Just as only half the yellow bile went to the gall bladder, while the other half combined with the venous blood, so for black bile only half went to the spleen while the other half mixed with the blood in the veins. Thus the fluid carried by the veins was considered by all writers to be a mixture of pure blood, yellow bile and black bile, and by some (such as Qusṭā) to include phlegm. Phlebotomy would extract from the body at least three humours (if not four), not simply one, and therefore it could not be used as a way to adjust the volume of one humour vis-à-vis the other three. With the fourth humour, phlegm, matters appear slightly more straightforward in that phlegmatic discharge from the lungs did not usually include the other humours (though blood was sometimes also present); however, phlegm (*balgham* بلغم) was often interpreted as any viscous moisture or mucus that could be seen in various discharges from the body (including blood, according to Qusṭā), in which case the isolation of it in terms of the other humours again becomes difficult if not impossible. This inability to isolate – and hence rebalance – one humour is evident throughout the literature.

To return to Qusṭā's treatise, because his patron loathed bloodletting (and that was the preferred method of treating a plethora of humours), Qusṭā was compelled to recommend purgatives. But that also is complicated, for purgatives, he says, act by heating the body, and, since heat expands matter, employing heat on an over-full, plethoric body could be dangerous. It was for this reason that bloodletting was considered the best way to cure an overfilled body. Thus, therapeutics was a complex matter involving the maintenance of an approximate total volume of bodily fluids and the balancing of bodily temperature.

Another example – from a treatise composed three hundred years later – again illustrates the complexities and difficulties of treating diseases caused by humours. In this instance the text was composed by a Jewish physician and avowed Galenist by the name of Yaʿqūb ibn Isḥāq al-Isrāʾīlī (d. c. 1202). He had practised for many years in

Cairo, but then moved to Damascus for a while, only to then return permanently to Cairo. After his return he wrote a diatribe concerned with the mistakes made by physicians in Damascus. Given the diatribe written at about the same time by the Cairene al-Sulamī against Damascene physicians (mentioned above), we might be justified in concluding that there was a tradition amongst physicians in Cairo and Damascus (the two most important medical centres during the twelfth and early thirteenth centuries) of trashing each other's medical practices. But that is another topic for discussion. This is what Ya'qūb ibn Isḥāq al-Isrā'īlī has to say about the treatment of diseases caused by the putridity of humours:

> I say: Diseases that come about because of the putridity of humours are obstructive diseases – which is to say that obstruction is often the cause of humoral putridity, although an obstruction which does not suppress heat and residues is not necessarily associated with putridity. Any treatment for putrid humours must aim at fighting the putridity as well as opening the obstruction; evacuation follows [only] after that. You should know, brother, that this is the rule [*qānūn* قانون] of how to treat putridity of humours. Yet the physician must always be aware that this condition has two sides, and that if he concentrates on one of them [only], the other will become stronger. Know also that putridity is treated through cooling, whereas obstruction is treated through heating. Thus, the treatment for putrid humours is complex, and the physician must concentrate on the dominant aspect of the condition without neglecting the other, or else he himself might become the cause of a major calamity! ...
>
> So we repeat: The treatment for putrid humours must involve cooling, moistening, opening, and finally evacuation of the bad humour [*al-khilt al-radī'* الخلط الردي]. And this is why the relevant drugs are so often taken with water. Water, however, may be drunk either hot or cold – when hot, it opens the obstruction, moistens, clears, and causes the matter to descend, but it does not quench the thirst that comes with the fever; cold water, on the other hand, constipates, and it does not relieve or moisten in the same way as hot water and it retains the matter ...
>
> We have made it clear that yellow-bilious fever – let alone the other kinds – requires cooling the putridity and opening the obstruction. Therefore in the treatment of fevers it is best to combine the drugs with small amounts of cooling substances such as saffron, or fennel seed, or spikenard or the like ... This is why cold water which is mixed with a little bit of wine has a stronger capacity to cool than cold water on its own. (Isrā'īlī 2000: 37–38, 55–56)[5]

Here again, the procedures advocated by Ya'qūb ibn Isḥāq al-Isrā'īlī are applied to all the humours, and the balance aimed at is one of balancing the potency of the drugs and adjustment of the primary qualities of the drugs and the fever.

With both these examples (Qusṭā and al-Isrā'īlī), it is evident that the therapeutic regime was dominated by balancing hot and cold, and dry and moist, through medicaments, food and the immediate environment, and/or the retention and evacuation of all, or most, of the humours by means of bloodletting (since three or even four were present in the blood) or purging. Even in the case of jaundice (*yarqān* يرقان), which is associated causatively with yellow bile, the best therapy was said to be the consumption of a purgative medicament (aimed at the elimination of no particular humour) and then the extraction of blood, which took off at least three of the humours (Ullmann 1983: 32). There is no attempt to rebalance the four humours, or remove a specific humour that is in over-abundance.

A similar pattern is found in the treatment of melancholia, whose explanation was usually couched in terms of black bile (said to be 'abundant' or sometimes 'burnt'), but which was also attributed to excessive yellow bile or to non-humoral causes such as a neglect of some of the six non-naturals (Ullmann 1978: 66; Dols 1992: 62–91; Pormann 2008). While there were different theories as to the cause, all therapy for melancholia consisted of purging and/or bloodletting along with the adjustment of the six non-naturals (surrounding air, food and drink, sleeping and waking, exercise and rest, retention and evacuation, and mental states).

Of all maladies, fevers were the ones most commonly associated with one of the four humours. More often than any other category of therapeutic procedure, their proposed therapies involved at least the mention of the imbalance of a specific humour. Certain types of fevers are associated with certain humours in terms of cause: tertian fevers with putrefied yellow bile, for example, or quartan fever with the putrefaction of black bile; quotidian fever with the putrefaction of phlegm (Isḥāq ibn Sulaymān 1981; Ibn al-Jazzār 2000; Pormann and Savage-Smith 2007: 57). Therapy, in virtually all cases, is an attempt to reduce the heat through various measures (drugs, cold compresses and such) also accompanied often (but not always) by general evacuation of bodily fluids, either through bleeding or purgatives. In the case of quotidian fever, attempts were also made to induce expulsion of phlegm, and it is only in the latter case that we have what might be interpreted as a distinctly humoral approach to therapy.

The irrelevance of humoral theory to basic therapeutics, and the complexities of trying to balance temperaments, is illustrated by the following harsh words that Cyril Elgood had for therapeutics in the Safavid Empire of Persia in the sixteenth and seventeenth centuries:

> Pathology taught that Pleurisy was caused by pure bile or by bile mixed with blood and there was even a type due to phlegm ... But who cared? Cough and pain in the side pointed to Pleurisy and Pneumonia, whatever the humour involved might be. It is clear that in many cases the diagnosis of the disease was easier than the diagnosis of the cause. Indeed, the multiplicity of remedies suggests that in most cases (as is too often the case today) the treatment was symptomatic and of the 'grape-shot' type ... Just as the patient and the disease had each his own temperament, so had all drugs. Not only had every drug its own specific temperament, hot or cold, wet or dry, but each of these temperaments was subdivided into degrees. Thus, a drug was said to be hot in the first, second or third degree. This gave rise to innumerable combinations and, as it was necessary to give the patient a drug with a temperament suited to his temperament, the difficulty for the treating physician was enormous. It will be remembered by readers of *Hajji Baba* [the popular picaresque novel of 1824 by James Morier entitled *The Adventures of Hajji Baba of Ispahan*] how the European doctor cured a case of colic brought about by over indulgence in raw cucumbers by means of a dose of mercury and the comment that the Persian doctor made upon such treatment: 'Whoever heard of mercury as a medicine? Mercury is cold and lettuce and cucumber are cold also. You would not apply ice to dissolve ice. The ass does not know the first rudiments of his profession'. (Elgood 1970: 16–17)

The Four Primary Qualities in a Therapeutic Context

By and large, however, it is evident throughout the medieval medical treatises and the recorded case notes that the balance that was to be reinstated during the restitution of health had to be centred not on the balance of the four humours but on the balancing of the four primary qualities (through the use of medicaments which could be quantified and ranked in terms of the primary qualities and in terms of potency), and also through the balancing of the environmental, non-humoral, elements known as the six 'non-naturals'. Thus, the overriding therapeutic principle was one of balancing the four primary qualities (hot, dry, cold, wet) and the 'non-naturals', rather than the balancing of the four humours.

To illustrate this further, and to encapsulate the general role of the concept of 'balance' in medieval Islamic medicine and therapeutics, I wish to return to the *Key to Medicine and a Guide to Students* by Ibn Hindū, with which I began this chapter. Ibn Hindū's definition of balance in the body:

> *al-i'tidāl* [الاعتدال, balance]: This term applies to three conditions:
> (1) Equality of constituents. For example, when an ointment consists of ceruse, wax, verdigris and oil, in four equal quantities.
> (2) Equality of potency. For example, increasing the level of bitterness in a moderately bitter substance and, if that is not possible because you have taken equal amounts of sharp vinegar and water, to increase the water relative to the vinegar. This is because the potency of a small amount of vinegar is equal to the potency of a large amount of water when tasted.[6]
> (3) The balanced state prevailing within a particular species. For example, the balanced state of a lion is one in which heat dominates. The balanced state of a rabbit, however, is one in which cold dominates. The former is the balanced state of the leonine species, while the latter is the balanced state of the species of rabbits.
> *Sū' al-mizāj* [سوء المزاج, abnormal temperament]: This means deviation from balance. When an abnormal temperament takes over the entire body, or a whole organ, and there is no sensation of pain, the abnormal temperament is called 'equable' [*mustawan*, level]. However, as long as the organ continues to feel pain, the abnormal temperament is not described as 'equable', but is then known as 'divergent' [*mukhtalif*]. (Ibn Hindū 2010: 97–98)[7]

We can see from Ibn Hindū's treatise addressed to medical students that the notion of 'balance' was fundamental to medicine, but that it did not refer to the four humours. In the same chapter Ibn Hindū also supplied a concise summary of the components of therapeutics, in which it will be seen again that the four humours play no role:

> *Banāt al-isṭaqisāt* [بنات الاسطقسات, lit. 'daughters of the rules'] and *banāt al-arkān* [بنات الاركان, lit. 'daughters of foundations']: These are the things by which a doctor works out what treatment is necessary. They are seven: the

patient's temperament, his age, his habits, his occupation, his strength, the time of year, and the temperament of the country in which he lives.

Take, for example, a patient suffering from an acute illness. If his natural temperament is cold, he requires for treatment extra cooling because, if it hadn't been for the fierceness of the heat that burned in him, it [the heat] would not have triumphed over his cold temperament.

On the other hand, if the patient's natural temperament is hot, he needs a moderate level of cooling, because a person with a hot temperament needs only a small amount of heat to warm up his temperament, and a small amount of heat will produce a hot illness in him. It is a similar case if the patient is a young man, or if he is used to eating spicy food, or his home is in a hot country, or his occupation is heat-producing, such as blacksmithing which employs fire. Hot diseases are less potent in these cases, and vice versa.

Similarly, if the patient is weak and requires bloodletting, the doctor refrains from bloodletting. But, if he does go ahead with it, he takes only a small amount. If the patient happens to be robust, the doctor embarks on phlebotomy boldly, without much care. Since these are basic matters upon which treatment is based, they are regarded as the foundations of the body and are given the name *banāt al-arkān* ['daughters of the foundations', that is, derivative principles]. (Ibn Hindū 2010: 97)[8]

Closing Remarks

The case I have tried to make in this chapter is that, in the medical practice of the medieval Islamic world, the four humours played a lesser role than has commonly been assumed by the description of medieval medicine as 'humoral pathology'. The concept of 'balance' on the other hand, was foremost in the therapeutic thinking of the day – but the balance was one of the four qualities (hot and cold, moist and dry) and the six 'non-naturals' rather than of the four humours.

If that was the case, and I believe that further examination of the sources will support that contention, then are we justified in speaking of humoral pathology to describe medieval therapeutics? The term 'humoral pathology', it should be noted, was invented by Europeans, with the first recorded use occurring in a letter of Thomas Beddoes written in 1793 in which he referred to 'the loose analogies of the humoral pathology'.[9] Its employment by the influential historian of science William Whewell, who in 1858 wrote of 'the humoral pathology of the ancients',[10] no doubt encouraged its widespread adoption by modern historians of medicine.

Are we, however, correct in glibly using 'humoral pathology' as a description of medieval medicine in general, as if that expression says all that needs to be said about both its theory and its practice? In other words, should not the adjective 'humoral' be restricted to the nosology and aetiology of the period – that is, to the classification of diseases and the theories of causation – and another sought to designate the qualitative balance that dominated therapeutic care.

Notes

1. In the eastern provinces, two brothers, Abū 'Attab Allāh and al-Ḥusayn, sons of Bisṭām ibn Sābūr, composed such a treatise drawing upon the authority of Shī'ite imams, while about the same time Ibn Ḥabīb (d. *c.* 853) composed in Muslim Spain an essay using *ḥadīth*s as a major source. For the former, see Ispahany and Newman (1991), and for the latter see Álvarez de Morales and Girón Irueste (1992). See also Pormann and Savage-Smith (2007: 71–6, 150–1) and Stearns (2007, 2011).
2. The name of his home town might also be read as Hinduwān, the former citadel of the city of Balkh. On Hinduwān, see Barthold (1984: 26–28).
3. For the original text, in a section entitled 'Terms Related to the Principles of Medicine', see Ibn Hindū (2002: 131–32). See also Khalīfat (1995).
4. Author's translation, based on Masīḥī (2000: i: 528–30) and a manuscript version (Bodleian Library, Oxford, MS Hunt. 202, fols.186a, 186b).
5. The passage follows the translation of Oliver Kahl, amended in places by the author.
6. The meaning of the last sentence is obscure.
7. For the original text, in a section entitled 'On Bits of Wisdom and Aphorisms Not Mentioned in Previous Chapters', see Ibn Hindū (2002: 204).
8. For the original text, see Ibn Hindū (2002: 203).
9. Beddoes, 'Letter to Erasmus Darwin', cited in the online version of the *Oxford English Dictionary*, s.v. 'humoral', 1.c. Retrieved 14 May 2012 from: http://ezproxy.ouls.ox.ac.uk:2277/view/Entry/89403?redirectedFrom=humoral#eid.
10. Whewell, *History of Scientific Ideas*, cited in the online version of the *Oxford English Dictionary*, s.v. 'humoral', 1.c. Retrieved 14 May 2012 from: http://ezproxy.ouls.ox.ac.uk:2277/view/Entry/89403?redirectedFrom=humoral#eid.

References

Álvarez de Morales, C., and F. Girón Irueste. 1992. *Mujtaṣar fī l-ṭibb = compendio de medicina*. Madrid: Consejo suprior de Investigaciones científicas, Instituto de Cooperatión con el Mundo Árabe.

Álvarez-Millán, C. 2000. 'Practice versus Theory: Tenth-century Case Histories from the Islamic Middle East', in P. Horden and E. Savage-Smith (eds), *The Year 1000: Medical Practice at the End of the First Millennium* [*Social History of Medicine*, 13 (2000)]. Oxford: Oxford University Press, pp.293–306.

———— 2010. 'The Case History in Medieval Islamic Medical Literature: *Tajārib* and *Mujarrabāt* as Source', *Medical History* 54: 195–214.

Barthold, W. 1984. *An Historical Geography of Iran*, trans. S. Soucek, ed. C.E. Bosworth. Princeton, NJ: Princeton University Press.

Dols, M.W. 1992. *Majnūn: The Madman in Medieval Islamic Society*. Oxford: Clarendon Press.

Elgood, C. 1970. *Safavid Medical Practice, or The Practice of Medicine, Surgery and Gynaecology in Persia between 1500 AD and 1750 AD*. London: Luzac.

Gutas, D. 2003. 'Medical Theory and Scientific Method in the Age of Avicenna', in D.C. Reisman and A.H. al-Rahim (eds), *Before and After Avicenna*. Leiden: Brill, pp.145–62.

Harbī, K. 2006. *Kitāb al-Tajārib li-Abī Muḥammad ibn Zakarīyā al-Rāzī ma'a dirāsah manhāj al-baḥth al-'ilmī 'inda al-Rāzī* [The book of experiences by Abū Muḥammad ibn Zakarīyā al-Rāzī, with a study of al-Rāzī's scientific method]. Alexandria: Dār al-Wafā' li-Dunyā al-ṭibā'ah wa-al-Nashr.

Ibn Hindū. 2002. *Miftāh al-ṭibb wa-minhāj al-ṭullāb*, [The key to medicine and a guide to students], ed. 'Alī Manṣūrī. Beirut: Mu'assasat al-Balāgh.

———— 2010. *The Key to Medicine and a Guide to Students*, trans. A. Tibi, rev. E. Savage-Smith. Reading: Garnet.

Ibn al-Jazzār. 2000. *Ibn al-Jazzār on Fevers*, trans. and ed. G. Bos. London: Kegan Paul.

Ispahany, B., and A. Newman. 1991. *Islamic Medical Wisdom: The Ṭibb al-a'imma*. London: Muhammadi Trust.

Isḥāq ibn Sulaymān. 1981. *Kitāb al-Ḥummayāt li-Isḥāq Sulaymān al-Isrā'īlī (al-Maqāla al-Thālitha: fī al-sill)*. Isaac Judaeus: On Fevers (The Third discourse: On Consumption), *I*, trans. and ed. J.D. Latham and H.D. Isaacs. Cambridge: Pembroke Arabic Texts.

Isrā'īlī. 2000. *Ya'qūb ibn Isḥāq al-Isrā'īlī's 'Treatise on the Errors of the Physicians in Damascus': A Critical Edition of the Arabic Text Together with an Annotated English Translation*, trans. and ed. O. Kahl. Oxford: Oxford University Press.

Khalīfat, S. 1995. *Ibn Hindū: sīratuhu, ārā'uhu al-falsafīyah, mu'allafātuhu: dirāsah wa-nuṣūs* [Ibn Hindū: his life, his philosophical views, and his compositions], 3 vols. Amman, Jordan: al-Jāmi'ah al-Urdunīya, 'Imādat al-Baḥth al-'Ilmī, Kullīyat al-Ādab.

Langermann, Y.T. 2003. 'Another Andalusian Revolt? Ibn Rushd's Critique of al-Kindī's *Pharmacological Computus*', in J.P. Hogendijk and A.I. Sabra (eds), *The Enterprise of Science in Islam: New Perspectives*. Cambridge, MA: MIT Press, pp.351–72.

Maimonides. 2007. *Medical Aphorisms, Treatises 6–9: A Parallel Arabic-English Edition*, trans. and ed. G. Bos. Provo, UT: Brigham Young University Press.

Masīḥī. 2000. *al-Kutub al-miʾah fī al-ṣināʿah al-ṭibbīyah* [The hundred books on the medical art], ed. F. Sanagustin, 2 vols. Damascus: al-Maʿhad al-Faransī lil-Dirasāt al-ʿArabīyah.

Mohaghegh, M. 1999. 'Ibn Hindū and the Hellenic Medical Tradition', in J.A.C. Greppin, E. Savage-Smith and J.L. Gueriguian (eds), *The Diffusion of Greco-Roman Medicine into the Middle East and the Caucasus*. Delmar, NY: Caravan Books, pp.129–37.

Perho, I. 1995. *The Prophet's Medicine: A Creation of the Muslim Traditionalist Scholars*. Helsinki: Finnish Oriental Society.

Pormann, P.E. (ed.). 2008. *Rufus of Ephesus: On Melancholy*. Tübingen: Mohr Siebeck.

Pormann, P.E., and E. Savage-Smith. 2007. *Medieval Islamic Medicine*. Edinburgh: Edinburgh University Press.

Qusṭā ibn Lūqā. 2000. *On Numbness: A Book on Numbness, its Kinds, Causes and Treatment according to the Opinion of Galen and Hippocrates*, trans. and ed. L. Amjbörn. Stockholm: Almqvist and Wiksell.

Sanagustin, F. 2002. 'Le *Canon de la médecine* d'Avicenne, texte de rupture épistémologique?' in J.L. Janssens and D. De Smet (eds), *Avicenna and his Heritage*. Leuven: Leuven University Press, pp.297–311.

Savage-Smith, E. 2006. 'New Evidence for the Frankish Study of Arabic Medical Texts in the Crusader Period', *Crusades* 5: 99–112.

——— (forthcoming). 'The Universality and Neutrality of Science', in M.G. Morony (ed.), *Universality in Islamic Thought*. London: Routledge.

Stearns, J. 2007. 'Contagion in Theology and Law: Ethical Considerations in the Writings of Two Fourteenth-century Scholars of Naṣrid Granada', *Islamic Law and Society* 14: 109–29.

——— 2011. *Infectious Ideas: Contagion in Premodern Islamic and Christian Thought in the Western Mediterranean*. Baltimore, MD: Johns Hopkins University Press.

Sulamī. 2004. *Questions and Answers for Physicians: A Medieval Arabic Study Manual by ʿAbd al-ʿAzīz al-Sulamī*, trans. and ed. G. Leiser and N. al-Khaledy. Leiden: Brill.

Ullmann, M. 1978. *Rufus von Ephesos: Krankenjournale*. Wiesbaden: Harrassowitz.

——— 1983. *Die Schrift des Rufus von Ephesos über die Gelbsucht, in arabischer und lateinischer Übersetzung*. Göttingen: Vandenhoeck and Ruprecht.

Chapter 5
Complexio and *Experimentum*
Tensions in Late Medieval Medical Practice

Peter Murray Jones

In the half century between 1270 and 1320, scholastic medicine both achieved its most brilliant intellectual feats and made a great breakthrough in persuading governing elites in Western Europe of its critical importance in health care. Teaching medicine in the universities of Italy, France and England was less than a century old by 1300, so this double triumph of the doctors was the culmination of a meteoric rise. The great scholastic medical authors, Taddeo Alderotti, Arnald de Villanova, Pietro d'Abano, Bernard de Gordon, and Henri de Mondeville, to name the most famous, were university teachers but also medical practitioners of high repute, employed by popes, kings, nobles and city communes. The medicine these doctors espoused had assimilated the medieval scholastic method of analysing texts and applied it systematically to a corpus of ancient writings newly translated from Arabic and Greek. On the basis of this textual scholarship, the medical scholastics claimed to have re-established the rational medicine championed by Galen and to be better prepared to maintain or recover the health of the individual than any other kind of practitioner.[1]

And yet one of the foremost modern historians of medieval scholastic medicine can ask this rhetorical question: 'In the entire history of universal culture, is there any other field that has more aptly served as a symbol of sterility of thought than that of scholastic medicine?' (Jacquart 1998a: 197). Danielle Jacquart has argued that this dismissive attitude to medical scholasticism has roots that stretch far back in time but which also run forward to the present day. The reputation of scholastic medicine has never recovered from the assaults of Renaissance humanists and later exponents of so-called 'experimental' science; for these groups, scholastic medicine represented unquestioning obedience to corrupted texts of the ancient authorities, and disputatiousness over mere words instead of attention to the results of observation and testing. Just as damaging, the reputation of the scholastics as practitioners of medicine has been almost entirely negative. The best that is usually claimed for them is that by applying the tenets of humoral theory in advising their patients on regimen and diet, they did at least attempt to tailor their prescriptions to the individual constitutions and circumstances of their patients. It is usually assumed otherwise that in medication and surgery the effects of applying a humoral theory of the body's working to practice was to obfuscate any real understanding of the effects of medicine or surgical intervention, and to encourage a promiscuous polypharmacy of herbs, animal parts and minerals, alongside an unfortunate, and often lethal, enthusiasm for purging and bloodletting.

How could scholastic medicine later become such a byword for intellectual futility and practical incompetence, and yet achieve hegemony over theory and practice in late medieval Europe? One way of explaining the surprising success of scholastic medicine in the later Middle Ages might be to argue that its imposing intellectual credentials disposed people to overlook its ineffectiveness or downright dangerousness as a technology for healing. In this perspective, medical practitioners were so much in thrall to the ideology of scholastic medicine, based on respect for ancient authoritative texts, that they could persuade themselves and their patients that the treatments they offered were the best to be had, when in fact they did no good. This was in fact essentially the line taken by one of the very few contemporary critics of scholastic medicine, Nicholas of Poland, who had studied medicine at one of the great centres of scholastic teaching, Montpellier, but rejected the classical authority of Hippocrates and Galen. About 1270 he returned to Cracow in Poland, took up practice at his Dominican monastery, and based his own treatments on the attribution of marvellous healing virtues to ordinary, indeed contemptible, things like the flesh of serpents and frogs. His remedies were collected, and circulated, as *Experimenta*

magistri Nicolai (Eamon and Keil 1987). *Experimentum* was in fact
a term that was well known to the scholastics – after all, the first
and most famous of the aphorisms of Hippocrates begins *Ars longa,
vita brevis, tempus acutum, experimentum vero fallax, iudicium
difficile* ('Life is short, and Art long, opportunity fleeting, experience
perilous, and decision difficult'). This text was the most heavily
commented at the hands of the scholastics of all those handed
down by ancient authorities, and was overwhelmingly interpreted,
following Galen, as a critique of empirical remedies (*experimenta*,
sometimes alternatively described as *empirica, mirabilia* or *secreta*)
that had no basis but their apparent success in use. It would seem
that Nicholas of Poland's defiance of the scholastics took the form
of embracing the use of *experimenta* and rejecting a medical system
that based itself on analysis of the textual tradition of Hippocrates
and Galen. As we shall see, the relationship between scholastic
medicine and *experimenta* was in fact much more complicated than
Nicholas's critique would allow.[2]

Complexio and *Experimentum*

The most important idea on which scholastic medicine was based
was that of *complexio* or *temperamentum* (Latin terms translating
the Greek *krasis*), in English, 'complexion'. What was understood
by this was the idea of a mixing or interplay of the four primary
qualities: hot, cold, wet and dry. This could be applied to a great
number of natural things, from medicinal herbs to the human body,
or even to planets. Health in the human body was the proper balance
or 'tempered' mixture of the qualities, hot, cold, wet and dry. This
applied to the body as a whole but also to each of its organs or
parts, and the appropriate mixture of qualities was affected by age,
gender, climate and other factors (Jacquart 1984). Note that strictly
speaking this *complexio* was not a balance of the humours but of the
qualities; nevertheless, most scholastic medical writers seem to have
thought of *complexio* as a balance of humours on occasion.

In this they were encouraged by Galen's development of the
scheme of the four humours that was part of the Hippocratic
tradition. Each of the humours – reddish bile, blood, phlegm, and
black bile – possessed a different combination of two of the qualities.
The humours too were mixed in the body and their relative quantities

might be considered as preserving an equilibrium in health. If health was a fragile balance of the qualities (or humours) in the individual body, then disease was identified as the loss of that balance, or *mala complexio*. This imbalance was not an equal displacement of the natural complexion in all parts of the body simultaneously but was uneven in its effects. Once the imbalance became uniform, however, then the entire body was threatened with destruction. The different forms that disease took were usually seen as a result of the over-abundance of one humour within the body once the balance had been lost, leading to the 'corruption' or 'putrefaction' of that humour (these last concepts deriving from Aristotelian natural philosophy). The task of the practising physician was then to use his knowledge of the human body, and the external environment that acted on it, knowledge derived from the texts he had studied, to maintain that complexional balance in the healthy body or restore it once lost.

Complexio and *experimentum* stood in stark opposition as competitive visions of medicine, or so it would seem. One was the keystone of a philosophical medicine that understood all disease as a balance of the qualities or humours, the other an empirical and even superstitious commitment to the test of experience alone in treating disease. But if we ask ourselves the questions how did those who subscribed to scholastic medicine act as practitioners, what treatments did they use and what was the rationale that lay behind these treatments, we will not find things to be so clear-cut. Of course even asking these questions immediately raises a real problem of method. If medical practice itself comes to be redefined by the scholastics as a branch of *scientia* or science, as a style of reasoning or a way of thinking about phenomena, it will loom very large when the historian looks for evidence of how humoral medicine influenced practice, and may obscure what we want to know about the mindset of the healer actually faced with patients. We are faced with hundreds of texts in thousands of surviving manuscripts, but overwhelmingly these have to do with teaching, not doing. We can address this problem in two ways. Firstly we should follow the hints given by the most sophisticated of the university theorists themselves, who attempted to map the boundaries of the heuristic approach to the practice of medicine. Secondly we should try to find those relatively scarce sources that bring us closer to those healers operating face to face with patients outside the university teaching milieu.

The subordination of practical to theoretical medicine claimed by the scholastics had its limits, limits explored by the scholastics themselves. Working in the 1290s and 1300s, the great Montpellier-trained author and practitioner Arnald de Villanova read newly available texts by Galen (García-Ballester 1982) in such a way as to underwrite what Arnald's editor Michael McVaugh has called 'medical instrumentalism' (McVaugh 1990: 75–84). Medical instrumentalism distinguishes the certain knowledge available to philosophers from that useful knowledge available to doctors of medicine. Truth for the physician is reasoned knowledge that can be to be shown to be effective in bringing about health, whether or not it conforms strictly to the necessary truth of natural philosophy. One application of this medical instrumentalism – set out most clearly in Arnald's influential *De intentione medicorum* of the early 1290s – was that medicines be judged not on their complexion (the balance of qualities that belonged to them as things composed of natural objects) but by their effect on the body to be healed. It followed that however sophisticated the analysis of the blending of the qualities of ingredients of medicine as reflected in the resultant *complexio* (complexional balance) of that medicine – and nobody did more sophisticated analysis in this area than Arnald himself –this could be discounted in practice if the compound medicine brought about certain recognized healing effects. Medical instrumentalism of this sort created a conceptual latitude for the scholastic medical practitioner to take account of observed effects on patients that might not accord with what humoral theory predicted, and to carry the treatment that caused those effects over into his practice if the effects were on the whole beneficial, even though he could not account for why they worked in this way (McVaugh 1990; Villanova 2000).

Arnald de Villanova himself took advantage of this conceptual latitude, so far as we can judge from his own writings on *experimenta*, known from a text of that name to be found today in a single manuscript in Salamanca. *Experimenta* in this context means simply information taken from experience in certain cases treated by the doctor, and Arnald's seventy-three *experimenta* record successful treatments he undertook on named individuals in the circles of the papal court at Avignon between 1305 and 1311. In recording these treatments Arnald diverges markedly from the elaborate remedies described in his more scholastic works on practical medicine. His

111

repertoire of medicines in the *experimenta* is much smaller and he uses hardly any of the elaborate compound medicines that feature so prominently in his other scholastic writings. Michael McVaugh judges that, 'Occasionally the *experimenta* presuppose the ... interpretation of illness as an imbalance or a corruption of the four humours', but more often they do not (McVaugh 1971: 111). Moreover some of the conditions treated are not those we might expect to be the province of a learned doctor of medicine – for example, soothing haemorrhoids, expelling fleas, mending a fracture, treating an unexplained aposteme or swelling. McVaugh has posed a question in relation to these *experimenta*: were the scholastics like Arnald actually involved in two kinds of medicine, 'one learned and formal, carefully prepared and polished for circulation among his professional colleagues or for presentation to royalty, and one more empirical or, in Arnald's own sense "experimental", practised as a matter of daily routine when scholarly learning was not required'. McVaugh does not in the end determine this question: 'it is impossible to be sure how to interpret these peculiarities. For the moment it must be enough to recognize that they are present' (McVaugh 1971: 111–12; see also McVaugh 1976).

Looked at in comparison with the *experimenta* of Nicholas of Poland, we might say that Arnald gives himself licence by means of his understanding of medical instrumentalism to make a collection of trusted remedies of his own. Arnald is by any account an exceptional case, as one of the greatest scholastic authors on medicine, but we can see that for him a sophisticated understanding of the workings of *complexio* does not inhibit a medical practice that can proceed without complexional theory applying in the particular case.

Three English Practitioners of the Fifteenth Century

Our second method of addressing the difficulty of the scholastic understanding of practice in heuristic terms, and its domination of textual production, is to get as close as possible to late medieval medical practitioners themselves, and to try to see in what ways maintaining or restoring complexional balance was important to them. A number of English practitioners of medicine in the fifteenth century left textual traces that do not belong to the scholastic genres of writing. It is very likely that similar documents might be found for practitioners in France, Italy, Germany or Iberia, but I will confine myself here to English examples. The kinds of document produced by the English practitioners might best be described as commonplace books kept in note form, or collections of memoranda relating to their medical practice written out by individual practitioners. These collections were not designed for scholarly circulation but may have been intended for personal use by the practitioners themselves, or by those they designated as heirs to their practice. There are in fact very few surviving documents that can be identified as having been compiled for practical purposes by the practitioners themselves, rather than as copies of texts in circulation (and thus a part of the scholastic textual economy of medicine). As such they can bring us closer to the face-to-face interactions of practitioner and patient than any other kind of document.

Of course these commonplace books are not transparent windows on to medical practice in this era for they are still texts. Much of the difficulty of interpreting them is to understand what may be left out or taken for granted: how far, for instance, do notions of complexional balance underlie the recipes prescribed as remedies for named disorders? Because a recipe does not mention qualities or humours does not mean that consideration of these factors played no part in determining what substances would be prescribed for use on the patient. Nevertheless, the commonplace books do provide real opportunities to interrogate late medieval medicine from the practitioner's or observer's perspective. There are three individuals who kept these medical commonplace books that will be examined here. They are quite different in most ways. Thomas Fayreford practised in rural north Devon and Somerset in the second quarter of the fifteenth century; John Argentein (*c.*1443–1508) was a royal physician, Fellow and later Provost of King's College, Cambridge; and William Worcester (1415–*c.*1485) was a learned man with antiquarian interests, an indefatigable traveller and ex-secretary to Sir John Fastolf (famous today for his prominent role in the letters of the Paston family of Norfolk). Of these three only John Argentein followed the conventional scholastic medical career, moving between university and court circles.[3]

Nevertheless there are certain features of the collections of remedies they assembled in their books that these men have in common, and which take us outside the self-contained world of scholastic medical texts. First and perhaps most important, their memoranda allow us to see individual practitioners as members of an information community that extended far beyond the scholastic world. These are men for whom remedies are objects of exchange, of purchase, or of the distribution of gifts and favours. In this perspective we can see how the individual remedy acquired value as it circulated amongst a community of lay health practitioners. This exchange of information in the form of remedies, identified often explicitly as *experimenta*, was facilitated by the development of a lay medical literacy that flourished outside university circles. This lay medical literacy was also witnessed in the creation of a new literature which adapted scholastic medical theory to new kinds of readers (Voigts 1989; Demaitre 1998; Jones 1999; Taavitsainen and Pahta 2004).

Secondly, we will see reflected in the books written by these practitioners the impact of epidemic disease. The demand for a medical response to epidemics directed attention to processes of corruption and putrefaction going on in the body, and to remedies that counteracted what were perceived as poisonings of the whole body or principal organ. This meant that promoting cure by contraries on the humoral model was less important. Nevertheless we will find that, thirdly, a fondness for *experimenta* of this new type, culled from a variety of sources, lay and scholastic, was still compatible with a continuing respect for diagnostic and prognostic skills predicated on humoral theory. It was also compatible with an interest in advice on regimen and diet that takes into account the complexion of the so-called 'noble' patient.

Thomas Fayreford and the Exchange of Remedies

We will begin with the commonplace book of Thomas Fayreford. Fayreford listed over one hundred cures he performed on named or identifiable patients, specifying the complaint of which they were cured. He also collected his proven remedies or *experimenta* in two texts, one medical and one surgical.[4] Both were organized under disease headings written at the top of the page in the book; *experimenta* were added under these headings at different times by Fayreford himself. Many of these remedies are quoted from those transmitted in scholastic texts like those of Avicenna, Bernard de Gordon or Gilbertus Anglicus, to which presumably Fayreford

114

had access for consultation purposes, and the skills necessary to decipher and copy. On the other hand, many *experimenta* come from patients rather than scholastic authors. A Lady Poyninges gave him a remedy written out in Middle English for 'demigreyne', a form of headache. Fayreford also testified to his own success with certain 'experiments' he tried for himself, and sometimes he witnessed the cures of others, for instance one performed by Nicholas Colnet in Oxford. Other sources of *experimenta* are less respectable: Fayreford also made it his business to record as many as forty-three healing charms, making no distinction between a charm for epilepsy and a 'rational' remedy for the same complaint (Olsan 2003; Jones 2007). Indeed some of his sources for remedies are identified as those whom scholastic medical authors usually condemned: ladies and country-dwellers. Of a cure for rotten teeth he says, 'take a green frog that leaps in trees on sacred ground, and anoint any tooth that you wish to fall out with that green substance'. He goes on to tell us that this is 'one of my secrets ("privityes") that barbers have given me silver for'. This suggests Fayreford was an active trader in the exchange of remedies that might on occasion not just be bartered but transacted in a monetized economy (Jones 1995, 1998).

Fayreford's method of collecting remedies under disease headings assumes a ready-made classification of the illnesses he confronted. It takes for granted that the healer can identify these illnesses in the patient and can apply specific remedies to patients suffering from them without any explicit reference to their individual complexional balance. However, at the same time disease headings on the page are usually immediately followed in Fayreford's book by definitions employing complexional terminology and following scholastic authority. The text offers something of a disjunction on each page between the scholastic definitions and diagnoses and the grab-bag of remedies that follow. The list of cures at the beginning also testifies to a certain incongruity between terms that would have been recognizable in a scholastic medical text on diagnosis and a rough-and-ready approach to describing the individual patient. Fayreford tells us about his most significant patient that, 'Lady Poynynges had frenzy and syncope and quinsy and suffocation of the womb all at once and in three weeks she was properly cured with God's help'. The names of each of her ailments as described by Fayreford would have been recognized by scholastics, though they would have been confused by the failure to distinguish the illness or *morbus* from its symptoms. Thus syncope would have been classed as a symptom of suffocation of the womb rather than as a distinct *morbus* in its own right (Jones 1998: 170–72). Further, the scholastics decreed that each *morbus* should be understood in terms of complexional imbalance, but there is no evidence that Fayreford thought in these terms. Fayreford goes on to offer in his commonplace book a number of treatments for suffocation of the womb, Lady Poyninges' ailment, and several of them are praised as having proved successful for him personally. They mostly involve herbal fumigations to draw out or drive noxious humours down from the womb, as would have been standard in a scholastic textbook of practical medicine, though Fayreford does not offer any suggestion as to how or why they should work. Implicitly, the rationale behind these therapies is that they are tested by experience, his own or others, many of whom are named in the book. We may note the importance he attaches to recollecting the sources of his *experimenta*, and to the warrant of experience (he uses *probatum est*, and similar expressions to convey this).

So Fayreford operated as a practitioner within a busy network of people exchanging and circulating remedies, sometimes in return for cash or kind, at other times because of relations of obligation or for charitable reasons. Fayreford swapped recipes with Lady Poyninges, whom he treated successfully for suffocation of the womb. This kind of network presupposes that people like Lady Poyninges had already developed a kind of functional medical literacy that would enable them to read and write down recipes. Passing on information about remedies was an extension of the charitable role that ladies and religious played in their local community by providing medical services to others. The barbers who were willing to give him silver for his green-frog recipe, and his patient Lady Poyninges, were also the sort of people in search of medical information for whom a lay literature of medicine was being created in late medieval England.

The later fourteenth and fifteenth centuries saw an explosive development in England of this lay literature of medicine. One aspect of this development was the enthusiasm for translating Latin scholastic medical literature into the vernacular, not just into English and Anglo-Norman but into all of the other European vernaculars as well. Between 1375 and 1500 we see the creation of an English vernacular medicine, complete with discourse forms adapted from

Latin scholastic literature and a new English technical vocabulary to create equivalents for scholastic terminology. This translation effort of course included as a priority the most practically oriented texts – such as surgeries, recipe books, texts explaining diagnosis by urine analysis – but also a surprising amount of theoretical literature, texts of Galenic or Arabic origin dealing with the four humours (Taavitsainen and Pahta 1998, 2004).

Just as significant as the vernacular translations (and at the present far less studied) was the proliferation of copies of Latin texts on medicine also designed for a new readership outside the universities. Here a bias towards the literature of medical practice is even more evident, whether expressed in the production of handbooks and compendia, recipe books or in short guides to diagnosis, prognosis and bloodletting. Most of these new Latin medical texts were not copied at or for the universities but were transmitted by lay scribes who wanted the texts for their own use, or were writing them for their clients, medical practitioners or householders with an interest in gathering information to guard or restore their own health.

These developments, and the increasing social prestige of scholastic medicine amongst those who could afford the services of doctors, ensured that humoral medicine, far from being eclipsed, was extending its reach throughout literate society. The effect of spreading lay medical literacy was not confined to those who were literate either. By means of reading aloud in households and local communities, the communication of medical knowledge reached out to those who could listen but not read. Many of these listeners must have been female, excluded from reading Latin or even English by gender biases in education. Through these channels of communication we can assume that the basic tenets of humoral medicine reached out for the first time well beyond the minority who could read Latin, Middle English or Anglo-Norman (Getz 1990; Jones 1994).

John Argentein and a Changing Disease Ecology

The second theme that emerges from study of the commonplace books of practitioners has to do with the disease environment of late medieval Europe. The disease crisis of 1348 to 1350 that we know as the Black Death, and the repeated subsequent impacts of epidemic disease that so marked the fourteenth and fifteenth centuries by comparison to what had gone before, had a profound impact on attitudes to healing (Benedictow 2004). The new diseases did not give healers time for prolonged treatment because of their lethality, and were not readily susceptible to the characteristic scholastic attention to *complexio* in the individual because their epidemic character did not distinguish between subtle differences in humoral balance. They posed a severe challenge to the orthodoxies of scholastic medicine confronted with such an emergency. It was widely agreed amongst scholastic doctors that certain ailments, most notably epidemic diseases labelled as *pestilentia*, required a new therapeutic approach. These epidemic diseases were not responsive to therapies which relied simply on adjusting the body's qualitative or humoral balance, using the orthodox Galenic approach of allopathy, countering an overabundance or deficiency in the body by corrective medication. Allopathic remedies could be relied on to deal with most of the familiar ailments described by ancient and modern physicians alike, but not with the challenge of new and deadly diseases (Arrizabalaga 1994).

The workings of pestilence were commonly seen as a process of the poisoning of the whole body system via the heart, not a problem of humoral balance. This would help in the eyes of medieval doctors to account for their swift action and frequent fatality. Theories of poison went back to classical times and had always required antidotes that were exceptional when compared to the use of herbs, spices, animal parts and minerals that made up the staple medicines used by the humoral doctor. It is no surprise to encounter the popularity in writings on pestilence of remedies that were complex, costly and mysterious in their effects like the ancient antidotes, theriac and mithridatum. But alongside these were new therapeutic agents that acted against poison by what scholastics would call their 'specific form', rather than by the effects of the compounding of their elemental qualities. Remedies of this kind included potable gold and various elixirs, but also those alchemical newcomers, 'quintessential' remedies derived from the writings of the Franciscan Jean de Roquetaillade (Johannes de Rupescissa) and the author now called Pseudo-Lull but known in England at the time as 'Raymund'. Whether or not these could provide a 'cure' for epidemic diseases, quintessential remedies and elixirs of life might in extreme cases delay the fatal outcome of a fast-acting pestilence long enough for the priest or confessor to administer last rites to the patient (Pereira 1989; Crisciani and Pereira 1998; DeVun 2009).

In this development of the quintessence for medical purposes we can link the interest in new alchemical remedies acting against poisoning of the heart or the whole body system to changes in the disease ecology of late medieval Europe. While this is not the place to develop the argument in detail, it may be that the same crisis in therapeutics caused by epidemic disease also helps to explain the growing enthusiasm amongst physicians for astrological aids to prognosis and healing, and for magical rituals and amulets that would counteract sudden-acting poisons. All three kinds of occult science – alchemy, astrology and magic – were increasingly fashionable in fourteenth- and fifteenth-century Europe. They did not displace the orthodoxies of humoralism amongst the scholastics but they did provide alternative sources of explanation for illness as well as new therapeutic devices (Jacquart 1990).

We can see the impact of epidemic disease at the level of the individual practitioner by looking at a second English medical commonplace book, that of Dr John Argentein. Argentein was a Fellow of King's College, Cambridge, who in the 1470s went off to Ferrara in Italy to complete his medical studies. On his return to England he took up the practice of medicine and emerged as an extremely successful court physician, becoming doctor to the sons of Edward IV (the last person to see them alive), and to Arthur, the eldest son of Henry VII. In his commonplace book he copied material from an encyclopaedic medical text called the *Tabula medicine*, originally compiled by Franciscans or Dominicans in England between 1416 and 1425. What he copied on each page under its disease heading were remedies from the *Tabula medicine*, to which he added whenever he came across them other remedies derived from his own experience, what he had observed or heard from others, as well as information extracted from authoritative medical texts. Essentially he compiled in the same way that Fayreford had done, and for the same purpose – to record remedies that worked irrespective of whether they derived from book reading, his own experience, observation or word of mouth. By comparison with Fayreford's modest use of alchemical remedies, Argentein was deeply committed to alchemy, which he seems to have learnt largely

119

in Ferrara, though England had a strong tradition of Pseudo-Lullian alchemy of its own in the fifteenth century.[5]

There is one feature of the Pseudo-Lullian approach to quintessential medicines that made it easier for scholastically trained physicians like Argentein to integrate them into their practice. By recommending not just the quintessence of wine obtained by fractional distillation but its use in alliance with quintessences drawn from the distillation of other substances, for instance herbal simples, this kind of alchemy effectively offered a means of amplifying the accepted medicinal effects of those substances. As Pseudo-Lull put it 'quintessence works a hundred times better [than the simples]' (Llull 1542: 102). Instead of using, for example, the plant peony itself to treat timidity and weakness, the text of Pseudo-Lull, *De secretis nature* (a revised version of Johannes de Rupescissa's work), recommends the use of quintessence of peony, together with the quintessences of other plants often used in treatment of these ailments. Thus the quintessence functioned not as a single panacea, which made all other medicines redundant, but as part of the physician's armoury which could be used alongside other non-alchemical remedies. Thus quintessences yield hundreds of times the power of the ordinary herbal medicines that were used by scholastics to alter the complexional balance of the patient. In this way claims for miraculous and perfect cures, based on the power of the quintessence to reverse corruption in the human body, did not mean that the quintessence effectively replaced or made redundant other therapies.

In addition to his enthusiastic embrace of alchemy, Argentein promoted the use of magical cures for certain ailments. These magical remedies derived from the Latin *Picatrix*, originally an Arabic magical work, and translated in the thirteenth century, possibly via a Spanish intermediary (Pingree 1986). Argentein drew on Book 3 of the *Picatrix*, and seems to have been particularly fond of those remedies he found there that make use of human or animal excrement. Argentein was also keen on the use of charms for diseases of the throat, for childbirth and menstruation, for spasms and for stopping the flow of blood. Remedies derived from magical texts, or from the oral and written tradition of charms, have the same standing within Argentein's commonplace book as alchemical and Galenical remedies. Argentein sees no conflict in recording treatments using alchemical or magical means alongside those derived from treatment by contraries under the orthodox Galenic and complexional model. And this made it a lot easier for Argentein when he was collecting remedies that were known to work against particular diseases – none of these alternative non-complexional approaches to treatment committed the practitioner to abandoning complexional medicine, either as an intellectual philosophy or as an instrument of therapy in the form of long-established herbal, animal part or mineral treatments.

William Worcester and the Most Valuable Goods in Medical Currency

This phenomenon of the coexistence of the complexional and experimental in medical practice was not confined to those who made their living from medicine. A third example of an English medical commonplace book exposes this in the relationship between very different texts within the book. The book belonged to William Botoner, or as he is better known William Worcester, who is often identified as a pioneering topographer and antiquarian. First employed as secretary and agent for Sir John Fastolf, a military hero and landowner, after Fastolf's death in 1459 Worcester spent much time travelling, examining manuscripts in libraries, and talking to local informants. His interests ranged very broadly and he recorded information in notebooks of a peculiar long thin shape adapted to being carried in a saddlebag. One of his fields of interest was in medicine and alchemy, and he left one notebook specifically devoted to memoranda he had gathered about medicine. He also owned other manuscripts of a more conventional format that he copied himself or acquired, containing texts relating to medicine and alchemy. The peculiarly shaped medical notebook that survives in the British Library reflects what he made of the fruits of his reading and of his wide-ranging contacts with individuals with medical information to impart. We cannot tell for sure whether William Worcester ever tried to practice medicine, though his remarks on the health of his former boss Sir John Fastolf suggest he certainly took more than simply a speculative interest in it. It is characteristic of William Worcester that he took great care to record who, what, where and sometimes when in making his memoranda.[6]

He records in this particularized way a remedy headed 'A medicine against a sickness in the mouth called canker and by others erispula or noli me tangere, and for instance Thomas Plummer the scribe died of this illness at London'. Worcester then gives the recipe, a medicinal water made from pure alum cooked with the juices of sage, fennel and woodbine. He tells us, 'I learnt it from an old apothecary living in Bowyer Row in London in 1465'. Other informants like the friar John Wellys of Bridgewater in Somerset are credited with a number of different *experimenta* of this type. But just as characteristic of William Worcester's recording of *experimenta* is his habit of the precise citation of manuscripts he has inspected, notably in Cambridge and London but sometimes found in other libraries on Worcester's wide-ranging travels. For example, 'these recipes for one-day fevers following I found as marginal glosses to an old text of the *Isagoge* of Johannitius in the library of St Paul's in London'. These *experimenta* of William Worcester, even when copied out of academic medical manuscripts, make no explicit mention of the four humours or the notion of complexional balance. They are extracted from their textual setting and presented as if their standing as *experimenta* was exactly on a par with the testimony of John Wellys or the old apothecary of Bowyer Row. Yet Worcester also copied out passages on specific diseases that do draw explicitly on humoral pathology.[7]

There is another important feature of his notebook that deserves to be compared with his notes on *experimenta*. The longest single textual unit in the notebook is copied into it by a scribal hand (not that of William Worcester), and is perhaps the single most important evidence for English scholastic medicine of the fifteenth century. It is the text of the *Dietarium*, written by Gilbert Kymer for Humfrey, Duke of Gloucester (his patron and patient), in March 1424. The *Dietarium* was the work of fifteenth-century England's most prominent and successful doctor, later twice Chancellor of Oxford University, and addressed to England's Protector, as the duke was styled at that time, being guardian of the infant Henry VI. It constitutes undoubtedly the most ambitious bid for the authority of scholastic medicine made in England. The *Dietarium* itself is a specimen of scholastic medicine's most eye-catching product, the regimen or guide to health addressed to a prominent lay patron by his doctor and designed to give the patron both bodily and spiritual guidance. As such it reflects Kymer's understanding of the duke's personal *complexio* or balance of humours, and most of the chapters are devoted to what the scholastics called the non-naturals, the various interfaces (Kymer listed ten) between the humoral body and its worldly environment. The standard Galenic list of non-naturals on which Kymer expanded included air, food and drink, sleeping and waking, motion and rest, excretions and retentions, and dreams and the passions of the soul. Since the body humoral and the body politic are so closely identified in the case of the Protector of England, Kymer is in effect engaged in designing a regimen for a kingdom as well as for its head. The fact that, a few months after the presentation of the text of the *Dietarium* to the duke in 1424, Humfrey's ambitious military expedition to enforce his wife's claim to rule the Low Countries ended in fiasco may be why the text never got the circulation or acclaim that Kymer must have hoped for (see Hardingham 2004).

The fact that William Worcester's notebook contains a copy of this *Dietarium* text, and that all around it in the book are found his *experimenta* culled from various sources, bring us close to the heart of an apparent paradox. In fifteenth-century England, humoral medicine was achieving unprecedented success in promoting itself to the highest in the realm, and through vernacular translations and short Latin texts for household use was also reaching a wider audience than ever before, well beyond the confines of the court and universities. But those who practised medicine, or perhaps aimed like William Worcester at collecting what were the most valuable goods in medical currency, were putting together collections of remedies that made little or no reference to the scholastic ideal of tackling illness as an expression of *mala complexio*, the disrupted balance of the humours.

Conclusion

Some part of the explanation for this paradox must be located in developments I have already discussed – the scholastics themselves endorsed a form of medical instrumentalism that put a high priority on the proven efficacy of remedies even when the humoral basis for that success was not understood. The challenge of epidemic disease meant a new interest in explanations of illness that prioritized processes of corruption and putrefaction of 'peccant' humours over imbalance of the humours, or even sidelined qualities and humours altogether by concentrating on poisoning of the principal organ, the heart, or the whole body system as causes. This development promoted remedies that worked by 'specific form' or occult principles, elixirs and quintessences, over the use of medicines compounded from simples and analysable into qualities of hot, cold, dry and moist. The flourishing of networks of cultural exchange by which remedies proved by experience and warranted by authority circulated in manuscripts or by oral transmission meant that practitioners and householders alike relied less on the patient-centred tailoring of medicines to individual *complexio* and more on 'off the shelf' remedies applicable in all cases of a named illness.

But all of these things did not mean that *complexio* was challenged as a framework for understanding the working of the healthy or sick body. Indeed, the areas of diagnosis and prognosis that the scholastic doctor claimed as his particular province of expertise were not threatened by the developments outlined above. Diagnosis and prognosis claimed to be based on a rational understanding of the workings of the qualities and the humours in the individual. Accordingly, these sources of scholastic authority for the medieval doctor were not subverted by the inroads of *experimenta* in the area of therapeutics, or even by the existence of a body of prognostic tests of the same kind. Whether a sick person would live or die could be ascertained by the analysis of the progress of their illness but also by this kind of test: 'take a new hatched egg, put it in the client's urine, wait for an hour and break the egg: if the egg is corrupt he is incurable, if it is still sweet he can be cured'. Both kinds of prognostic are found together in manuscripts used by practitioners like Fayreford and Argentein.[8]

What is more, even in therapeutics a lack of mention of humours or qualities in the recipes prescribed by the *experimenta* cannot in itself be regarded as a rejection of complexional thinking. A recipe that is in effect a purgative we might assume has a rationale that is humoral because it implies there is some peccant humour that is to be purged, even if no mention of humours is made in the text (Ogden 1938: xviii). Such recipes commonly do not state their justification in humoral terms; instead they move straight from the indication ('For gout ...') to composition, preparation, application and a statement of efficacy. These different parts of a recipe leave out their relation to humoral theory but we must not assume that there is no such relationship. With this point in mind, the whole matter of the rationale of medieval remedies becomes an extremely difficult one to assess even tentatively because silence on the matter of *complexio* does not necessarily imply indifference. In most cases we have to conclude the reasoning behind the use of a particular recipe in response to a named illness is not spelt out for us. A useful if necessarily cautious assumption might therefore be that remedial balancing of qualities or humours is only one of the overlapping rationales that propped up late medieval medication.

Late medieval practice was not a steady retreat from the rigour and certainties of early fourteenth-century medical scholasticism into incoherence or occultism. The complexional understanding of illness was not pushed aside by the growing interest in *experimenta*, and the tension between the two was never stretched to breaking point. But a proper appreciation of that tension will help us to understand better a period that is sometimes represented in terms of a failure to maintain intellectual standards or an over-refined method of analysis collapsing under its own theoretical weight. Instead I think the evidence from the practitioners themselves shows flexibility and willingness to adapt to new developments in disease ecology, and to borrow approaches from related sciences like astrology and alchemy. Vernacularization of medical texts and the increasing availability of paper and ink meant also that new kinds of literate practitioners were able to flourish despite not having had a university medical education. A culture in which *experimenta* could be exchanged as gifts or for financial reward was not one that rejected complexional medicine but one in which the tension between *complexio* and *experimenta* could be a source of practical creativity.

Notes

1. See McVaugh (1993), Jacquart (1998a: 197–240; 1998b) and O'Boyle (1998). Four of the leading medical scholastics of the fourteenth and fifteenth centuries are the subject of the following monographs: Demaitre (1980), Siraisi (1981), French (2001) and Pesenti (2003).
2. For discussion of the relationship between *experimentum* as a knowledge of particulars and *experimentum* as a remedy tested by experience, see Agrimi and Crisciani (1990); see also the remarks of Olsan (2003: 347–49). There was a long tradition of textual circulation of medieval *experimenta* that is described in Thorndike (1923).

3. Biographical entries for all three men can be found in the *Oxford Dictionary of National Biography*.
4. Fayreford's book is British Library, Harley MS 2558. Quotations in this paragraph are from ff. 76, 82.
5. Argentein's medical commonplace book (Bodleian Library, Oxford, Ashmole MS 1437) is discussed in Jones (1994, 2008, 2011). On English fifteenth-century alchemical medicine, see Getz (1992).
6. For studies of Worcester, see McFarlane (1981), Richmond (1996) and Wakelin (2005). Worcester's medical notebook is to be found in the British Library (BL), London, Sloane MS 4.
7. See BL, Sloane MS 4, ff.51v, 57r.
8. See Bodleian Library, Ashmole MS 1437, p. 62 (Argentein).

References

Agrimi, J., and C. Crisciani. 1990. 'Per una ricerca su *experimentum-experimenta*: reflessione epistemologica e tradizione medica (secoli XIII–XV)', in P. Janni and I. Mazzini (eds), *Presenza del lessico Greco e Latino nelle lingue contemporanee*. Macerata: Università di Macerata, pp.9–49.

Arrizabalaga, J. 1994. 'Facing the Black Death: Perceptions and Reactions of University Medical Practitioners', in L. García-Ballester et al. (eds), *Practical Medicine from Salerno to the Black Death*. Cambridge: Cambridge University Press, pp.237–88.

Benedictow, O. 2004. *The Black Death, 1346–1353: The Complete History*. Woodbridge: Boydell.

Crisciani, C., and M. Pereira. 1998. 'Black Death and Golden Remedies: Some Remarks on Alchemy and the Plague', in A. Paravicini Bagliani and F. Santi (eds), *The Regulation of Evil: Social and Cultural Attitudes to Epidemics in the Late Middle Ages*. Firenze: Sismel-Edizioni del Galluzzo, pp.7–39.

Demaitre, L.E. 1980. *Doctor Bernard de Gordon: Professor and Practitioner*. Toronto: Pontifical Institute of Mediaeval Studies.

——— 1998. 'Medical Writing in Transition: Between *Ars* and *Vulgus*', *Early Science and Medicine* 3: 88–101.

DeVun, L. 2009. *Prophecy, Alchemy and the End of Time: John of Rupescissa in the Late Middle Ages*. New York: Columbia University Press.

Eamon, W., and G. Keil. 1987. '"Plebs Amat Empirica": Nicholas of Poland and his Critique of the Medieval Medical Establishment', *Sudhoffs Archiv* 71: 180–96.

French, R. 2001. *Canonical Medicine: Gentile da Foligno and Scholasticism*. Leiden: Brill.

García-Ballester, L. 1982. 'Arnald de Villanova (c.1240–1311) y la reforma de los estudios medicos en Montpellier (1309): el Hipócrates Latino y la introduccíon del Nuevo Galeno', *Dynamis* 2: 97–158.

Getz, F.M. 1990. 'Charity, Translation, and the Language of Medical Learning in Medieval England', *Bulletin of the History of Medicine* 64: 1–17.

———— 1992. 'To Prolong Life and Promote Health: Baconian Alchemy and Pharmacy in the English Learned Tradition', in S. Campbell, B. Hall and D. Klausner (eds), *Health, Disease and Healing in Medieval Culture*. New York: Macmillan, pp.141–50.

Hardingham, G. 2004. 'The *Regimen* in Late Medieval England', PhD dissertation. Cambridge: University of Cambridge.

Jacquart, D. 1984. 'De *crasis* à *complexio*: note sur le vocabulaire du tempérament en Latin médiéval', in G. Sabbah (ed.), *Textes Médicaux Latins Antiques*. Saint-Etienne: Université de Saint-Etienne, pp.71–76.

———— 1990. 'Theory, Everyday Practice, and Three Fifteenth-century Physicians', *Osiris* 6: 140–60.

———— 1998a. 'Medical Scholasticism', in M.D. Grmek (ed.), *Western Medical Thought from Antiquity to the Middle Ages*. Cambridge, MA: Harvard University Press, pp.197–240.

———— 1998b. *La médecine médiévale dans le cadre Parisien (XIVe–XVe siècle)*. Paris: Fayard.

Jones, P.M. 1994. 'Information and Science', in R. Horrox (ed.), *Fifteenth-century Attitudes*. Cambridge: Cambridge University Press, pp.97–111.

———— 1995. 'Harley MS 2558: A Fifteenth-century Medical Commonplace Book', in M.M. Schleissner (ed.), *Manuscript Sources of Medieval Medicine: A Book of Essays*. New York: Garland, pp.35–54.

———— 1998. 'Thomas Fayreford: An English Fifteenth-century Medical Practitioner', in R. French et al. (eds), *Medicine from the Black Death to the French Disease*. Aldershot: Ashgate, pp.156–83.

———— 1999. 'Medicine and Science', in L. Hellinga and J.B. Trapp (eds), *The Cambridge History of the Book in Britain*, Vol. 3: *1400–1557*. Cambridge: Cambridge University Press, pp.433–48.

———— 2007. 'Amulets: Prescriptions and Surviving Objects from Late Medieval England', in S. Blick (ed.), *Beyond Pilgrim Souvenirs and Secular Badges*. Oxford: Oxbow, pp.92–107.

———— 2008. 'The *Tabula Medicine*: An Evolving Encyclopaedia', *English Manuscript Studies 1100–1700* 14: 60–85.

———— 2011. 'Mediating Collective Experience: The *Tabula Medicine* as a Handbook for Medical Practice', in F.E. Glaze and B. Nance (eds), *Between Text and Patient: The Medical Enterprise in Medieval and Early Modern Europe*. Firenze: Sismel-Edizioni del Galluzzo, pp.279–307.

Llull, R. 1542. *De secretis naturae*. Venice: Peter Schoeffer.

McFarlane, K.B. 1981. 'William Worcester: A Preliminary Survey', in K.B. McFarlane, *England in the Fifteenth Century: Collected Essays*. London: Hambledon, pp.199–224.

McVaugh, M.R. 1971. 'The *Experimenta* of Arnald of Villanova', *Journal of Medieval and Renaissance Studies* 1: 107–18.

———— 1976. 'Two Montpellier Recipe Collections', *Manuscripta* 20:175–80.

———— 1990. 'The Nature and Limits of Medical Certitude at Early Fourteenth-century Montpellier', *Osiris* 6: 62–84.

—— 1993. *Medicine before the Plague: Practitioners and their Patients in the Crown of Aragon, 1285–1345*. Cambridge: Cambridge University Press.

O'Boyle, C. 1998. *The Art of Medicine: Medical Teaching at the University of Paris, 1250–1400*. Leiden: Brill.

Ogden, M.S. (ed.). 1938. *The 'Liber de Diversis Medicinis' in the Thornton Manuscript (MS. Lincoln Cathedral A.5.2)*. London: Early English Text Society.

Olsan, L.T. 2003. 'Charms and Prayers in Medieval Medical Theory and Practice', *Social History of Medicine* 16: 343–66.

Pereira, M. 1989. *The Alchemical Corpus Attributed to Raymond Lull*. London: Warburg Institute.

Pesenti, T. 2003. *Marsilio Santasofia tra corti e università: la carriera di un 'monarca medicinae' del Trecento*. Treviso: Antilia.

Pingree, D. 1986. *Picatrix: The Latin Version of the Ghāyat al-Hakīm*. London: Warburg Institute.

Richmond, C. 1996. *The Paston Family in the Fifteenth Century: Fastolf's Will*. Cambridge: Cambridge University Press.

Siraisi, N.G. 1981. *Taddeo Alderotti and His Pupils: Two Generations of Italian Medical Learning*. Princeton, NJ: Princeton University Press.

Taavitsainen, I., and P. Pahta. 1998. 'Vernacularization of Medical Writing in English: A Corpus-based Study of Scholasticism', *Early Science and Medicine* 3: 157–85.

—— (eds). 2004. *Medical and Scientific Writing in Late Medieval English*. Cambridge: Cambridge University Press.

Thorndike. L. 1923. *A History of Magic and Experimental Science*, Vol. 2. New York: Columbia University Press.

Voigts, L.E. 1989. 'Scientific and Medical Books', in J. Griffiths and D. Pearsall (eds), *Book Production and Publishing in Britain 1375–1475*. Cambridge: Cambridge University Press, pp.345–402.

Villanova, A de. 2000. *Tractatus de Intentione Medicorum: Arnaldi de Villanova Opera Medica Omnia*, Vol. 1, ed. M.R. McVaugh. Barcelona: Universitat de Barcelona.

Wakelin, D. 2005. 'William Worcester Writes a History of his Reading', *New Medieval Literatures* 7: 53–71.

Chapter 6
Yunani *Tibb* and Foundationalism in Early Twentieth-Century India
Humoral Paradigms between Critique and Concordance

Guy Attewell

Although there are countless discussions of humours in Arabic, Persian and Urdu sources on *tibb* (medicine) there is no autochthonous construct of a humoral theory or pathology as representative of this stream of medical thinking before it appears in Urdu and English at some point in the nineteenth century. Humours (*akhlat*) are but one dimension of a matrix of the so-called 'foundational principles' (*usul al-tibb* or *usul-i tibb*, or *kulliyat*).[1] Yet, there is scarcely a book, article or website on the history or practice of Yunani *tibb* which does not refer to the theory of four humours as one of its defining characteristics.[2] In representations of *tibb*, humoral theory and its related concepts have been largely assumed to be central to practice, and the place of this theory is often assumed to exist outside time and socio-political context as a cornerstone of aetiology, diagnosis and therapeutics. This perspective is not peculiar to Yunani medicine. Equally, a variant on this humoral paradigm – *tridosha* – is also widely understood as fundamental to other codified and state-supported Indian medical systems, such as Ayurveda and Siddha.[3] However, considering the transformations in medical knowledge and practice that have taken place through the twentieth century, there is good reason to reflect on how *hakims* (practitioners) have interpreted and negotiated foundational theories, and how, in doing so, the nineteenth-century invention of 'humoral theory' has been accorded a quasi-deterministic quality that endures today.[4]

This chapter discusses how foundational concepts have been framed in the context of the formation of a professionalized, institutionalized Yunani medicine. It hinges on a paradox: just at the time when it became important for those *hakim*s who were intent on mobilization within the ambit of the state to emphasize the alignment of their practices within a theoretical grid, roughly around the turn of the twentieth century, it was conversely also the time that many of the foundational constructs of Yunani *tibb* (the elements, the humours, the temperament of the lived body and notions of judicious balance) began to be explicitly questioned or realigned by certain *hakim*s themselves.

The first part of the chapter sets out the terrain for discussing the question of continuity and change in foundational concepts. The second part examines the reification of theory through a process suggested in the term 'foundationalism', which we can think of as taking place through a desire or a constraint, under certain conditions, to essentialize streams of medical knowledge and healing through their foundational theoretical conceptions.[5] I see this process relating to a rhetoric of authenticity in the cultural politics of how India's medical traditions were made and remade from the late nineteenth century. The third part shows that the attention to theoretical foundations was not unproblematic, in the sense that the formation of Yunani *tibb* was predicated ideologically not only on its differentiation from other 'indigenous' healing practices, but also on a revival in the light of new sciences (especially, at this time, the disciplines of chemistry and bacteriology) and the engagement, in their terms, of *tibb-i qadim* (old medicine, Yunani *tibb*) with *tibb-i jadid* (modern medicine).

The chapter identifies two principal ways in which *hakim*s have negotiated this problematic: concordance and critique. The place of 'balance' within a humoral system, and the importance of identifying derangement and restoring it, is not an absolute and timeless underlying principle as has frequently been assumed. Furthermore, as will be shown, the desire to tie theory and practice to a foundational paradigm should not be misapprehended as secularization, or 'resecularization' in Charles Leslie's formulation (Leslie 1998: 360), since the invocation of God as the font of healing, in the act itself, was not displaced during newly professionalizing trajectories. Apart from discussing divergent representations of fundamental concepts, the chapter points to the instrumentality of foundational thinking (with regard to temperament, appropriateness, balance and moderation) in a broader socio-political arena. The invocation itself of theoretical constructs has been a mode of practice embedded in the politics of health in a manner often taken for granted by researchers and commentators on India's medical traditions.

The Foundational

In the *tibb* of the Indian subcontinent there is a centuries' long tradition of textual production and transmission associated with centres and networks of Indo-Muslim power and noble, scholarly and religious elites (Jaggi 1977; Speziale 2003, 2010; Alavi 2008). In these works we can find elaborate, sophisticated doctrines on the causation and progression of illness and there is a canonical literature in *tibb* long before the British began their territorial occupation of India in the late eighteenth century. The existence of an authoritative corpus of textual knowledge in Arabic from West Asia and in Persian texts compiled in India from the thirteenth century onwards provided a common reference point for these articulations down to the twentieth century, even if there is a very considerable spectrum of difference between texts and genres across time and place in the name of *tibb*.

With regard to a canonical literature, we have to note in this regard the prominence of sayings attributed to eminent figures, Ibn Sina (frequently just *al-shaikh*, the master), Jalinus (Galen) and Buqrat (Hippocrates), and the many commentators and abridgers of Ibn Sina's *al-Qanun* (among them, Ibn al-Nafis, Nafis ibn Iwad, Aqsarai, Ali Gilani). *Tibb*, or its other main appellation, *hikmat*, were marked for distinction by their practical application, which was intertwined with other streams of healing knowledge and practice in the subcontinent (Speziale 2010). *Tibb* or *hikmat* were also known as *ilm* (knowledge, which encompasses both the practical and theoretical), and for their association with other scholarly disciplines, especially *mantiq* (logic), *falsafa* (philosophy) and *akhlaq* (ethics). We find that many of the Persian texts on various aspects of *tibb* composed in the Mughal era, widely considered in the twentieth century as the apogee of Indo-Muslim medicine, were not necessarily written by physicians but by courtiers and the nobility. This underlies the sense in which *tibb* could be embedded in the pursuit of higher learning by a refined gentleman. There was indeed a special sense that *tibb* was a noble pursuit within Islamicate cultures. First, healing was principally in the service of humankind (*ashraf al-makhluqat*, the noblest of creation) in the Qur'an; it could thus be considered a noble art (*fann-i sharif*). Second, healing was given the sanction of the Prophet and his interpreters, as is attested by the *tibb al-nabi* (traditions of prophetic medicine; see Savage-Smith, this volume).

The second half of the nineteenth century saw the beginnings of a flourishing of printed works on *tibb* in Urdu (discussed in more detail below), including the translation of major Persian and Arabic works which drew on precepts attributed to Hippocrates, Galen and their successors. In addition to this canonical literature, there were also a wide variety of other discussions of health and disease published in Urdu, some of which drew on varieties of medical practice that bore the imprint of the dissemination of Western medical ideas and practices during colonial rule (from works on sanitation, relatively mainstream Western surgery, chemistry, pathology and therapeutics, to homeopathy, mesmerism and chromotherapy), as well as reformed versions of transregional streams of healing (such as *tibb-al nabi* and Ayurveda).

Amid this tremendous variety of late nineteenth-century accounts of healing, scholarly expositions on the body in health and illness within a stream of *tibb* were underpinned and cohered through a theoretical matrix based on the interplay of potencies derived from the four elements (fire, water, earth and air) and the importance of maintaining or restoring balance (*i'tidal*) in the body's economy. This conceptual terrain structured discussions on concepts of disease and their systematic inter-relatedness to organic function, on causes of disease, on people's predispositions and body types, on appropriate foods and drinks, on sexual behaviour, on the body in its lived environment (in terms of habitat and seasonality), on notions of correct comportment, on modes of diagnosis and prognosis, on appropriate modes of therapy, on methods of preserving health (*hifz-i sihhat*), and so forth.

It is important at this point to note that the concepts of judicious balance between opposing forces or substances and ways of living were long established in *tibbi* literature, but they also articulated with an aesthetic of moderate comportment among elite social reformers from the late nineteenth century.[6] Moderation (*i'tidal*), along with culture, piety and moral example, were key standards in the late nineteenth- and early twentieth-century 'noble' (*sharif*) Indo-Muslim reformist agendas on the Gangetic plains (Metcalf 1982). The language of bodily illness, weakness and corruption conveyed through the humorally oriented concepts of temperament (*mizaj*), excess (*kusrat*), depletion (*qillat*) and corruption (*fasad*) resonated with a reading of the ills of contemporary society in the throes of great social upheaval and political mobilization. For instance, at the turn of the twentieth century, the Sunni reformer Maulana Ashraf Ali Thanavi described Muslim women's ignorance of Islamic doctrines as a ruination (*tabaahi*), for which he struggled to find a cure, but which had spread to everyday matters, to their children and even to affect their husbands – and this resonated with the plague that was then raging in northern India, and could be captured in the humoral language of weakness and corruption (*fasad*) (Metcalf 1990: 47).

Within *tibb*, the concepts of *anasir* (elements), *mizaj* (temperament) and *akhlat* (humours) have formed a central part in elaborations on the body in health and illness. We can refer, for instance, to an authoritative and well-disseminated Urdu manual on Yunani medicine of the late nineteenth century, the *Tibb-i Ihsani* by Hakim Ihsan Ali Khan, for a representation that is framed by theoretical doctrines resonating with the *Qanun fi al-Tibb* of Ibn Sina and its later abridgements and commentaries.[7] In the 1911 edition of *Tibb-i Ihsani*, the numerous marginal glosses explaining Arabic terms and amplifying on the technical language of *tibbi* doctrine underline that this edition (at least) was aimed at the non-specialist. Ihsan Ali describes in this text the processes by which the four humours, vital spirits, bodily faculties and the *mizaj* (temperament) are produced in the body. From this perspective, digestion is understood as a process of cooking, rarefaction and the production of wastes that, at every stage, are fundamental to the ways that the body functions. It is nourished in optimal states and harmed when, for instance, there is insufficient heat or too much heat in the stomach, which either burns the food or leaves it unassimilated in the body. Ihsan Ali describes the qualities (*mizaj*) associated with the dominance of one humour. For instance, a *mizaj* dominated by *safra* (yellow bile) is 'hot

133

and dry, essence: fine, taste: bitter, colour: yellow', and the qualities (*kaifiyyat*) of the dominance of *safra* on the body are: the tongue is bitter and yellow, the stool is burning and yellowish, the body is restless and alert, the pulse is rapid and continuous (Khan 1911: 7). We can see from this brief example that the notions of elemental embodiment, inclusive of references to *ruh* (soul, vital spirit), could be fully manifest as physical signs and implied techniques of diagnosis.

Within *tibbi* literature, however, there is unequal treatment of foundational concepts (elements, humours, temperaments) across genres. I do not go into detail here, and leave an analysis of this question in pre-nineteenth-century material to others, but we can illustrate this point through a highly regarded therapeutic manual and *materia medica* produced by a *hakim* who flourished in the late nineteenth and early twentieth century. The 1926 eight-volume *Khaza'in al-adviya* (The treasury of medicinal substances) by Hakim Najmulghani Khan (1859–1932) of Rampur can be seen as an illustrious early twentieth-century example of the therapeutic interpreted within the Galenic-inspired stream of Indo-Muslim *tibb*, but in which discussions of elements and temperament were more dominant than humours. Najmulghani Khan was the nephew and pupil of the renowned scholar-physician Hakim Azam Khan, who was employed by nobility in the semi-autonomous Princely States of Bhopal and Indore during British rule. Several Princely States, which were nominally sovereign entities under British paramountcy, either maintained or initiated new forms of patronage for *hakims* and *vaidyas*, practitioners of *tibb* and Ayurveda. In addition to detailing the uses of each *materia medica*, Najmulghani Khan elaborated on how the properties and effects of medicines could be understood as the operation of their temperament (*mizaj*). For instance, he combined detailed expositions on the types of *mizaj* with simple clarifications, such as 'if one says that a medicine is hot, it is to be understood that this medicine produces heat in the body which is in excess and separate from the body's own heat' (Khan 1926, i: 94).

As was conventional in *tibb*, he and other authors on *materia medica* graded simple medicinal substances on a scale of four, according to the dominance of an elemental quality (hot, cold, dry, wet) where the first degree represents dominance in a mild form, and the fourth in a potentially injurious one. The leaves of the famed *azad diracht* tree (which Khan identified as neem, conventionally *Azadirachta indica*), with a wide range of applications in medicine, were considered hot in the second or third degree and dry in the first or second degree (Khan 1926, i: 325). This is a convention going back to the application of mathematics to pharmacology by the ninth-century polymath al-Kindi, who also provided a means of computing the overall quality of a polypharmaceutical compound based on the qualities of each individual ingredient. In theory, the grading of potency is an attempt to quantify the potential effect of a given substance on the state of the body. Determinations of potency may have been arrived at through a process of observation and of analogy (*qiyas*) with other substances and their effects on the body. The grading of substances is present in a majority of texts on pharmacy in Persian and Urdu down to the present, even if we should not assume equivalences of method for determining temperament or the stability of attributions made over time.[8]

In practice, it may be suggested that the use of a medicinal by *hakim*s may not by necessity have borne any direct relationship to a conception of the state of the body couched in the language of humours and temperament found in the textual streams of *tibb*, but rather to a specific picture of affliction or symptom and its customary use as such. The point that will be made in this case is that the relationship between the humoral or temperamental conceptions and the applications of a remedy in medical practice were consciously unhinged in the reflective and often critical debates about Yunani *tibb* that marked realignments of the profession in the early twentieth century. As we will see, this renegotiation of Yunani theory began at a time when the foundational underpinning of Yunani medicine gained new valorization and instrumentality among elite practitioners.

In Need of Theory: A Rationale for Recognition

From the late nineteenth century, elite Yunani *hakim*s were engaged in the quest to create a platform for legitimacy and the valorization of knowledge at the level of theory and science, something we also see happening at this time regarding Ayurveda.[9] Practitioners' projects for the revival of 'the science and art of *tibb*' (*ihyaa-i ilm o fann-i tibb*) were

135

many and diverse. One of the animating dimensions of these projects for reform-minded practitioners was to make *tibb* 'rational', which layered a complex negotiation with Western medicine and science, and with other local practices (Leslie 1998). Socially and politically influential families of physicians in northern India were major actors in this process, which was driven by a very active Urdu and vernacular print culture and a changing political economy of medical practice. *Tibb* had become all the more accessible to those who had no pedigree, instruction or association with established physicians, and provided new economic avenues (Attewell 2007; Alavi 2008).

A pivotal figure in the zones of engagement through which a 'revived', or newly invented, Yunani *tibb* emerged was Hakim Ajmal Khan (1863–1927), a member of the influential family of physicians who set up a school, the Madrasa Tibbiya, in Delhi. Ajmal Khan was frequently referred to as *muhi-i tibb* (the reviver of *tibb*) or *mujaddid-i tibb* (the renewer of *tibb*). In his capacity as the founder and president of the only professional organization to represent Yunani and Ayurvedic physicians under one umbrella (the All India Vedik and Yunani Tibbi Conference, AIVYTC), Ajmal Khan and his organization pushed themselves to the centre of a crucial debate, initiated in the Imperial Legislative Council of the British government of India in 1916, over whether 'indigenous systems of medicine' could be 'placed on a scientific basis', and therefore warrant consideration for state support.[10] Over the following year, the government of India conducted a massive country-wide survey of its health officials, administrative personnel and even police, who provided information on the kinds of practice which went under the names of Ayurveda and Yunani, the modes of education and the regard in which people held them. The summary of this survey concluded: 'It is practically impossible to place the indigenous systems of medicine on a scientific basis. The systems are a survival of a state of medical knowledge which once prevailed in Europe, but has been superseded by a series of scientific investigations and discoveries extending over several centuries'.[11]

Several dimensions of the negotiation of science at this time have already been discussed in the literature (e.g., Liebeskind 2002), so it is not necessary to rehearse them here. Ajmal Khan's representation on behalf of the AIVYTC against the findings of the survey denied the incommensurability of what he termed 'indigenous medicine' and science. No practitioners of indigenous medicine had been consulted in the survey, and the representation of their skills in the survey was almost universally negative. The central issue for our discussion is the way that Ajmal Khan identified 'humoral theory' as the distinguishing feature of 'indigenous systems' which, although being partly 'superseded since the rise of germ theory of disease', should not be rejected as a 'clog on medical science' without a 'hearing'.[12] And as a final point he made an appeal to experience (*tajriba*) and the art of medicine, which any serious practitioner of any medical formation would undergo during their interactions with the sick. No one, not even the most ardent British (or Indian) critic of the so-called backward and ignorant *vaidya* or *hakim*, could deny that these practitioners, especially those of established families and lineages that had practised over generations like Ajmal Khan's, had experience. Here Ajmal Khan was valorizing the experiential domain of practice beyond any particular theorization of the body in health and sickness.

God Gave Us Reason

An emphasis on the 'rational' core of Yunani medicine during this process might be expected to support the proposition that the professionalization of indigenous medicine was characterized by increasing secularization. We can indeed find explicit negotiations of what was considered the proper domain of *tibb* in interchanges in some of its most prominent journals that distinguished divine from secular causation. For instance, in debates about appropriate treatments for plague in the 1910s, we can see how certain practitioners insisted that *Rafiq al-Atibba* was a Yunani journal, and that discussion of treatments should be confined to medical principles (*usul-i tibb*) rather than promoting divine causes drawn from Islamic scriptures for the plague's visitation (Attewell 2007: 85–88). The fact that Yunani *tabibs* proposed variant causative models itself points to heterogeneity and non-consensuality. But equally, there is evidence to suggest that articulations of foundational theory need not dispense with the divine, which would subtly corroborate a myth of the inevitable conjuncture of rationalization and secularization. Two works of the early twentieth century can illustrate this well, of which I present one at more length here, the *Amaliya-i Jalinus* (Galen's practical knowledge) by Hakim Ashuftah Ajmali Lakhnawi (Ashuftah n.d.).[13]

Hakim Ashuftah settled in Hyderabad after moving from his native Lucknow and the city's famous centre of Islamic learning, Farangi Mahal. In Hyderabad he taught at the *tibbi* college set up by the ruling dynasty of the Princely State. His connection to these scholarly and powerful circles is evident in the addresses that preface his work: two are in Arabic, one from a religious figure, Maulana Abdulmajid Farangi Mahali, and the other by Hakim Ajmal Khan, and there is an encomium of the work from the then chief Yunani physician in Hyderabad, Hakim Maqsud Ali Khan. The *Amaliya-i Jalinus* was an eminently practical work. The narrative is stripped to a tabular form, with names of diseases, the *tabi'at* (dynamic force) of the disease, the kind of pulse and stool associated with it (for diagnosis), the elemental qualities of the prescribed food, whether bloodletting is indicated, prescriptions from 'Galen's own practice' and other prescriptions from the 'treasure-house' of family records of eminent physicians, including the author's own.[14] Thus, for instance, *falij* (paralysis) has a cold and moist nature; the pulse is very hard (*mutawattir jiddan*); the stool is white and difficult (*shakhsin*); bloodletting is strictly forbidden; the treatment attributed to Galen includes *hiera* (*habb iyaraj*) and the other treatment is from a renowned Hyderabadi *hakim*, Hakim Bina, which also involves *habb iyaraj*, with a list of ingredients for making it.[15]

In the preface to his work, Ashuftah critiqued the foundational theories of Yunani *tibb* for their incompleteness compared to Western medicine, as well as for the relative lack of a spirit of research: 'Compared with the discoveries of other kinds of medicine, all the theories of our *tibb* are baseless and worthless, while even the minutiae of other medicines are scientific (*sa'intifik*), from one perspective this objection can be raised against us, that every branch of *tibb-i* Yunani is incomplete and wanting, especially in research' (Ashuftah n.d.: 3). If research, and also the continued support of the rulers of the Deccan (the Nizams of Hyderabad) were part of the solution, the preface also strikes a different, but in his view complementary, tone. *Tibb-i* Yunani is glossed as *tibb-i ilahi* (divine healing); Ashuftah praises as a gift of God the faculties (*quvvaton*) and powers of reason and of the brain to seek out the antidote (*tiryaq*) for the illnesses of people (Ashuftah n.d.: 1). He goes on to say that he hopes people will benefit from the proved prescriptions (*mujarrabat*) in this book. But more important than anything else (including his own tabular notation on illnesses and their causes), he considers that the healer should possess divine force (*taqat*), and that the healer's human faculty (*bashari quvat*) should be yearning to reach this state, in order to be able to treat illness (Ashuftah n.d.: 5). The value of reason was worked through an overarching sense of the power of the divine in the effectiveness of treatment.

Ashuftah is but one example of a *hakim* who rose high in the changing professional environments of *tibb* in the twentieth century and whose writing reveals that generalizations about an inevitable secularizing trajectory for professional Yunani *tibb* do not stand up to scrutiny. May we then posit that the foundational for some practitioners did not comprise theoretical foundations but the presence of the divine in the healing act itself?

Revisiting the Foundational

Debates about the nature of the elements, humours and the temperament, how their existence could be proved or defended, how they informed therapeutics and how they could be understood in the light of new theories and knowledge, are testament to their centrality in the elaboration of a rationally grounded Yunani identity. We will speak here of two ways that *hakim*s negotiated the theoretical, which we will loosely organize under the headings of critique and concordance. Frequently, representation of the foundational theories of Yunani occupied several strands of critique and desire for reconciliation with science.

Before embarking on the discussion of those, let us briefly address a methodological problem intrinsic to any study of medical practice. Take the example of the 'question and answer' sections, common to several Yunani medical journals of the first half of the twentieth century, in which sufferers were requested to detail their complaints in order to seek professional advice on treatment. These windows on to physician–patient communication scarcely involved the patients in revealing their humoral temperament (*safravi, dammavi, balghami* or *saudavi*, and their permutations), and this was no impediment to the prescription of remedies. Much more central to interactions between patients and their physician interlocutors were descriptions of the symptoms of illness (weakness, pains, cramps and so on), and at times descriptions of feelings of heat (*garmi*) or cold (*sardi*) that

139

speak to an expression of imbalance and disorder in the body in terms of elemental qualities and, albeit indirectly, humours. This style of thinking about excesses of heat and cold and their many effects on the lived body, both as causes of illness and indicators of appropriate ways of living and medical interventions, transcends any of the elite, textual traditions and can be considered as falling in the domain of the everyday in India.

The methodological problem is evident: the absence of terminology on humours or temperaments does not in itself indicate the absence of a humoral or temperamental logic in the prescription, which may be implied and tacit knowledge.[16] But it is notable that physicians' prescriptions were guided by the remarks of the patients in which the scholarly apparatus (in terms of individual temperament and so forth) was not in evidence. We can take from this brief example that the concept of restoring balance for health need not be predicated on the formulaic descriptions that we find in much of the contemporary and antecedent *tibbi* literature.

Critique

In written documentation on *tibb*, in my research at least, direct critique of the theoretical structures of Yunani *tibb* by *hakim*s themselves is less visible than questioning only certain aspects of theory and attempts to reconcile *tibb* with science. But critique there is.[17] A penetrating engagement with *mizaj* (temperament), with considerable weight given to applications in practice, may highlight this. It was provided in a series of articles on *mizaj* published in one of the most widely circulated Yunani journals of the early twentieth century, *Rafiq al-Atibba*, published in Lahore. In an introductory essay to these articles, the editor of the journal, Hakim Ferozuddin, clearly spelt out the redux version of the importance of *ta'dil* or *i'tidal* (equipoise, balance)[18] between the elemental constituents of the humours and temperament in Yunani *tibb*:

> There has been a lot of agreement [among indigenous practitioners] on
> the restrictiveness [*inhisar*] of the treatment methods in Islamic (Yunani)
> *tibb* and *vedik* [Ayurveda] in which each person, each part of the body and
> every entity among the plants, minerals and animals of this world has a
> temperament, and that if any one of the elements constituting the *mizaj*
> is lacking, in excess or is corrupted, then illness will ensue. (Ferozuddin
> 1912: 10)

The fact that Maulvi Ali Hyder Tabatabai, a *hakim* from Lucknow, argued against the foundational theories of Yunani *tibb* in the ensuing articles (Tabatabai 1912a, 1912b), led Ferozuddin to further comment that this could mean the destruction (*hasti hi munhadam ho ja'e*) of *tibb* and Ayurveda.

Tabatabai's arguments juxtaposed the writings of (principally) Ibn Sina and his commentators with research in chemistry. He argued that the concept of *mizaj* was based on false assumptions and knowledge. Elements, in the form understood in Yunani *tibb*, do not materially exist, and the qualities (*kaifiyyat*), which they are believed to generate in the body, cannot be proved (except for the 'element' fire). Among the many arguments that he makes, Tabatabai writes that what the ancients considered as indivisible elements (*anasir-i basit*, earth, and so on) have been shown to be compounds of numerous elements (such as water, oxygen and hydrogen). Conversely, the experiments of 'foreign physicians' have demonstrated that most minerals are simple (and indivisible), while the ancients thought them to be compounds – that is, comprised of the elements, like plants and animals. This fairly straightforward reasoning was backed up by an in-depth treatment of the intricacies of the theories of the two kinds of qualities (*kaifiyyat*), passive and active, and their relationship with the elements.

Tabatabai's arguments extended to treatment and the use of medicinal substances. He cautioned against the new medicines of *daktari* (Western medicine), many of which were chemical compounds not found in nature: 'Any element which is not found in the human composition will be harmful to it, because it is not "natural" [*ghair tab'i*]' (Tabatabai 1912b: 13), 'natural' meaning in this context that it was commonly consumed and not considered harmful. For this reason he espoused the practice of what he understood to be the characteristic treatment methods of the respected *hakim*s of Lucknow: to treat ailments primarily with foodstuffs, including, grapes, plums, raisins, wild figs, salep, wood apple (*bael*) pulp, *jamun*, *amla*, honey, apple jam, purslane, a decoction of *mung dhal* (a green gram preparation with barley), or by adding foodstuffs to medicines which were not 'natural'. He noted that medicines in *daktari* (Western medicine) had such specific properties, but because they were acidic (*tezabi*), in his estimation, they would harm the functioning of the body.

Tabatabai's idea of successful treatment hinged on there being a relationship between a disease and the specific (therapeutic) property of a medicine (*dava dhu'l-khasa*), that is, one which was not based on a restorative model of elements (in the Yunani sense) and individual temperament (Tabatabai 1912b: 13). If we want to expand our pharmacopoeia, he said, we need to search out these medicines, which have these curative properties. 'Uncivilized peoples' (*vahsh qaumon*) possessed knowledge of amazing (*ajib va gharib*) medicinal plants, and there was no limit to the variety of medicinal plants, but, he said, we have very little knowledge of their properties: 'Regarding cure, scholastic knowledge (*ilm*), *hikmat* [humours] and philosophy have nothing to do with it (*kuch kam nahin ata*). If you have diagnosed a disease, and the healer does not know of the specific property of the medicine but prescribes a medicine based solely on analogy (*qiyas*), then the prescription will mostly be useless' (Tabatabai 1912b: 13).

Tabatabai was arguing that the theoretical component accounting for the activity of remedies was an overlay. From this perspective, it would be fruitless to work from the level of theorizing illness and the quality or potency of a remedy to its application in practice. Only once a remedy had been used and known could its *mizaj* and qualities be theorized – a pointless venture, as far as this *hakim* was concerned.

This repositioning of the dominant theoretical framework of *tibb* might not have been so revelatory for practising *hakim*s, and hence it comes as no surprise that his articles do not seem to have influenced the debate. It is conceivable that practising *hakim*s in a sense already knew that their art did not depend on abstract formulations of types of *mizaj*, even if aetiology, diagnosis and therapeutics could be presented accordingly. After all, the very strong emphasis on tried-and-tested (*mujarrab*) remedies for specific conditions, mostly irrespective of individual temperament, runs through the pages of these journals, and is indeed a long established genre of therapeutics in its own right within Arabic-Persian-Urdu medical literature.

While there are limits to what can be inferred from textual sources about humours and temperaments in clinical practice, we can nevertheless see that the theoretical foundations of Yunani *tibb* had a discursive reality, as markers of distinction, since they have conferred on *tibb* its place as a viable and identifiable system of medicine. For this reason, attempts to make the theoretical foundation of *tibb* accord at some level with science have been much more commonplace than critique during the twentieth century, as practitioners have sought recognition in the wider scientific community. In so doing, the idea of the importance of readjusting imbalance for health has been largely sidelined or taken in new directions.

Concordance

Hakim Kabiruddin was a major figure in new professional and institutional currents in *tibb* for which germ theory was the dividing line between Western and Eastern approaches to medicine (Liebeskind 2002; Attewell 2007: 91–93). Kabiruddin wrote at some length on this apparent division as part of a submission to a report on indigenous systems of medicine for the colonial government of the Madras Presidency, which considered supporting indigenous medicine in the early 1920s. Kabiruddin's submission was the only one by a *hakim* that was translated from Urdu into English, which attests to the importance it was given. He wrote:

> [Germ theory] does not differ in essentials from the theory of the humours inculcated by the unani system. The followers of the latter system hold that diseases are caused by the putrefaction of humours and the resultant deleterious matter, while the allopaths contend that diseases are indirectly produced by bacteria and directly by the poisonous matter (toxin) engendered by them. (GoM 1923, i: 90)

For Kabiruddin the distinction was a matter of degree of perception, not order of perception. Microscopy had made visible a deeper level in the diseased body, enabling the viewer to see organisms in 'what was previously called matter'. In practice, Kabiruddin argued, this distinction was of little consequence since practitioners of both groups sought 'to neutralize' either the germs or the poisonous matter. This discussion was very much of the moment – the Spanish influenza outbreak of 1918/19 had brought widespread death in the Indian subcontinent.

Kabiruddin's effort to reconcile the humoral with the biomedical was an erasure of ontological and epistemological distinction in favour of a linear progressivist view of historical change, in which technological advancement and terminological change could account for the apparent divergence. This kind of flattening of difference may seem strained, but it has actually been deployed quite often to account for the possibility of reconciling *tibb* and biomedicine. Moreover, Kabiruddin's insistence on it only underlines how, in a government report (with all of its implications for state support), he was intent on presenting the case for a scientific rationale within *tibb*. If this was a politically charged moment for Kabiruddin, and indeed for Yunani *tibb*, we can also see many other examples of how the conceptual boundaries between *tibb* and biomedicine have been collapsed, or at least made to correlate in a variety of other contexts through to the present.

Conclusion

The starting point of this chapter was to show how expositions of foundational theory in *tibb*, in which concepts of balance and restoration occupied a central place, articulated with socio-political dimensions of practice in the early twentieth century. Priority has been given to drawing attention to a variety of enactments of the foundational in order to emphasize that the theory is itself multiple in the ways that it has been consolidated, reworked, contested and applied through different media with different implications. Practice, then, is viewed as attention to production. I have attempted to show ways in which foundational theory could be considered fundamental to the 'survival' (pitched in this term) of *tibb*, but also problematic, marginal and even irrelevant to the practice of healing.

Not all enactments of the foundational have, however, been equal. The humoral has done work and continues to do so in contemporary thinking about the differentiation of streams of health-related knowledge and practice. This instrumentality can be seen as simultaneously an envelopment of the physiological and the socio-political.

Notes

1. The 'humours' are conventionally, *dam* or *khun* (blood, hot/wet), *balgham* (phlegm, cold/wet), *safra* (yellow bile, hot/dry) and *sauda* (black bile, cold/dry). There are different interpretations among writers on *tibb* prior to the nineteenth century about how they combine with their elemental qualities to form a person's *mizaj* (temperament); on this, see Azmi (1995). The 'foundational principles' are five in number: elements (*anasir*,

arkan), temperament (*mizaj*), humours (*akhlat, banat al-arkan*), pneuma (*ruh*) and the body's dynamic force (*tabi'at*). In addition, and of central importance, are six exogenous factors, the regulation of which is necessary for averting illness or restoring health: the 'six non-naturals' (*asbab al-sittah al-daruriyah*): air, food and drink, action and rest, mental activity and rest, sleep and wakefulness, retention and elimination of wastes. These are a resource for contemporary formulations within Yunani *tibb* of appropriate guidance for living in harmony and ecological balance. In such cases, balance is evidently invested with a different set of meanings and applications than in prior formulations. See also Savage-Smith, and Jones (this volume).

2. Among the many possible sources, there are some useful in-depth standard accounts on the fundamental principles in English, especially Khan (1986), Ahmed and Qadeer (1998) and Sheehan and Hussain (2002).

3. *Tridosha*: there are conventionally three *doshas*: *vata, pitta* and *kapha* (or *slesma*). See Mukharji (2007, 2009) for differing views on the constitution of *doshas* in late nineteenth- and early twentieth-century Bengali medical literature; see also Langford (2002) on conceptualizations of the *doshas* in contemporary Ayurvedic practice in parts of western India. Scharfe's (1999) take on the origins of the *doshas* in Siddha and Ayurveda demonstrates how twentieth-century debates on antiquity and authenticity beyond Yunani medicine have also revolved in part around foundational principles. I am grateful to Roman Sieler for an exchange about *doshas* in Siddha medicine (personal communication, April 2011).

4. In studies on therapeutics in India, claims about the foundational place of the humoral paradigms, broadly conceived, have been mostly restricted to discussions of the 'scholarly traditions' of Ayurveda, Yunani and Siddha. Anthropological studies in which humoral concepts are not given primacy relative to other dimensions of healing include Nichter and Nordstrom (1989), Lambert (1992) and Sax (2009).

5. There is no intention to connect it in this context with the philosophical approach of the same name, although there are evident overlaps.

6. We can note here works on maintaining health produced by women for women, such as the ruler of the state of Bhopal, Sultan Jahan Begum (1916), in which she described hygiene, moderation (*i'tidal*), daily exercise and keeping regular timings as the four walls of health. See also Muhammad Sajjad Mirza Beg Dihlavi (Mirza Beg 1906), in which the author emphasized reason, duty, the cultivation of ethical principles and obedience to the principles of health.

7. The demand for this work can be gauged from the number of editions it went through, mostly printed in Delhi and Lucknow. I have located eight editions of the Urdu text by 1879. Vanzan (2000: 8) states that the work was written in Persian. Alavi (2008: 222–28) refers to Ihsan Ali Khan's works in Urdu, published between the 1860s and 1911. She sees *Tibb-i Ihsani* as 'steering Unani even further away from its "secular" mechanistic stance, as here [Hakim Ihsan Ali] sees illness in terms of the relationship

between the body and the soul' (Alavi 2008: 224). She reads into this text an inflection of medieval Sufi healing practices. It is unfortunate that this interpretation rests on her understanding of *ruh*, which can indeed mean soul, but also specifically means *pneuma* or vital spirit, one of the *arwah* (vital spirits) of the scholarly Yunani tradition going back to Ibn Sina and others. Its appearance in Ihsan Ali's text is thus thoroughly conventional, precisely, for instance, where Alavi discusses it: in the production of various kinds of *ruh* in the body.

8. One among many other prominent texts of the early twentieth century that could be cited for comparison of elemental qualities by degrees is Kabiruddin (2000).
9. See Mukharji (2009) and also Langford (2002).
10. Proceedings of the Home Department for 1919 (Medical), no. 29, July, 'Question of Placing the Ancient and Indigenous Systems of Medicine on a Scientific Basis', manuscript housed at the British Library (BL), African, Asian and Pacific Collections (AAPC), P/10595.
11. Proceedings 1919, no. 29 (BL/AAPC, P/10595).
12. Proceedings 1919, no. 29 (BL/AAPC, P/10595).
13. The other work, the *Tajdid-i Tibb* (The revival of *tibb*) is a collected volume of Hakim Abdullatif's journal articles and speeches of the 1920s (Abdullatif 1972), published under the auspices of a memorial society set up in his name. It identifies a correlate role for the divine in effecting cure over and above the refined formulations of foundational theory, which, as Liebeskind (2002: 66) notes, characterize his work.
14. The *tabi'at* is another concept that has been defined in various ways from foundational texts in Arabic to contemporary authors, including nature, the source of movement and rest in the body, and as a form of bodily governance that allows for the proper functioning of the body, which it is the healer's duty to aid. According to Azmi (1995: 134), many contemporary Yunani physicians correlate *tabi'at* with the immune system, although he distances himself from this view.
15. These do not conform with the ingredients for the *hiera picra* and *hiera cum agarico*, cited by Cox and Dannehl, who note: 'Hiera was a commonly used name in ancient medicaments' (Cox and Dannehl 2007: s.v. 'Hiera cum agarico – Hl'). It probably referred to a species of drug rather than a specific formulation.
16. See Zimmermann (this volume), who offers strong support for this point.
17. The most recent critical analysis of Yunani theory is by Altaf Azmi, from Jamia Hamdard, Delhi, who advocates rejecting the idea that the humoral doctrine has a role in disease causation, but does not accept that this imperils Yunani medicine's integrity (Azmi 1995: 106).
18. Other terms conveying balance in Urdu are *tasawi*, *tawazun*, and the more colloquial *miana ravi* (also meaning moderation).

References

Abdullatif. 1972. *Tajdid-i Tibb*, ed. Syed Zillurrahman. Aligarh: Tibbi Academy.

Ahmed, J., and A. Qadeer. 1998. *Unani: The Science of Graeco-Arabic Medicine*. New Delhi: Lustre Press.

Alavi, S. 2008. *Islam and Healing: Loss and Recovery of an Indo-Muslim Medical Tradition, 1600–1900*. Basingstoke: Palgrave.

Ashuftah, A. n.d. *Amaliya-i Jalinus*. Hyderabad.

Attewell, G. 2007. *Refiguring Unani Tibb: Plural Healing in Late Colonial India*. Hyderabad: Orient Longman.

Azmi, A. 1995. *Basic Concepts in Unani Medicine: A Critical Study*. New Delhi: Jamia Hamdard.

Cox, N., and K. Dannehl. 2007. *Dictionary of Traded Goods and Commodities, 1550–1820*, Wolverhampton: University of Wolverhampton Press.

Ferozuddin, M. 1912. 'Mizaj aur Tahqiqat Qadim va Jadid [Editor's note]', *Rafiq al-Atibba* 10(4): 10.

GoM. 1923. 'Report of the Committee on the Indigenous Systems of Medicine, Madras', 2 vols. Madras: Government of Madras.

Jaggi, O.P. 1977. *Medicine in Medieval India*. Delhi: Atma Ram.

Jahan Begum, S. 1916. *Hifz-i Sihhat*. Agra: Steam Press.

Kabiruddin, M. 2000 [1937]. *Makhzan al-Mufradat, al-ma'ruf Khavas al-Adviyah*, 2nd edn. Delhi: Daftar al-Masih.

Khan, I.A. 1911. *Tibb-i Ihsani*. Lucknow: Munshi Naval Kishor.

Khan, M.S. 1986. *Islamic Medicine*. London: Routledge and Kegan Paul.

Khan, N. 1926. *Khaza'in al-adviya*, 8 vols. Lahore: Barqi Press.

Lambert, H. 1992. 'The Cultural Logic of Indian Medicine: Prognosis and Etiology in Rajasthani Popular Therapeutics', *Social Science and Medicine* 34: 1069–77.

Langford, J. 2002. *Fluent Bodies: Ayurvedic Remedies for Postcolonial Imbalance*. Durham, NC: Duke University Press.

Leslie, C. 1998. 'The Ambiguities of Medical Revivalism in Modern India', in C. Leslie (ed.), *Asian Medical Systems: A Comparative Study*, 2nd edn. Delhi: Motilal Banarsidas, pp.356–78.

Liebeskind, C. 2002. 'Arguing Science: Unani Tibb, Hakims and Biomedicine in India, 1900–1950', in W. Ernst (ed.), *Plural Medicine: Tradition and Modernity, 1800–2000*. London: Routledge, pp.58–75.

Metcalf, B. 1982. *Islamic Revival in British India: Deoband, 1860–1900*. Princeton, NJ: Princeton University Press.

——— 1990. *Perfecting Women: Maulana Ashraf Ali Thanawi's Bihishti Zewar*. Berkeley: University of California Press.

Mirza Beg, M. 1906. *Hikmat-i Amali* [Practical wisdom]. Hyderabad: Qasim Press.

Mukharji, P. 2007. 'Medicine and Modernity in Colonial Bengal', PhD dissertation. London: University of London.

——— 2009. *Nationalizing the Body: The Medical Market, Print and Daktari Medicine*. London: Anthem Press.

Nichter, M., and C. Nordstrom. 1989. 'A Question of Medicine Answering', *Culture, Medicine and Psychiatry* 13(4): 367–90.

Sax, W. 2009. *God of Justice: Ritual Healing and Social Justice in the Central Himalayas*. Oxford: Oxford University Press.

Scharfe, H. 1999. 'The Doctrine of the Three Humors in Traditional Indian Medicine and the Alleged Antiquity of Tamil Siddha Medicine', *Journal of the American Oriental Society* 119: 609–29.

Shankar, D., and P. Unnikrishnan (eds). 2004. *Challenging the Indian Medical Heritage*. New Delhi: Foundation Books.

Sheehan, H., and S. Hussain. 2002. 'Unani Tibb: History, Theory and Contemporary Practice in South Asia', *Annals of the American Academy of Political and Social Science* 583(1): 122–35.

Speziale, F. 2003. 'The Relation between Galenic Medicine and Sufism in India during the Delhi and Deccan Sultanates', *East and West* 53(1–4): 149–78.

——— 2010. *Soufisme, Religion et Médecine en Islam Indien*. Paris: Karthala.

Tabatabai, A. 1912a. 'Mizaj aur Tahqiqat' [Research on temperament], *Rafiq al-Atibba* 10(4): 10–15.

——— 1912b. 'Mizaj aur Tahqiqat', *Rafiq al-Atibba* 10(7): 11–14.

Vanzan, A. 2000. 'Medical Education of Muslim Women in Turn-of-the-Century India: The 9th Chapter of the Bihishti Zewar', *Journal of the Pakistan Historical Society* 48(1): 3–8.

❖

Chapter 7

Hot/Cold Classifications and Balancing Actions in Mesoamerican Diet and Health

Theory and Ethnography of Practice in Twentieth-Century Mexico

Ellen Messer

Introduction

Humoral-based understandings of food, health, environment and cosmology have a controversial history in Latin America. Disagreements centre on whether humoral ideas, which have been reduced to the hot/cold idiom, are indigenous or European-introduced, and how central these ideas are to nutrition, preventive medicine and curing practices. Most historical and ethnographic studies of diet, health and healing find evidence of the utilization of the hot/cold principle and classifications in diagnostics, health maintenance and therapeutics. Hot/cold reasoning enters also into evaluations of human body states and pathologies, foods and medicines, all of which are related also to the hot/cold dynamics of the larger natural and social environment. Yet analysts persistently disagree over how connected diet and medicine are to other domains that may also be classified in hot/cold terms, and also whether individuals draw on sensory evidence, abstract symbolic referents or both when incorporating hot/cold reasoning in practice.

As a corollary, some insist users share principles of hot/cold classification, whereas others assert they share only rote classifications of particular items. Opinions also vary on the extent to which the ideal or practical dynamics of eating, healing and social behaviours prioritize the balancing of hot/cold opposites, or instead privilege other analogical frames, such as the sweet-versus-bitter taste of hot-versus-cold herbs, or additional forces, such as 'airs' or 'witchcraft' that are believed to cause illnesses of a hot or cold quality. Even where hot/cold reports from contemporary Mesoamerica discuss diagnoses of bodies out of balance, therapeutics that aim at restoring balance, and the idea of balancing opposites around some equilibrium point or points, commentators do not always agree whether the desired quality of a healthy balance is essentially neutral, slightly warm or cool, or in modern contexts, 'healthy'.

Mexican ethnohistorians and ethnographers since the 1970s have developed a corpus of texts that emphasize the autochthonous origins of hot/cold reasoning within a 'dual cosmovision', which is all-pervasive and widely shared across indigenous systems of thought (e.g., Lopez Austin 1975, 1980; Ortiz de Montellano 1980, 1990). Their findings contrast with certain ethnographic and historical analyses, mostly by US anthropologists, who assert this dual cosmovision is something altogether separate from the hot/cold classifications that they consider to be a result of European introductions of humoral medical reasoning from the sixteenth century onwards.[1] All these accounts, however, find that both indigenous and Spanish (Mestizo) understandings of the body in balance reduce the European hot-wet, hot-dry, cold-wet and cold-dry combinations to a hot/cold quality, occasionally combined with a wet/dry dimension, but never an equilibrium of different humours. Illness situations labelled and associated with 'blood' and 'bile' do appear in these New World medical discussions, but not in roles comparable to Old World humours. Nor do *materia medica* ordinarily carry any wet/dry classification, although this wet/dry dimension is connected to an indigenous cultural discourse about internal (body heat) and external influences (such as the heat of the sun or a cooking fire) on the hot/cold state of the human body.

An additional area of theoretical and practical interest is how hot/cold knowledge is structured and shared and systematically undergoes diminution or change in particular cultural settings (e.g., Messer 1978, 1981, 1996). People in Latin America are far from isolated; they are exposed to a variety of new and old medical systems and influences, and can choose and mix medicaments and procedures drawn from different authorities and vendors. A practical implication, of special interest to modern health practitioners, is how a patient's cultural ideas of hot/cold therapeutics may (positively) influence health and healing or (negatively) interfere with prescribed Western pharmaceutical regimens (e.g., Harwood 1971).

Below, after a brief review of the historical controversies, the dynamic notion of hot/cold balance is considered from the ethnographic perspectives of indigenous Nahuas and Popolucas in the Mexican state of Veracruz (Chevalier and Sanchez Bain 2003) and of Spanish-Zapotec speakers in the pluralistic Valley of Oaxaca (Messer 1987, 1991), drawing insights from the ethnography of medical practice (see Low and Hsu 2008). These Mexican ethnographic sources show that traditional patients and practitioners also extend the hot/cold idiom to geographic, social, political-economic and spiritual and mythological realms that Spanish physicians or friars would never have countenanced or possibly imagined. They also consider interpretations of how hot/cold knowledge is transmitted but also changes. The final section brings these ideas together to suggest why hot/cold or related idioms, used to describe balance in nature, might continue to contribute to healing practices, even as people have access to modern medicines.

Latin American Hot/Cold Controversies

Indigenous peoples have lived in what is now Latin America for some 14,000 years, where, over the past 500 years, most have experienced European, African, Asian and transnational influences. Not surprisingly, in their particular cultural contexts, populations have responded to exigencies of health and disease through some combination of indigenous and introduced concepts and procedures. In this process, local and regional (culture-area wide) medicinal systems have experienced both internal and external trajectories of change, and their interactions, producing syncretisms that employ elements from each contributing culture but also mix them up in new combinations.

In Mesoamerica, a culture area that encompasses modern-day Mexico, Guatemala and Central America, most cultural populations

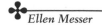

use hot/cold, and to a lesser extent wet/dry, terminology to relate the domains of the body, specifically health and nutrition, to the larger social and natural environment. They describe human development over the life cycle, and also in traditional maize-based agricultural societies the life cycle of the maize plant and field, in hot/cold and wet/dry terms. Hot/cold terminologies are just two of many dichotomies that appear in the dual cosmovision, which is widely shared among indigenous Latin American cultures, and the cultures that have come into contact with or descended from them.

Latin Americanists divide into two camps regarding the historical dimensions and significance of humoral or hot/cold classifications and reasoning in Latin American health and healing cultures. To the first belong Mexican ethnohistorians and ethnographers, particularly those studying Aztec (Nahua) and nearby cultures in the central valley of Mexico. They assert that the hot/cold concept and idiom are indigenous to Latin American thought and actions on the world, the opposition containing just two of the multitude of elements, conceptualized as dichotomies, that organize and order the world, which in addition to hot/cold also includes wet/dry, down (lower)/ up (upper), mother/father, female/male and other paired opposites. Among the most compelling translators, compilers and commentators on Aztec medicinal cosmology are Lopez Austin (1975, 1980) and Ortiz de Montellano (1980, 1990), who illuminate the operation of hot/cold principles through human actions and reactions to natural, magical and divine forces in the world. In their analyses, hot/cold is indigenous, pervasive, and aims toward a healthful (or not-harmful) equilibrium, which can be maintained by each individual's attention to ritual duty, socially appropriate work and sexual behaviours, and proper diet.

Hot/cold is also a critical part of their understanding of two distinctive Mesoamerican health and illness concepts: the association of healthy soul substance with 'heat' (*tonalli*) and the association of a dangerous cluster of debilitating illnesses with the rain god complex, Tlaloc, and his emissaries and associates, including rain dwarfs who inhabit the earth, underworld, rivers and caves. In this reasoning, human health is an integral part of this cosmos and subject to its forces, which include the heat of the sun, exertion from work, fire, and intrinsic properties of classes, categories, specimens and items in the physical, biological and spiritual world. Recent ethnographic texts further elaborate at least three principles involved in hot/cold classifications among modern Nahua and Popoluca: the balancing of hot/cold opposites, including the avoidance of extremes and clashes between them; cyclic motion, as in diurnal cycles of night followed by day, and annual cycles of dry season followed by rainy season; and heliotropic sun-led growth based on the life-giving heat of the sun, which transforms cool and wet infants and maize seedlings, over their life cycles, into predominantly hot and dry, mature human beings nourished by maize in its final seed stage (Chevalier and Sanchez Bain 2003). Together, these hot/cold processes aim toward a harmonious state that is a dynamic balance and less of a static equilibrium, dependent on all of the above natural, human and super-human forces. All these scholars reason that hot/cold ideas and the health and healing actions associated with them are so pervasive that they must be indigenous to New World peoples and cultures.

By contrast, US anthropologist George Foster and disciples (see Foster 1994), who worked among Mexican coastal and Tarascan (western central Mexican) peoples, reach the opposite conclusion. They assert that hot/cold food and medicinal classifications, while pervasive in New World cultures, are not indigenous but a Spanish introduction. This nutritional and medicinal reasoning, based on hot/cold, wet/dry humoral concepts, was subsequently simplified into hot/cold classifications and employed almost exclusively in the nutritional-medical domain. They furthermore assert that hot/cold is divorced from indigenous New World cosmological vision and theory and applies only to the realm of diet and medicine. They do not deny that there exists an indigenous dual cosmovision, but they assert this constitutes a separate domain and is not part of medicinal analysis. An additional point is that hot/cold balancing aims toward equilibrium, or a 'neutral' state, by manipulation of known hot/cold qualities of foods and medicines.

In their ethnographic findings, Foster and his students assert that there is an ideal equilibrium, of neutral quality, which is the harmonious goal of health, and also encourages the addition of new items of neutral quality. The hot/cold qualities of older items are inherited knowledge, and learned by rote, not by cosmological or experimental reasoning. They reach this conclusion based on findings in interviews, using checklists, that the hot/cold qualities of close to 300 foods and medicines have assigned qualities, which show widespread agreement. This interpretation also favours Foster's position that hot/cold ideas were introduced by Spanish personnel, and then passed down intact, generation to generation. They conclude that dual cosmovision is something altogether different, as are applications of hot/cold terminologies to non-food and medicinal items, such as prayers.

Regarding ideas of balance, Foster notes that hot/cold reasoning is used primarily to validate (after the fact) rather than to guide curing behaviours, with the aim of dietary, health and healing behaviours being to maintain or restore a balanced state. Between the classifications of (very) hot (*irritante*) and cold (*fresco* or *frio*), a neutral (*templado*) category allows people to incorporate new food items and nutritional information to maintain a healthy dietary balance. As noted above, however, Foster's position does not match the wider ethnohistorical and ethnographic findings, which show that cosmological dualities and complex juxtapositions of hot/ cold, growth/rot and other pairings of opposites are characteristic of all systems of Latin American indigenous thought, cosmological orientation, health and healing practices.

To be sure, there is no ideal, abstract, neutral harmony or equilibrium but always a 'moving equilibrium' or 'dynamic balance', depending on life stage, work history and other factors, such as diet, exposure to illness agents, satisfaction in work or love versus overwork or excessive leisure or overindulgence in food or sex, or denial and deprivation of either. In this larger cosmovision, atmospheric, weather and climatic conditions are important, as are cycles in reproduction, work, social well-being and social 'stress'. Moreover, in the context of accumulative heat and dryness over the life cycle, there is a slight preference for coolness and moisture, especially in mature years, where heat and dryness accumulate and may present themselves as illness and suffering. There is also a general avoidance of extremes of cold or heat during infancy and early childhood, when too much wetness and coolness or too much heat are both extremely harmful and treated with medications that seek to moderate this delicate childhood condition. Below, additional ethnographic evidence demonstrates how dualistic cosmic classification enters into many aspects of health and healing regimens, even in modernizing, pluralistic dietary, health and medical contexts.

Dynamic Balance in Mesoamerican Ethnographic Practice

Latin American indigenous populations continue to reason in terms of hot and cold in their management of diet, nutrition and health, but the extent to which they consciously reflect on pre-Columbian divinities, superhuman forces and disease complexes varies very much by place and individual context and personality.

Veracruz: Pervasive Dualism in Humans and Maize

Chevalier and Sanchez Bain (2003) provide a recent comprehensive ethnographic account of hot/cold practices in contemporary Mexico, based on intensive observations and interviews among indigenous Nahuas and Popolucas in the state of Veracruz. Drawing also on sixteenth-century documentary sources, they argue that contemporary practice shows the survival of pre-Hispanic beliefs and practices, along with multiple types of syncretism with later philosophical, medical and ritual introductions. Their main point, repeated over and over again in examples, is that, in this indigenous system, hot/cold balance is a moving target, not an absolute fixed equilibrium point; the hot/cold balance is inherent in the cyclic motion of hot/cold diurnal and seasonal cycles, and cumulative sun-led growth over the life cycle of humans and maize. They thus allude to a concept of 'dynamic balance', as advocated throughout the present volume.

These hot/cold dynamics form part of a larger dual cosmovision, which incorporates elements juxtaposing cosmic and bodily dimensions of up/down, above/below, sun/moon, male/female, lowlands (hot)/highlands (cool), and also various pairings of divine forces, conceptualized in pre-Columbian mythologies. The ethnography captures the interdependent relationship between humans and maize in theory and practice. It describes the conceptual interplay of hot (the sun, the heavens) above in cyclic flow with cold (water, Earth, youth) below, and all the ways that the daily cycles of sun's heat, seasonal heat or cold, rainfall (moisture) or drought (dryness) affect the growing child, mature adult and human body of reproductive age, and also the annual growth cycle of maize plants in cultivated fields (*milpa*).

Individual chapters treat ordinary cases of illness (diarrhoeal disease, acute respiratory infections), special cases of illness (love-

155

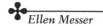

sickness, fear of death), dangerous times in the life cycle (childbirth, special illness vulnerabilities among young children), and finally, hot/cold dimensions in the life cycle of the maize plant and maize-related mythology. The human cases demonstrate the many ways individuals in these traditional settings use hot/cold analysis and terminology to diagnose signs of harm – such as fever, worsening illness, reddening wounds – all signifying that the normal flow has been disrupted by hot/cold clashes or excesses; and then how individuals counter such disturbances through the introduction of medicinal herbs, foods or other remedies of the opposite, or balancing, quality, or through changes in behaviour, such as rest if the hot/cold imbalance stems from overwork, or abstinence in diet or sex if the imbalance stems from overeating or sexual overindulgence.

In curing, topical applications as well as the ingestion of medicaments influence hot/cold dynamics. Such hot/cold practices transcend the material versus metaphorical distinction that has sometimes been used to describe hot/cold qualities, because medicinal choices and actions involve both. For example, women hot from labouring in the maize fields or kitchen, or experiencing the normal heat of menstruation, pregnancy or childbirth, will cool their bodies with rest, or cooling evening food or drink at home, or drink warm water or teas prepared from medicinal herbs classified as moderately hot. They will also try to avoid 'cold clash' with water, air or cold foods. Should they nevertheless experience a harmful, cold body state, whose sign may be diarrhoea or lethargy, they will counter it with dietary changes, warm clothing and applications of hot herbs, such as mustard and holypalm leaves.

In these particular cases, principle and practice favour juxtaposition, or a balancing of opposites, and also avoidance of extremes through the maximum separation of hot and cold. So, as a precaution applied to breastfeeding, a working mother will try to 'cool down' and wash her breast, and extract the first 'hot' milk before feeding her infant, who is naturally cold. Neither coolness nor warmth are preferentially favoured, although people express a desire for freshness (that is, young and green, cool and moist), which leads them to avoid or counter extremes of heat and its drying actions, both in general and also in the treatment of specific illnesses, such as watery diarrhoea, which involves multiple remedies. After self-diagnosis of too much heat, one also avoids consuming hot foods, such as chilli, or spicy or oily foodstuffs, or cold beverages, such as water, cold milk and coconut water, and also cold foods like pineapple that could deliver a shock. Diarrhoea that is hot and drying is related to an aetiology that may be attributed to drinking cold water instead of a warm maize beverage; cold water will stop up the blood and prevent normal cooling, especially after hot work in the fields. Hot diarrhoea may also be tempered by a cool plant remedy, such as an extraction of *guayaba* bark or leaves, boiled and filtered (Chevalier and Sanchez Bain 2003: 57, 70, 77).[2] Another remedy is to drink a cool or fresh herbal brew, like corn-leaf tea, to counter heat piling up in the body. However, the treatment does not consist of herbs and potions only. A diagnosis of adult diarrhoea, attributed to excessive heat, may lead to additional causal analysis that may point to the ingestion of too many hot foods, a period or lifetime of too many hot activities (working long hours in the sun or in front of a hot fire), socially disruptive quarrelling, or smoking or drinking too much while not eating sufficient healthy food in a timely fashion. The suggested remedies include multiple changes in diet and behaviour, plus cooling herbs.

Reproduction is also an extremely dangerous time, when beliefs and practices address the 'hot' status of pregnancy and the *post partum* period (following birth), with its attendant loss of blood. As in other Mesoamerican cases, the natural status of the newborn child is cool and wet (watery). The mother, meanwhile, is deemed hot because she has lost all the cool wetness of the newborn child (Chevalier and Sanchez Bain 2003).[3] Attendants try to facilitate the restoration of a moderate temperature by avoiding overly hot foods or medicines. Procedures may also involve sweat baths or soak baths and herbs to restore a protective hot/cold balance in the mother, who must also protect her child.

In short, life is a constant balancing act for those who care to reflect and adjust balance and the pace of life accordingly. To avoid extremes or clashes, and so avoid untimely illness or death, one must constantly remain aware of natural hot/cold cycles (youth/old age, night/day, rest/work, hunger/eating, sexual tension/sexual relief and reproduction), and try to behave with moderation in all matters (Chevalier and Sanchez Bain 2003: 78–79). Both overwork and laziness are extremes that predispose one toward illness, as dangerous to the person's healthy balance as the evil eye, lovesickness or soul loss, which are all classified as hot ailments, and in particular cases involve additional diagnostic factors. The significant principle is balance rather than whether equilibrium in the hot or cold direction is either good or bad, or whether the causal agent is what Western scholarship would term natural (life stage, work), magical (sorcery, the evil eye) or divine (connected to ancient beliefs associated with attributes and the cult of the rain god, Tlaloc). One or more agents may work in combination, and Mesoamerican traditional illness ideas and herbal remedies associated with soul loss, which can involve all three classes of causal agents, suggest the difficulty of applying these categories in traditional Mesoamerican medicinal settings.

People combine traditional and modern nutritional and medical ideas to varying degrees. Chevalier and Sanchez Bain's work provides case studies by curers and commentaries by others, but does not speculate on how widely the information and procedures are shared and used. Moreover, some of the respondents, in integrating new information, also reach some troubling conclusions. For example, some assert that chlorinated water and bottle feeding are harmful because they destroy water's natural motion (one explained chlorinated water is 'not alive'), which means it is moderately warming or cooling, depending on the situation.

Models of Syncretism

Chevalier and Sanchez Bain, after expounding the contemporary persistence of hot/cold usage in a local Mexican setting, with critical commentaries on historical parallels, suggest three basic syncretic processes for further studies: the nomadic, the hegemonic and the global. The first, 'nomadic', is a process whereby Latin American travellers adopted and used ideas and *materia medica* from those with whom they came into contact. These accretions were inserted, added and integrated to greater or lesser degrees, depending on the predilections of the individuals exploring their larger environment and doing the integrating. Given that there are both commonalities and differences within and between Latin American socio-cultural environments, this process of change in any particular location would have involved incorporation not only of Spanish ideas but also of those of other indigenous and mixed cultures.

The second, 'hegemonic', model envisions a more powerful agent, enjoying a higher religious or secular position or prestige, which imposes medical ideas on a subject (or subject population). This authority decides what can or cannot be admitted from the pre-existing culture, which then declines or goes underground and is marginalized. Chevalier and Sanchez Bain suggest that sixteenth-century Spanish religious beliefs were subject to this same central-versus-peripheral (marginalizing) processes, as Spanish sorcery and witchcraft ideas and rituals became integrated into local indigenous cultural ideas of the world but never became part of official, central medical practice, which was simultaneously adopting medical materials from indigenous elites.

The third process, which continues today, involves global forces that continually introduce new ideas and types of medicine. These global medical ideas are mostly in the allopathic, techno-scientific realm, but also include whole systems of alternative medicine, including global herbal pharmacopoeias, homeopathy, spiritism and spiritualism, and certain dietary regimes.

In any Latin American settlement, large or small, one can see all these local-to-global systems coexisting, as people combine the ideas of the past, which have been passed on to them by older generations, with scientific or alternative medical ideas of the near present and present, which are communicated through schools, radios, markets, and state or private health systems.

The Valley of Oaxaca: Avoiding Imbalances at Critical Stages in the Life Cycle

Descriptions of hot/cold usage in Veracruz suggest that pre-Hispanic customs and knowledge connected with maize agriculture and the cult of Tlaloc are represented much more so here than in the Valley of Oaxaca, where Zapotec-speaking populations are declining, and maize agriculture is giving way to weaving and other crafts, as well as tourism. The Oaxaca area exhibits an exhilarating medical pluralism, including local herbal medicines, patent medicines, modern pharmaceuticals and transnational healing cults.

As in the Mesoamerican cases described above, the hot/cold status of women during pregnancy and immediately afterwards is considered to be delicate and carefully managed with herbs, baths and diet. In the Oaxaca area, women in the 1970s described how a mother, who was usually although not always classified as 'hot' from childbirth, was bathed in water, and additionally struck with leafy herbs, such as *chamizo*, characterized as 'cool' because they grew near the river (though, according to their sensory perception, these switches 'burned like fire'). Whether a woman's *post partum* condition was initially classified as extremely hot or cold, the therapeutic practice used the same herbs and procedures, and was conceptualized as an act to return her to a desirable, less dangerous state, and not introduce either too much heat or cold through diet, work or social activities.

Hot/cold reasoning was also very evident in protecting and dosing young children, especially in the management of diarrhoea. Young children, as in the Nahua and Popoluca cases, are classified as predominantly cool and thus especially vulnerable to excess cold and in need of special protection. One mother of three young sons described in loving detail how she had observed and learned to integrate and act on hot/cold knowledge, not when she was first exposed to such information but when she actually had to use it. Although she had previously been exposed to bits of information from her parents when they discussed hot/cold qualities of illnesses and herbs, she had paid little attention; the information was not yet relevant. With three young children, however, hot/cold observations and thinking took on new significance. She began to observe that their episodes of diarrhoea followed a pattern; they occurred after they had eaten certain foods, such as thin black beans or grapes, both classified as cold, or had drunk Coca Cola. Infant diarrhoea might also follow having eaten certain foods herself, such as avocado, classified as cold. Putting together the information she had learned from her parents that children are cool and that cold foods can make them ill, she concluded that hot/cold diagnoses and remedies could be used to explain and treat her children's ailments. More careful dietary precautions could also prevent future episodes of cold diarrhoea. For both children and more mature individuals, she had observed that hot teas of *yerba buena* and oregano relieved stomach ailments, such as *dolor*, classified as cold. This provided additional confirmation that her hot/cold interpretations were correct, and so the hot/cold classification of illness symptoms, remedies and the principle of opposites became part of her own curing knowledge and practice. Afterwards, she had paid greater attention to the hot/cold qualities of foods in the family's diet; she became more careful in preparing meals for the children, and knew what herbs to administer when they became sick. The hot/cold ideas that she had heard as a youth and rejected as hearsay had become a guide for her dietary planning, food preparation and home remedies.

Remedies, in addition to herbs, also included store-bought patent pharmaceuticals, such as fizzy Alka Seltzer (hot) or its alternative (Sal de Uvas, cold), which allowed the curer and patient to experiment and re-diagnose an ailment's hot/cold quality. In one telling case, again from the 1970s, a young mother described diagnosing and dosing her young son. She started out by giving him Alka Seltzer, reasoning that the diarrhoea was cold, given his age and tendency to drink (cold) water and eat (cold) foods, but when the remedy failed to produce relief she switched to Sal de Uvas (literally 'grape salt'), used analogously to Alka Seltzer, but classified as cold because it contains grapes (which are cold). The end of the child's diarrhoea was associated with the second remedy, so the mother concluded that the diarrhoea had been hot, and re-analysed what the child might have eaten or done.

The sudden onset of diarrhoea was never treated as a random occurrence, but instead invoked an illness aetiology that considered the possible hot/cold body state of the patient and particular foods that had been recently ingested and might have triggered an excess. As indicated above, an evaluation of the hot/cold state of the body considered age, reproductive status, immediate and also cumulative heat or cold from work activity, social-psychological states related to immediate or longer-term social relations, as well as diet and other illnesses. An elderly farmer (male), who considered himself hot from his many years of toiling in the sun, observed what foods made him ill (such as chocolate and pork), which he classified as hot, and what foods he digested easily (cooked leafy greens, for instance), which he classified as cool. He concluded that cool foods for him were harmless, and that he could prevent digestive disorders by avoiding hot foods like chocolate or foods that are highly spiced with hot chilli peppers. Coincidentally, the modern medical doctor he consulted had urged him to avoid fatty and spicy foods, which led him to conclude that the doctor also understood his illness in hot/cold terms.[4] This same individual classified pharmaceuticals as hot if they did not relieve his own symptoms of painful indigestion. Some elderly people, both men and women, indicated they drank bitter herbal tonics as an additional measure to strengthen their bodies, which are hot and dry. In general (but there are exceptions), sweet herbs were classified as hot or heating, whereas bitter herbs were classified as cooling (in Spanish, *fresco*; in Zapotec, *nyel yuh*, refreshing, cool and wet).

For the general population, diarrhoeal diseases, which might be more or less watery and include blood or mucus, came respectively in hot or cold categories, based on the observed colour (red/black or white/green) and consistency of the stool, as well as *post hoc* dietary and behavioural diagnostics. Traditional remedies for hot diarrhoea involve complex herbal preparations including the white inner bark of the *guayaba* and its green fruit, which are classified as cool; curing cold diarrhoea by contrast, might mean employing herbs or pharmaceuticals, such as terramycin, which was increasingly used instead of more complex herbal remedies, whose traditional usage appeared to be dying out.

For all kinds of aches and pains, people would try one remedy after another until something worked. Home remedies usually involved *post hoc* diagnoses based on observations of which hot or cold herbs or other medications relieved or failed to relieve symptoms, the timing of symptoms (in relation to day versus night – itself a hot/cold opposition – and the seasons, being rainy or dry, winter or summer), and the social context (anger can produce hot indigestion or diabetes in extreme cases, which is furthermore associated with thirst and a sensation of dry heat). All these interpretations followed the general rule of treatment by the principle of opposites.

Hot/cold reasoning also entered into the therapeutics of illnesses attributed to soul loss due to fright, the evil eye, sorcery or witchcraft. Soul loss due to fright (*espanto*, *susto*) encompassed a number of digestive and emotional symptoms, including lack of appetite, a yellowish complexion and general lethargy. It could be diagnosed and treated at any age, although in adults it was more likely to be diagnosed in females. The name of the most important herb for treating this condition derived from the condition itself, and was known in Spanish as *yerba de espanto* ('fright herb'), and equivalently in Zapotec as *shkwan jehb* (*Loeselia mexicana*). Frothing into a sudsy green liquid, it was considered to be very fresh, and so to transfer an important cooling dimension to those suffering from soul loss, which leaves the body hot. Administration of this herb through ingestion or by enema comprised part of a larger soul-restorative ritual, which featured multiple hot/cold elements. These included calling forth the soul by means of a gourd, from the four corners of a house, and also from a place below (such as a well). The curing ritual also involved spit-spraying (*soplar*, 'blowing') the patient with water, alcohol (cold) or mescal (hot),[5] an action that could be classified as either cold or hot, depending on the liquid. The effective impact of the action was to startle patient who gasped with a sharp intake of breath, so provided a context, analogous to the original fright during which the soul escaped, for the soul to re-enter the body. The ritual also included moments of 'talk therapy', during which the patient would describe possible contributing events or frightening contexts, such as family fights, a close encounter with a bull or a moving vehicle, floodwaters, or death. This confessional stage was facilitated by the curer's encouragement and divination using ritual incense, which was burned on a palm cross in water. Cosmologically, ritual incense could be both protective and connective; it allowed the healer and patient to reach a new plane, connecting Earth to both the heavens and the underworld, where the errant soul might be located and attracted back into the patient's body.

Soul loss was also closely identified with diabetes, which was classified as hot and drying, because the aetiology of the onset in specific cases was associated with hot 'extreme anger' (*muina*) or aroused bile (*bilis*). Diabetes was treated with extremely bitter herbs, which were classified as cold or very cold. Beverages prepared from them would be imbibed very early in the morning, before the sun came up and while the dew still freshened the earth. These bitter brews caused shivering ('like an ice cold shower'). Moreover, bitter was opposed to sweet, as cold is to heat, and diabetes was associated with too much sugar (sweet) in modern medical diagnosis. Punishing thirst and loss of water (excessive urination) also indicated that diabetes was hot and dry, and so required cool, refreshing remedies. In sum, people combined the diabetes aetiologies of modern medical doctors with traditional beliefs and practices, to treat the bodies and souls of diabetics.

Hot/Cold Terminologies, Translations and Transitions

The Valley of Oaxaca, the context of these observations, was pluralistic in medical systems, language and culture. Zapotec speakers recognized, discussed and labelled a total of seven hot/cold terms,

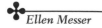

ranging from very cold, cold and cool to warm, hot and very hot. Both Zapotec and Spanish terminologies distinguished cold from cool, which combines cold and wet, but only Zapotec distinguished between the warming internal heat of the body and the external heat of the sun, which were both glossed 'hot' in Spanish. These terms were used to describe and distinguish the hot/cold qualities of foods and medicines, which especially with regard to digestion were related to their functional effects, namely, whether they were digestible or made one ill, and whether they had been observed to cure ailments of the opposite quality. These judgements, in any particular instance, involved an iterative process of reviewing all the evidence, including the evaluation of one's hot/cold body and emotional state, and prior experience.

In either language, terminologies also relied on cognitive judgements of similarity, including perceptive, functional, affective, nominal and fiat judgements (see Messer 1987). In the case of a herb judged and described as hot, for example, an individual might consider, first, attributes which are perceived as intrinsic to the herb: Is the colour red? Then this indicates hot. Or is it white? In this case it is cold. Second, what are the herb's perceptible extrinsic attributes? For example, hot herbs grow in the sun, cool herbs grow in moist soils. Because most herbs grow in the sun in the rainy season, this provides considerable latitude for classification. Next, the person moved on to intrinsic functional attributes – such as hot herbs cook uncooked food in a cold stomach – or extrinsic functional attributes – such as hot herbs are applied to cold headaches. Affective attributes assert emotional judgements – for instance, hot foods are 'bad' because they make you sick, or hot foods are good because they do not make you sick. These observational or experiential criteria contrast with nominal attributes, which attribute hot or cold qualities to a named category – for example, a herb is classified as hot because it is known to belong to the hot category, or more simply by fiat: 'hot herbs are (simply) called hot'.

For purposes of assessing practice, however, even this more complete descriptive account leaves out the important question of whether or not people act on their reasoned knowledge. For diet, health and healing, and other behaviours, the pragmatics are the most significant: not only how individuals evaluate choices, but also what they subsequently do. Do they use items or procedures consistent with hot/cold qualities, and, if so, in what contexts?

Many garden and wild herbs had healing qualities but certain ones also had special virtues that made them good for healing evil diseases, such as the evil eye, sorcery, witchcraft or soul loss (as discussed above). Most of these syndromes were considered to be hot conditions, although young children were most vulnerable to the evil eye and witchcraft, so usually suffered diseases attributed to excess cold. As in the case of ordinary human diseases, which did not have an evil or super-human origin, the primary referent was the disease category, but the secondary rationale was in hot/cold terms.

The home curer who shared her discoveries of dualism in the simple observation that 'all things come in [hot/cold] pairs' that were part of God's created world order described in detail the paired hot/cold qualities of edible species (sheep and goat, cow and pig, chicken and turkey) and of the distinctive herbs that seasoned and balanced soups and stews. Other pairings included red versus white-leaved amaranth and castor beans, which also demonstrated the duality and balance of the universe. She revelled in the beauty of this understanding, but at the time I did not probe into whether this juxtaposition of opposites meant a kind of balance, equilibrium or dynamic tension.

Reflections

My research in the 1970s focused on how knowledge is structured and how it changes. I focused on food systems and food plants, and added medicinal plants and health and healing practices to my study because they were integrally tied into diet. My conclusion in that study was that variations in the hot/cold classification of individual items was widespread, discussed and significant. However, over and above such variations, people shared a common system or way of thinking about the world, which was widely shared, although in decline from generation to generation.

If I were to continue these investigations today, following Mintz (1996) I would probably adopt the conceptual and rhetorical outsider–insider scheme.[6] Outsider dimensions include political-economic, environmental, commercial and biological forces beyond the control of any individual, household or cultural community.

Insider dimensions consider local cultural understandings and internal dynamics of culture change. In this case, insider dimensions include factors that affect the decisions that people make regarding dietary and health-promoting and health-restoring choices and structures. They also emphasize the ways particular items (foods, medicines, healing practices) are integrated into everyday life and cultural meanings, and people's inclination to embrace hot/cold knowledge leading to actions as a means of trying to attempt to understand and assert control over their health.

Notes

1. For a summary of these views, see Foster (1994).
2. The species *guayaba* refers to the tree and fruit of *Psidium guajava* and related species, known in English as 'guava'.
3. Among other cultures, however, such as the Guatemalan Maya, the mother may be classified as cold because she has lost a lot of blood (see, e.g., Cosminsky 1975, 1977). See also Galinier (2004).
4. Some doctors, knowing that people expect to be given a dietary regimen, happily provide one, such as the avoidance of fatty, piquant foods that are difficult for those who are ill and taking medication to digest.
5. Mescal (mezcal in Spanish) is a distilled spirit made from the juice of the roasted underground heart of the indigenous century-plant (*Agave sp*).
6. For use of this scheme, see Messer (1997).

References

Chevalier, J.M., and A. Sanchez Bain. 2003. *The Hot and the Cold: Ills of Humans and Maize in Native Mexico*. Toronto: University of Toronto Press.
Cosminsky, S. 1975. 'Changing Food and Medical Beliefs and Practices in a Guatemalan Community', *Ecology of Food and Nutrition* 4: 183–91.
——— 1977. 'Alimento and Fresco: Nutritional Concepts and their Implications for Health Care', *Human Organization* 36: 203–7.
Foster, G. 1994. *Hippocrates' Latin American Legacy: Humoral Medicine in the New World*. Langhorne, PA: Gordon and Breach.
Galinier, J. 2004. *The World Below: Body and Cosmos in Otomi Indian Ritual*, trans. P. Aronoff and H. Scott. Boulder, CO: University Press of Colorado.
Harwood, A. 1971. 'The Hot/cold Theory of Disease: Implications for Treatment of Puerto Rican Patients', *Journal of American Medical Association* 216: 1153–58.
Lopez Austin, A. 1975. *Textos de Medicina Nahuatl*. Mexico City: Universidad Nacional Autonoma de Mexico.

—— 1980. *Cuerpo Humano e Ideologia: Las Concepciones de los Antiguos Nahuas.* Mexico City: Universidad Nacional Autonoma de Mexico.

Low, C., and E. Hsu. 2008. 'Introduction', in E. Hsu and C. Low (eds), *Wind, Life, Health: Anthropological and Historical Perspectives.* Oxford: Blackwell, pp.1–17.

Messer, E. 1978. 'Present and Future Prospects of Herbal Medicine in a Mexican Community', in R.I. Ford et al. (eds), *The Nature and Status of Ethnobotany.* Ann Arbor: Museum of Anthropology, University of Michigan, pp.137–61.

—— 1981. 'Hot/cold Classification: Theoretical and Practical Implications of a Mexican Study', *Social Science and Medicine* 15(2): 133–45.

—— 1987. 'The Hot and Cold in Mesoamerican Indigenous and Hispanicized Thought', *Social Science and Medicine* 25(4): 339–46.

—— 1991. 'Systematic and Medicinal Reasoning in Mitla Folk Botany', *Journal of Ethnopharmacology* 33: 107–28.

—— 1996. Review of G. Foster (1994) *Hippocrates' Latin American Legacy: Humoral Medicine in the New World, Journal of the Royal Anthropological Institute* 2(4): 741–42.

—— 1997. 'Three Centuries of Changing European Tastes for the Potato', in H. Macbeth (ed.), *Food Preferences and Taste: Continuity and Change.* Oxford: Berghahn, pp.101–13.

Mintz, S. 1996. *Tasting Food, Tasting Freedom.* Boston: Beacon Press.

Ortiz de Montellano, B. 1980. 'Las Hierbas de Tlaloc', *Estudios Culturales Nahuatl* 14: 287–314.

—— 1990. *Aztec Medicine, Health, and Nutrition.* New Brunswick, NJ: Rutgers University Press.

A Balance of What?

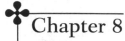

Chapter 8

Balancing Diversity and Well-being

Words, Concepts and Practice in Eastern Africa

David Parkin

Early Notions of Cosmological Balance

I argue in this chapter that many and perhaps most healing methods in sub-Saharan Africa are premised on an idea of relational balance. Some Muslim healers in Africa work from Arabic texts and some incorporate biomedical methods in their treatments. But many so-called indigenous healers in much of Africa work not from texts but from long-term experience and from knowledge and practices handed down to them by tutor healers, who are often family members. It is on these latter healers that I here focus.

Such healers will not therefore normally turn to texts for information on precise criteria of sickness and misfortune. They do sometimes explain illnesses in terms of broadly opposed elements such as the hot and cold, or dry and wet, properties of food, activities and patients' bodies. But they have to deal with sicknesses and misfortunes that do not lend themselves to explanation through set oppositions of this kind. The problems brought to them are not just those of the body or mind but are often of interpersonal conflict, loss of property and livestock and personal failures. When we translate

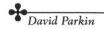

indigenous terms, we find that a broad notion of 'misfortune' usually covers this diversity of problems rather than the narrower 'sickness'.

This means that, in diagnosing and treating a problem, a healer has to judge whether it is caused by elemental imbalance of the hot/cold kind or by some other kind of imbalance, perhaps resulting from deviant social behaviour, of which witchcraft, sexual transgressions and broken prohibitions are the most common, or from what are regarded as physical disorders such as breech births or a club foot, which, Eurocentrically, might be called 'natural' imbalances.

It may well be that, in the absence of diagnostic texts, healers are given the scope to be more experimental in finding explanations and to reach novel conclusions. Healers have therefore to restore either elemental or social imbalance in order to remedy a problem. They are themselves having to balance their judgements of the causes of imbalance. The idea of balance here is as much a question of the healer juggling several factors as of finding an equilibrium between set pairs of elemental oppositions. Relational balance perhaps best describes this process. It presupposes flexibility of interpretation and so is well suited to taking into account the whole person of the patient being diagnosed, including their social circumstances.

The analytical notion of balance in African studies goes back a long way. An early anthropological volume explored comparatively the relationship between African cosmologies and forms of livelihood and subsistence (Forde 1954). In common with the theoretical thrust of functional holism at the time, chapters in that volume described the 'interdependence' of social, material and cosmological ideas and values, and that these were ideally to be kept in 'equilibrium' or balance with each other, lest misfortune arise. Other terms used to indicate the proper functioning of society and cosmology in balance were 'harmony', 'cooperation' and (mutual) 'adjustment' (Forde 1954: x–xvi). Balance ensured social continuity and the health and fertility of a society's people, land and livestock, while imbalance created misfortune, ranging from infertility to natural, social and personal disasters. Medicines and rituals were seen to be harnessed in the interests of securing the harmonious interdependence and balance of the cosmos and social behaviour.

The volume's editor, Darryl Forde, was however careful not to depict the African societies described in the book as static, even if a kind of dynamic homeostasis was implicit, with disruption 'naturally' reverting in due course to normality. He referred to the considerable social changes undergone by African societies, though this was a less-treated theme by his contributors, some of whom were to become senior figures in the subject. Forde also emphasized the basic similarity of view between African and European societies in the interdependence of cosmology and society: uncertain social conditions evoke fears of ruptured relationships between humans and the non-human spirit world.

Not acceptable today, however, was his view that, while similar in essence to those of Europe, African cosmological and social beliefs lack the analytical range and depth of European (*sic*) theories of causation and repair. Thus, 'Where they [African societies] have differed from the Europeans who have recently come among them has been in the depth and range of their collective knowledge of natural process and in the degree of control and security that they could thereby command' (Forde 1954: xi).

Nowadays, we would agree with Scott Atran, among others, who points out that many hunting, foraging and, in some cases, horticultural peoples of the kind found in Africa, Amazonia and elsewhere have more advanced understandings of botanical and zoological phenomena through complex systems of taxonomic classifications than many so-called First World peoples who, apart from their scientific specialists, are closed off to such knowledge through dependence on modern, urban technologies (Atran, Medin and Roos 2004).

The point of initially discussing Forde's compilation, written before the British, French and Portuguese empires in Africa had been removed and with contributions based on fieldwork carried out during the imperial period, is to show how a notion of balance or equilibrium was not only a theoretical starting point in anthropological analyses of the time, but was also believed to characterize the driving force in African society. It was given more prominence than other determinants such as the incursions of colonial depredation, the wage economy, migrant labour, land dispossession and redistribution, the imposition of over-defined ethnic boundaries, and the substitution of new forms of education for indigenous crafts and skills. At first, we might be inclined, therefore, to dismiss such interpretations as too moulded by colonial bias to warrant the idea of homeostatic balance as being at the root of such artificially demarcated 'tribal' societies and indigenous kingdoms as described in the collection.

However, later studies did modify such ideas by incorporating modern socio-economic influences, such as rural–urban migration. Victor Turner's classic studies of the Ndembu of Central Africa took account of their dependence on remittances from urban wage labour. He showed that, although a predominantly rural agricultural society tied to a cash economy, much of their cosmology derived from an earlier hunting-and-gathering ethos, in which ideas of and practices securing moderation were seen as the antidote to acts of excess or depredation, a kind of drive for social and ecological balance. His monograph, *The Drums of Affliction* (Turner 1968), was one of a number in which he provided instances of a dynamic drive for equilibrium, a theme encouraged by his mentor, Max Gluckman, and some other members of the so-called Manchester/Rhodes-Livingstone school of anthropology (Gluckman 1958). Later, John Janzen was to produce a significant book – called simply *Ngoma* (Janzen 1992), variously translatable as drum, dance, song, medicine and ritual – which built on Turner's interest in fundamental cosmological and social concepts, and focused on explaining core African ideas and practices of illness diagnosis and therapy in four areas. It went further in showing the semantic clusters associated with such ideas, or what Ardener called 'language shadows' which hint at but are not necessarily exactly isomorphic with them (Ardener 2007: 91). An earlier example is how cultural templates among the Luo of Kenya, shared with contiguous peoples, are partially expressed in key verbal concepts and phrases (Parkin 1978), cases to which I shall return.

So, contrasting with Forde and his contributors' undeniably sequestered view of African societies as discrete and self-contained, socially and cosmologically, there developed a view of them not as discrete but as constituting a large, overarching tradition of indigenous theories, philosophies, semantic clusters, beliefs and practices which have persisted across great areas of the African continent, often in partially overlapping ways. Extensive work on Africa by Luc de Heusch (1982, 1985) shows the range of key ideas and institutions that run up and down tracts of the continent, especially south of the Sahara, though not exclusively so. De Heusch is the counterpoint to Forde in the delineation of fundamental African concepts. While Forde proceeded from a view of societies in Africa that could be studied as relatively individually bounded and distinctive and whose differences and similarities could be displayed through comparison, de Heusch focused on the conceptual and institutional continuities and twists threading through the continent and its abundantly porous and fuzzy ethnic borders. Following de Heusch, I take the view 'that African philosophies and practices make up a long, tangled skein that stretch from any point in Africa to another' (Parkin 1990: 185), so precluding the sharp delineation of distinctive regions and societies and allowing us to speak of Africa as having its own pan-culture of orally transmitted concepts and institutions.

Moderation of Excess

Now, at first there appears to be little concern here with a concept of balance, which indeed seems irrelevant and even opposed to the characterization of Africa-wide institutions and beliefs as making up a tangled skein. This is not to deny the regional concentrations of language and custom that we roughly identify, in eastern Africa for instance, as Bantu, Nilotic, Cushitic and Sudanic. It is to argue that such concentrations are cross-cut by common strands.

However, I believe that this tangled skein comprises overarching, institutionally based ideas of relational balance that link different regions of African in sets of common understanding, and that such ideas of balance permeate notions broadly akin to those of humoral medicine. Devisch actually refers to certain symptoms addressed by the *mbwoolu* affliction cult among the Bantu-speaking Yaka of Congo as, among other things, 'lack of humoral balance' (Devisch 2007: 119–20), the humours in question being those of wet and dry. Among Bantu-speaking peoples and others it is remarkable how similar such notions are over large areas, connecting communities whose dispersal throughout Africa has resulted in diverse socio-political systems and variable linguistic distance. Here we may return to Janzen, who proposes six 'dominant ideas in African medical traditions' drawn from 'late twentieth century research and writing' (Janzen 2008: 524–26). They are often partly or wholly expressed through verbal concepts and cover diagnostic symptoms, purity, flow and blockage, contagion, causal dualism (illness caused by happenstance and perhaps attributed to a 'god' or those caused by a specific human, ancestor or spirit), and, importantly, the fact that, overall, balance and harmony determine health.

In fact, it could be argued that all the concepts relate in some way to the proposition that the body, cosmos and society need to be in harmony for the well-being of its occupants. Janzen (2008: 525) cites, for example, Davis's ethnography among the Tabwa of Congo (Davis 2000) on 'verbal concepts of order and disorder articulated as inside and outside, individual and society, and heat (the fire of passion, anger, and affliction) and coolness (of health, grace and harmony)', noting that these opposites need to be in balance to secure health lest, out of balance, they bring about disease (see also Janzen 1992: 64). Janzen acknowledges that in some areas influenced by Islam and humoral theory, a similar hot/cold equilibrium is necessary for health but does not suggest an Islamic or Greek provenance for all cases of hot/cold interplay. Indeed, my own impression (Parkin 1991: 145 et passim; cf. Krige and Krige 1954: 76) is that the African concern with balancing hot and cold in the treatment of ill health is pre-Islamic, as is that of wet and dry discussed by Devisch for the Yaka, being found almost everywhere and apparently long-standing, and, one may surmise, humanly intuitive though expressed in culturally diverse ways.

Janzen (2008: 525) talks also of the opposition between ritual human purity and the pollution that leads to sickness when human affairs become disordered, and of that between flow and blockage, as among the Rwanda (Taylor 1992), where normal bodily flows and social exchanges mutually constitute healthy individuals and society, and their blockage creates social malaise and sickness. 'Blocking the way', as it was once put to me by Luo, has the destructive quality of acts causing the pollution that creates disease. I was reminded of how an apparently metaphysical concept like this can have empirical support when, many years later in Zanzibar town, I noted how the profligate use of plastic bags blocked drains, created pools of stagnant rain water where mosquitoes could deposit their larvae, and so caused a marked increase both in malaria and, through effluent entering piped drinking water, cholera. A Swahili term (*mazingira*) was coined to capture the global sense of an 'environment' vulnerable to pollution in this way, alongside which the diseases were sometimes also blamed on religious (Islamic) impiety ('the wrath of God') as well as on bad environmental care (Parkin 2007: 201–3). Like polluting actions or substances, the effects of disease and even misfortune can spread. The notion of 'contagion' is indeed, as Janzen (2008: 525) suggests (following Green 1994, 2000; see also Arnold 1985; Parkin 1991), likely to be an ancient idea which long precedes modern microbiology. Among the Giriama of Kenya contagion takes various forms, of which a primordial one appears to be that which I have translated as 'deathliness' and which results from the death of a person. It has harmful consequences for others, not just through the contagion of a disease like tuberculosis from which the person may have died, but from the very fact of death itself, which may in some cases be regarded as a 'bad death' against which ritual purification is needed, such as removing the body from the community (Parkin 1991). Deathliness here shares something of the concept of pollution, as does the idea of contagion itself – that is, contagion from a polluting source. A 'bad death' is one which is premature, untimely, the result of an accident or caused by violence and, being a source of harmful contagion, requires that the body is buried outside the homestead. Similarly, a child born by breach birth, with a club foot, or with teeth which are already evident or which grow first at the bottom rather than the top, or a child allegedly already 'talking' or born physically marked or 'monstrous', is supposed to be destroyed by suffocation and left outside the homestead, again to prevent the ill effects affecting other members of the home. In some societies twins are also regarded as inauspicious, though in others the opposite is the case. What characterizes the sources of adverse contagion is the fact that they are not normally seen to be the direct result of human agency but as intrinsic evil, although *post hoc* reasoning may sometimes thereafter attribute blame to violated prohibitions or to malevolent or negligent humans ('witches'). Essentially, however, gross human abnormalities are juxtaposed to normal birth and death.

Contagion leading to pollution in Euro-American thought can be glossed as 'dirt' being harmfully contagious and needing to be removed, with dirt and cleanliness as natural opposites. But Douglas's definition of dirt as matter out of place (Douglas 1970) locates dirt as also to do with disorder and improper sequencing, an expanded definition which seems suited to semantic usage in eastern Africa.

Dirt is thus that which is wrongly sequenced or tangled and which needs to be straightened out. Dirt also blocks up things, and so again has to be removed in the act of cleansing. Cleansing and cooling often go together semantically in Bantu languages: the cool water restoring a state of normality, not only through the removal of 'dirt', however, but through the suppression of the agitation of heat. At a further remove, then, terms for 'cooling' sometimes shade into meaning 'cure', and there is certainly a pre-Islamic understanding among Giriama of certain diseases or afflictions being 'hot' and needing to be cooled (see also Janzen 1992). In this way, there is sometimes semantic overlap and similarity in the terms for cooling, curing, cleansing, and also clearing and whiteness, as among the Giriama, for instance.

It is true that these African ideas of disease and misfortune causation cannot all be fitted into neat dichotomies of the hot/cold and wet/dry kind, and so in this sense are part of the overall skein to which de Heusch refers rather than that of schematic humoral theory. On the other hand, there is clearly a strong theme that a relational or proportionate balance needs to be maintained between behavioural and existential extremes, lest misfortune, disease, death and infertility follow and even infect or pollute chains of 'innocent' other persons. It is often also the case that the cause and symptom of imbalance are regarded as the same phenomenon; thus, incest and the infertility it may cause can be referred to by the same term.

In some African societies, what may be translated as 'evil' is either one of two extreme notions: physical excess (great heat, fever, greed, incest, rape, child monsters, twinship, flooding); and physical imperfection or impoverishment (great cold, wasting disease, blocked flows, failed crops, dying livestock). Keeping matters between these two extremes is 'goodness'. Evil and goodness are thus both causative act and effect.

As I have analysed elsewhere (Parkin 1985), evil and goodness are often also each characterized respectively as 'ugly' or 'physically deformed', and 'beautiful'. The aesthetic is thus coterminous with the moral. Balancing matters so that they remain good is the same as ensuring that matters remain moderate, properly formed and physically and visually acceptable.

Among Giriama, as elsewhere, herbalists speak to leaves, roots or bark before plucking or taking them for medicinal usage. They promise the plant that it will only be used for the benefit of humankind and not for evil purposes. The allusion is to the recognition that herbs can be a force for evil as well as good: a moderate dose may suppress the malaria or diarrhoea symptoms, while an excess may exacerbate the condition and even poison the patient (Parkin 1991: 173–81). Violations of the potential for human benefit thus lead to evil which must be removed.

Removal of such ill-effects takes various, related measures: unblocking, disentanglement, cleansing or purification, and cooling. There is notable semantic similarity among Bantu speakers with regard to the terms denoting such features, which partially overlap with those proposed by Janzen and which evidently persist over time.

It is true that Islam has provided some African societies with humoral theories of causation and remedy derived from Arab (and thus Greek Galenic) connections, as among the Swahili of East Africa (Parkin 2000). It is important to recognize this actual or potential influence, which makes it all the more remarkable that, at a fundamental level, pre-Islamic concepts prevail. They may sometimes be embedded and expressed through Islamic (and Christian) theology, but they are more often than not separated out from this embeddedness by healers and patients as explanations of and remedies for misfortune and illness: such as the malevolence of spirits, other non-human agencies and of humans themselves, or as the result of transgressed behavioural and procedural prohibitions.

In other words, these causative and remedial ideas and practices generally remain distinct from classically derived humoral theories. But what do we mean by humoral balance and why have pre-Islamic ideas persisted? I would argue that what the Islamic humoral and pre-Islamic concepts have in common is a fundamental and perhaps universally human concern with concepts and practices of balance and restoration. They are kept separate because Islamic and Galenic ideas have been formalized and standardized through textualization with only minor local variations, while the non-Islamic concepts have been kept flexibly vibrant through overlapping usage among the many peoples linked through the essentially oral pan-culture of much of Africa, a part of which is evident in language usage.

A Flexible Eco-cosmology

Given that variations occur, how precisely framed by texts is humoral theory? A conventional scholarly view is that the theory presupposes relational balance among constituent elements, with imbalance causing, or manifested as, an absence of well-being. A notion of proportionate relationality is thus central, with the number of elements varying cross-culturally and, sometimes, situationally among a single people. Textualization may have fixed the elements and constituted them as a coherent system more than was the case before literacy: Were yellow and black bile, and blood and phlegm really so set as might be suggested by reliance on Galenic writings and South Asian Ayurvedic understandings of *dosa*? Were there not before textualization competing and/or overlapping theories of proportionate relations as being constitutive of health and well-being? This is asked because pre-textual African ideas of negative conditions requiring balance and restoration are indeed of a variety of types that do not constitute a set or fixed system.

So, when we read ethnographies of African metaphysics and healing processes, we are presented with a myriad of alternative ways of relating bodily effect and precipitating cause. With the notable exception, then, of those societies in Africa embracing or significantly influenced by Islam, no one system of proportionate relations dominates.

This is why I argue that, while some scholars might interpret much of Africa as therefore lacking the textually based so-called Great Traditions typical of much of Asia and Europe, it is in fact cross-cut by a web of overlapping concepts and practices which can be discerned as spreading in a variety of different directions across the continent. Africa's Great Tradition is in fact its diverse yet interlinked and widespread means of explaining sickness and misfortune, even if, as Janzen points out, medical practitioners are not normally aware of the overarching pan-African nature of many of the medical concepts with which they deal.

This is not to say that attempts have not been made by scholars wishing to apply a set system to particular African societies. Forde's pioneering volume, *African Worlds*, with which I began this chapter, provided numerous case studies on the mutual influence of cosmological and natural balance by, among others, Mary Douglas, Godfrey Lienhardt, Kenneth Little, J.D. and E.J. Krige, and Marcel Griaule and Germaine Dieterlen. The argument was that use of natural resources, livelihoods and the conduct of social relations both shaped and were shaped by beliefs in a god, spirit and humanly transcendental forces, with Mary Douglas (1954) arguing for the Lele of the Congo that it was their cosmic world-view which partly

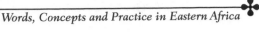

determined the people's choice of where and what to hunt. Balanced nature and cosmos made for successful living, while imbalance had to be repaired.

Although one would certainly question nowadays the extent to which cosmological ideas may be said quite so sharply to determine peoples' subsistence modes, rather than as being in a constantly changing two-way relationship, it is noteworthy how characteristic even nowadays the Durkheimian view is of Africa as embracing views of a cosmology whose order is premised on a corresponding social and material order.

Some years ago the expression 'eco-cosmology' was coined to describe this indigenous perception of the intertwining of material and spiritual ideas and practices, in a book about social and economic development (Croll and Parkin 1992: 22–27). The term eco-cosmology clearly presupposes a duality of cosmos on the one hand and material practice on the other, which is then compressed to show their interpenetration, and then almost dissolved in favour of the idea that to speak of nature is *ipso facto* to speak of the cosmological or spiritual, such that, for example, to venerate the land is also to conserve it and its forest. The dualism is, then, a useful heuristic fiction.

In fact crises occur when behavioural or procedural rules are violated, so plunging a community into deprivation and chaos and invoking the medico-ritual 'drums of affliction'. Insofar as there is a need for balance, it is in maintaining proper relations and restoring to normality those which go wrong.

The duality of cosmos and materiality has been a useful gloss in distinguishing African from Euro-American ideas of causality. Until recently a prevailing Euro-American view has been of the natural environment as inevitably and uncritically subject to human agency, in contrast to the alleged African view of the two as mutually involved and equally active on each other. This has changed in recent decades and ironically the two views, African and Euro-American, are closer together, as the prosperous part of the world, Euro-America, announces itself nowadays as eco-friendly in recognizing that a balanced ecology is intrinsic to human well-being.

However, we have to recognize that in Africa a sharp and overarching dualism of nature and cosmos never really existed and that this was the European way in which the cross-cutting interpenetration of diverse forces could be conceptually managed and written about. It may indeed have been a useful gloss, still much used in some circles, in counteracting the popularly held view in Euro-America of humankind dominating or in conflict with nature.

In fact this dualism of nature and cosmos was imposed on a variety of different and overlapping responses to crisis as experienced in Africa. The reality is that villagers suffering, say, the loss of their cattle to disease, or experiencing the death of young people, or confronting the wider threat posed by contagious sickness, do not normally phrase the problem in Manichean- or even Cartesian-like terms as one of grand cosmological and socio-material forces being in confrontational imbalance with each other. Rather, the misfortune comes from particular prohibition breaches, of matters having become out of sequence or order, of having become entangled, or of blockages of normal flows of blood, milk and life. It is true that, sometimes, as in the case of AIDS at present, the disaster may become viewed among Christians and Muslims dualistically as deriving from the wrath of a wronged high God bearing down on humanity, but even here, away from the pulpit, particular cases may be explained through more indigenously focused idioms – idioms which follow each other in the manner of trial and error. For instance, most or all Africanists know cases of a misfortune or disease being explained first through, say, spirit possession; next, perhaps, through breach of a sexual prohibition or non-sexual seniority rule; and then through witchcraft, with a so-called practical explanation possibly also fitted in, and not always in this order. This explanatory paradigm thus includes a variety of possible sources of affliction which serve as variable stages in diagnosis.

How does this explanatory paradigm lend itself to the kind of understanding as conveyed by humoral theories? In other words, what room is there in the plethora for explanation based on elemental balance and imbalance?

We can answer this not by requesting and then listing healers' reported understandings of health-through-balance but by observing the different ways in which they identify violation and imbalance in particular patients and how they bring about restoration. In other words, I argue that it is methodologically more fruitful to proceed from a consideration of individual cases of imbalance and its restoration to balance or normality rather than by asking healers how balance achieves health, as if asking a set text. After all, it is normally only the negatively marked issues of daily life, the imbalances and harmful consequences, that engage public attention, not the taken-for-granted flow of normality. For instance, cases of so-called 'evil', as with sickness, call forth action and comment, while everyday health evokes no comment or action. With imbalance and restoration-to-balance as my analytical starting point, let me return to my initial definition of humoral balance as to do with the maintenance and restoration of proportionate relationality. What I want to show ethnographically is that, while in non-Islamic Africa there is no single procedural system of set elements reinforced by textual instruction as in 'classical' humoral theories, the many restorative beliefs, techniques and precipitating actions in Africa do show similarity with ideas of balance and imbalance, including reversible ideas of bodily heat as sickness and coolness as cure, even if the precise equivalent of the three or four humours is absent outside Islam.

Semantic Overlap

So, what are the conditions ethnographically reported as giving rise to misfortune and disease, and what do people need to do in order to restore normality and well-being, that is, to remedy the imbalance?

I earlier identified the following as remedies for reversing the conditions causing sickness and misfortune: disentanglement, unblocking, cooling and cleansing. They partially overlap and are a semantic cluster. As I suggest below, a notion of entanglement or crossing boundaries seems to be fundamental in precipitating the imbalances requiring reversal.[1] It lends itself to cognitive spread and borrowing among both Bantu and non-Bantu neighbouring peoples, perhaps indicating a universal human proclivity to think of crossed lines, paths or boundaries as either inauspicious or a source of supra-human power. It is instructive to consider this semantic spread in order better to understand how the idea of entanglement or crossing boundaries appears to be easily taken up by peoples and becomes the basis of negative conditions requiring reversal or restoration to balance. I take the particular case of a widespread archetypal concept variously identified as *chira* or *kirwa* and many other renderings in different languages.

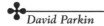

Chira and Related Concepts

Among the Nilotic-speaking Luo of western Kenya, the Bantu-derived concept of *chira* is a delict ranging from incest, incestuous adultery, to breach of seniority rules and even disrespect, and related to the idea of 'mixing bloods' in an improper manner or relationship (see Parkin 1978: 148–55), as distinct from the permissible blood mixing that occurs in, say, approved marriage.[2] *Chira* causes fatal bodily wasting, infertility and the death of a descent line, or the loss and sickness of children and livestock. Among Luo, something of a contrast to *chira* occurs in the form of *riwo*, which Geissler and Prince (2010: 12) gloss as 'mixing-through-sharing', including bodily and interactional merging, and as therefore conducive to socially approved marriage and reproduction when applied to bodily intercourse. *Riwo* is thus distinct from *chira* which is related to the idea of 'improper mixing of bloods' (Parkin 1978: 148–55). *Chira* derives from a sense of crossing or stepping over, as does *riwo*; but while *riwo* carries a benevolent connotation of merging through crossing, *chira* has that of transgressing, of crossing over too far. The idea of crossing over or transgression thus plays on a distinction between socially acceptable human engagement in which bodily boundaries may be transcended or merged, as in legitimate sexuality; and its opposite, when these boundaries or 'fences' (see also Geissler and Prince 2010: 205) are illicitly disregarded.

An interesting question is whether and how much the ideas behind the concept of *chira* have changed since the time I observed the use of the term (during the period 1962 to 1969) and the present (as observed in accounts made during and since the 1990s by Dilger and Geissler and Prince in particular). The question is raised because the earlier descriptions by Luo of the illness symptoms and effects of *chira* are uncannily similar to those of AIDS today, especially with reference to it as a 'wasting disease sometimes culminating in death' (Parkin 1978: 149), with only 'temporary remissions' rendering people 'weak and unable to talk and walk properly' (Parkin 1978: 155), and with 'haemorrhages and emaciation' ending in death and also resulting in a woman's barrenness (Parkin 1978: 157–58).

Of course such descriptions of 'wasting' and so forth might apply to individual cases of some kind of (genetically inherited) auto-immune systemic failure and not AIDS. However, not surprisingly, once AIDS became identified biomedically as a pandemic in the 1980s, many Luo rapidly came to refer to the affliction as *chira*. Are there then some differences in the referential uses of the term over the period? In the 1960s in Nairobi, Kenya, breaches of seniority rules figured as much as cases of illicit sexuality as causes of *chira*, though it is true that even some of the broken seniority rules involved sexuality, or at least, for example, brothers marrying in the wrong customary order or fathers sleeping in a son's house.[3] An impression drawn from speaking to Luo nowadays is that *chira* now refers more to excessive adulterous or promiscuous sexuality than broken rules of seniority. Geissler and Prince also talk of a shift of 'emphasis towards individual responsibility and sex' from that of concerns for lineage or group growth (Geissler and Prince 2007: 98). But broken seniority rules, often implying sexual violations, clearly do remain significant, for Dilger also gives an interesting case of *chira* arising from a dwelling being built in the wrong order with a father and his sons' houses in customarily reversed positions (Dilger 2008: 221–22).

In the 1960s, men bore most of the moral responsibility for afflicting a family or couple with *chira*, for it was men who were seen to be in charge of the proper conduct of rule-governed behaviour in Nairobi. In Dilger's and Geissler and Prince's data, it is women who seem to take on more of the moral blame and stigma for having incurred *chira* through their alleged adultery or promiscuous sexuality.

Another change arising from men's customary obligations is the increased ambivalence of views concerning customary 'ritual widow cleansing' (see Dilger 2006: 114–15). In the 1960s a fecund widow's inheritor, who would be a real or classificatory brother of her husband, had to have sexual relations with her in order to remove the contagion of death from her and her lineage: sex-as-life would remove the inauspicious effects of his death. The chosen heir might not want to take on the associated responsibilities and might ask another to fulfil the role instead. It was nevertheless regarded as imperative that some eligible agnate perform the ritual, for failure to do so would endanger the widow herself and her husband's patriline with infertility resulting from *chira*. By the 1990s, however, Luo were divided on the place of the ritual in modern life. Some continued to argue in customary mode that *chira* would result from not carrying it out. Others held that, given the possibilities that the husband had died from AIDS and that his widow might also be infected, she would transmit the disease to whoever was ritually obliged to perform sex with her and thence to his wives.

These comparative impressions must be treated with caution in view of the different locales of Luo communities for which the accounts were given: Nairobi in the 1960s (Parkin); Nyanza province in the 1980s and 1990s (Prince and Geissler); and Maro in Tanzania in the 1990s (Dilger). But, given the close intercommunication among Luo throughout East Africa, they may be pointers. What is noteworthy is the persistence of the underlying denotation and connotations of the term *chira*. Change may have occurred, though we cannot yet be sure how much, but enough of the semantic template continues to capture the changing conditions of sexual, family and lineage relationships. *Chira*-like or other terms used in other eastern and central African societies seem to show a similar persistence of underlying meaning.

Citing earlier observations (see Parkin 1978: 327–30), I note that there are other apparent Nilotic borrowings of versions of the Bantu concept. Crazzolara gives the Nilotic Acholi noun *kiir* as meaning, 'infringement of intimate social customs, mainly family, which require atonement in order to prevent ill luck of some kind', and *kiir*, the verb (also *kiire*), as 'to jump over' (Crazzolara 1938: 256), surely related to the Bantu *-kira*, to cross over. Ray Abrahams reported that among the Nilotic Labwor, who are an even more northerly Lwo-speaking group in Uganda, the noun *kir* refers to the disease afflicting people who have quarrelled with a spouse or close relative (and sometimes also afflicting a child related to them) after one of them has uttered an oath or curse against the occurrence of an event which nevertheless occurs, such as a mother refusing to countenance her daughter's marriage to a particular man and being attacked by *kir* on subsequently changing her mind even though she had previously cursed the prospect of the marriage during the quarrel.[4]

Abraham's informant further associated the term *kir* with the verb *kiro* 'to sprinkle', since one form of curative treatment involves being sprinkled with medicine. We may speculate that the phonetic similarity of the two terms, one of Bantu origin and the other Nilotic, and their use within a common medico-ritual domain, has associated them semantically. Among the Kenya Luo, too, the verb *kiro* can be used to describe the sprinkling of medicine (*manyasi*, another term shared with Bantu Swahili), which is required to cleanse and so reverse the effects of *chira*.

At this point we may simply note that the Acholi and Labwor (Lwo) term *kiir* (or *kir*) are to do with the breach, and the consequence of such breach, of close marriage, family and kin relationships. As I have indicated, this equates roughly with the broad range of meanings traditionally underlying the Kenya Luo term *chira* before its expanded sense in the age of AIDS.

When we turn to the meaning given by Crazzolara of the Acholi verb *kiir*, 'to jump over', we seem to find another phonetic and semantic convergence with the Bantu root term *-kira*, meaning 'to pass over' or 'cross over' and widely used to refer to breaches of customary behaviour. Thus, on the one hand the Acholi *kiir* (and Lwo generally) is surely morphologically and even semantically related to the even more northerly (Sudanese) Nuer noun *kier* (verb *kir*), meaning the removal of people from a dangerously impure state through sacrifice (Evans-Pritchard 1956: 227). On the other hand, the precise meaning in the Acholi *kiir* of 'to jump over' surely also derives from the Bantu root *-kira*, 'to pass over', possibly via Interlacustrine Bantu speakers in southern Uganda, who have influenced other key ritual and religious concepts among the Acholi and other Nilotes of northern Uganda (Southall 1971). Indeed, since the distant Nuer concept of *kier* 'has no meaning outside its sacrificial usage' (Evans-Pritchard 1956: 227–28), perhaps even it, like the Acholi *kir*, derives ultimately from the Bantu root *-kira*, though of course only reaching the Nuer at several removes through a succession of non-Bantu peoples.

My suggestion that the meaning of 'passing over' contained in the Acholi term *kiir* and similar Nilotic terms is largely borrowed from Bantu is supported by the fact that these Nilotes already have their own terms for expressing the idea of 'passing over': *kalo*, 'to jump or step over', *kato*, 'to pass over' (Labwor/Acholi), *kalo*, 'to cross' (as in a river or road), and *kadho*, 'to pass by or over' (Kenya Luo). These non-Bantu terms can also, like the Nilotic *kiir*, carry symbolic and ritual connotations. Thus, Labwor oath taking may involve stepping over objects, such as one's spear or clothing, for which the term *kalo* can be used. More strikingly, the Kenya Luo have a clearly developed *post partum* practice called *kadho imbo nyathi*, 'to pass over the child's umbilical cord' (Parkin 1973: 332–33), which refers to the act of sexual intercourse (nominally?) performed by husband and wife four days after the birth of a boy at his 'coming out' of seclusion. Other Nilotic peoples have the same custom, as do many non-Nilotes, though some reverse the respective number of days' seclusion for a boy and girl.

It seems then that among these Nilotes, the verbal concepts of (a) *kato* (*kadho*)/*kalo* and (b) *kir*/*kiir* are used alongside each other in semantically related symbolic and ritual domains. It may be that the different Nilotic cultures range these terms in relation to each other in contrasting combinations. Among the Kenya Luo, *kadho* in the example given in the preceding paragraph seems to denote a process of 'passing over' which moves someone from a dangerous to secure state. By contrast, the Luo *chira*, which is the closest approximation to *kir*/*kiir* among Labwor and Acholi, denotes a process in which a person has crossed over 'too far' – that is, has exceeded the proper bounds of and so has confused or tangled relationships. It is in this respect that the Luo concept of *chira* shares with neighbouring Bantu-speakers a similar sounding set of terms derived from the root term -*kira*, and semantically focused on problems arising from what we crudely translate as incest and adultery, or improper sexuality, nowadays stigmatized as the alleged 'promiscuity' producing the wasting diseases of AIDS.

The Kenya Luo term *chira* appears, then, to be of Bantu origin whose form is -*kira* or a variant. It was adopted by the Nilotic Luo, who have a number of Bantu-speaking neighbours in their home regions of Kenya and Tanzania. Other Nilotes in Uganda and Tanzania appear also to have borrowed a variant of this concept, possibly from Bantu speakers in southern Uganda, while at the same time having their own Nilotic terms for comparable concepts.[5]

The Bantu verb stem, -*kira*, appears to be an eastern and central African regional variant of the Guthrie starred proto-Bantu root, -*kid* (confirmed by Derek Nurse in a personal communication 1978), with the meaning of passing over extending to the idea of transgression, for which the passive, -*kirwa*, is also found in different variations but with the same sense among eastern Bantu. Janzen (1992: 63–65) identifies -*gido* (Guthrie 1967–1971) as the root term for ideas of interdiction or abstinence, and one wonders at the possible extension or link to a notion of transgression through the act of crossing or passing over – that is, excessively and hence transgressing.

Throughout Bantu society in east, central and southern Africa, there are cognate terms of the *kira/kirwa/chira* type denoting variations on the theme of transgression and its penalties. Neighbours of the Luo, known by the collective name of Luhya, have the term, *ishira*, which comes conceptually close to that of *chira* (Parkin 1978: 150; Whyte and Whyte 1981). Among the Ganda, on the other side of Lake Nyanza (Victoria) from the Luo, the term *amakiro* (*-kiro* again deriving from Bantu *kira*) refers to 'a disease caused by a pregnant woman committing adultery with many men' (Kisekka 1973: 156). The disease appears to take the form of nausea and general debility in a mother or child, and even their deaths. Formerly, adultery by either parent while the mother was pregnant or nursing might bring about *amakiro*. *Chirwa* and *kirwa* have a similar reference among the Swahili and Giriama of the Kenya coastal area, with, among the latter, two unrelated terms denoting similar ideas, *mavingane* and *vithio* (Parkin and Parkin 1973: 278–79). Among the Nkole of Uganda, *amakire* is a fatal respiratory disease among children which also results from adultery by either parent during a mother's lactation period (Mushanga 1973: 178). Among the Sukuma of Tanzania, 'an adulterous woman suffers from *lwikilo* (a child who wants to emerge from the mouth)' (Varkevisser 1973: 240) (*sic* but translation unclear); and Bösch, writing on the Nyamwezi, mentions the blindness or even death afflicting a child whose parents commit adultery, a sin referred to as *kumkira mwana* (to pass over the child) and, apparently, connected with pregnancy prohibitions (Bösch 1930: 269–70, 48). Bösch refers to the curative herbal medicine as *makile*, but Abrahams, working much later in the area, found the term referred to the prohibitions rather than the cure.[6] Among Bantu speakers in southern Africa, Wreford (2008: 23) cites Green (1999: 68–71) and refers to the concept of *isiki* as a group of sexually related illnesses, associated again with infidelity, the violation of sexual mores, and with improper conjunctions of blood and bodily fluids. As elsewhere, including among Kenya Luo, the similarity in symptoms is made between this traditional illness category and HIV/AIDS.

As in the contrast between Giriama and Luo, there is regional variation, with perhaps the Luo concept of *chira* the most severely salient and highlighted of the traditional Nilotic-Bantu *chira-kirwa* range. The underlying connotation, however, is that of entanglement, as in crossing prohibited generational, seniority and/or sexual boundaries (a man marrying before an elder brother, entering a place in front of his father, having sex with his brother's wife, and so on), which bring about the affliction. Incest and incestuous adultery among Luo, and adultery during pregnancy among Giriama, invoking *chira* and *kirwa* respectively, are prime examples of tangled states. Entanglement and the related idea of a 'trap' (*mutego* in Giriama, who sometimes also borrow the Swahili term *matatizo*) also inform ideas of witchcraft effects and its cure, and is used as an idiom in divination (Parkin 1979). Disentanglement occurs when, again classically, the drums, or rituals, of affliction aim to expurgate the whole community of the effects of the delict, even when caused by a single individual. In addition to meaning curative ritual, dance and song, medicines and associated spirits, the term for drum (*ngoma*) has recently in Zanzibar ironically come to mean AIDS (Beckmann 2009), this being a not uncommon case of semantic reversal used to denote crises, such that the affliction is referred to as the cure. Devisch also speaks of the Yaka healer's 'disentangling of whatever may be binding and disabling the body of the patient' (Devisch 2007: 126). Straightening or reordering the community is also captured in the very root term for 'cure', *uganga*. The term or similar is commonly found among eastern, southern and central Bantu-speaking societies to mean the operational techniques and practice of therapy, for which the practitioner is known as *muganga* or allied forms. It seems to derive from, or at least be related to, a root verb meaning to straighten, *ku-ganga*, by using a stick, as in the treatment of a broken leg with a splint (see Johnson 1939: 111 on Swahili). Among Giriama *ki-gango* refers to the hardwood ancestral memorial post set upright in the ground for deceased members of a secret society who, like other ancestors, are venerated for the well-being they bring but who may bring harm should their memorials be uprooted and sold, or negligently dislodged from their upright position (Parkin 1982). Thus, straightening, setting up and disentangling are cure and laying across and tangling are disorder or sickness.

Unblocking as a medico-metaphysical concept also occurs and, as noted above, is well documented for the Rwanda by Taylor (1992). But it is found elsewhere among Bantu and Nilotic peoples to varying extents. Among Rwanda it especially affects the flow of maternal milk, so harming the suckling child, and may also refer to the flow of other bodily fluids. Unblocking requires standard ritual procedures as described by Taylor (1992). The Luo, along with many other peoples, also talk about the 'way ahead' (that is, one's life course and progress) being blocked and needing to be unblocked (Parkin 1978: 157). The blocked way ahead is also said to need straightening, so showing overlap with the earlier concept. Straightening or unblocking may also relate to the idea of unhindered and free-flowing social reciprocity, which is in turn a feature of egalitarian balance. In many Bantu languages the reciprocal verbal suffix (such as *-na*) converts a standard active verb into one of interactive reciprocity. Thus, the Swahili verb *ku-pendana*, 'to love each other', is built on *ku-penda*, 'to love (someone)'; similarly, in both Giriama and Swahili, *ku-fanana*, 'to resemble or be equivalent to each other', is from *ku-faa* or *ku-fana*, 'to be suited (to something or someone)'.[7] While it would be speculative to assume that this grammatical form significantly shapes social relations, it is worth noting the sense of egalitarian balance in the reciprocal form of the verb.

Conclusion

The partially overlapping African ideas and practices summarized in English, and semantically identified in a range of eastern African languages, as disentanglement, unblocking, cooling and cleansing, are clearly attempts to remove obstacles to well-being and restore normal health and vitality to people, animals and crops. There is in such practices a highly developed sense of proportionate relationality as being at the basis of collective as well as – and, indeed, incorporating – individual well-being. Avoidance of incest, adultery and disrespect to seniors are common examples of maintaining proportionate relationality. Another common example, often reported in the ethnographic literature and observed in the field, is of persons who are bewitched being themselves sometimes blamed for causing the envy of the witch. As Middleton (1960) showed long ago for the Lugbara, a person passing by a group of neighbours enjoying a meal will understandably feel resentment at not being invited to join them. Morally, he has been wronged. Morally, also, he ought to contain his resentment, but sometimes he cannot and has the malicious thoughts about his unkind neighbours that result in the psychic harm to them that ethnographers have called with only minor local variations 'witchcraft'. Removal of witchcraft comes about through divination and confession on his part, but also through recognition by the greedy neighbours that they, too, played a part in causing their own misfortune. Witchcraft and its reversal, as in this kind of example, suggests moral balancing. It has been presented to me as such in the field. Sadly, moral balancing and restoration are not nowadays always the result of witchcraft beliefs and alleged practices, and even in Middleton's early work were challenged by the moral asymmetry which he called sorcery as distinct from witchcraft, and which characterized the use of harmful medicines by alien specialists for gain. Seemingly permanent imbalances are very much a feature of modern Africa, as numerous studies of the role of witchcraft in politics, power and the post-colony have showed. This does not, however, stop people seeking to remove evil and regain well-being in the idioms of straightening, unblocking, cooling and cleansing. As must often be the case with humoral practices, the theories persist despite thwarted consequences.

I have perhaps strayed from a conventional idea of 'balance' as equalization through even weighting, as in a set of weighing scales. But the line is surely a thin one between balance in this literal sense of equilibrium and balance as a metaphor for steering between extremes or reversing in proportionate measure the effects of some breach. Whether literal or metaphorical, I would argue that balance is a humanly intuitive way of promoting moderation, avoiding excess and ensuring that lineal continuity which we call survival. Agonistic rituals may rail against such moderation as we all do from time to time in exultantly rejecting the boredom and strictures of rule-governed behaviour. But the status quo of an uncluttered, disentangled middle road or line customarily reasserts itself as the desired ideal, so justifying to some extent those early portrayals of society as homeostatic, not as an objective measure of how society really is but as a standard way in which peoples live in the hope that insecurity may one day give way to a bearable normality.

Bearing such qualifications in mind, I conclude therefore that there are three processes making up my understanding of the semantic complex of balance, imbalance and restored balance in the African cases I have described: first, the archetype of crossing-over, comprising entanglement, blocking and disordered sequencing – that is, transgression; second, a collective response to such transgression, even though it is demonstrably an individual's behaviour which is responsible, through acts of reversal; third, social morality as the collective maintenance of space between such extremes as proper versus improper blood mixing (that is, acceptable reproductive sex versus illicit forms and 'incest'), respecting seniority rules versus their violation, and contagion through human abnormalities (bad death, breach births, and so on) versus their removal.

Malevolent human agents, so-called witches, may be blamed during the procedure to discern the cause, course and treatment of a disease or misfortune. But primary in the understanding of the metaphysics of disease and calamity are these three processes: the concept of the witch is a means by which they can be expressed; the witch is thus a product of these processes. Such metaphysics are intrinsic to being-in-the-world, which is commonly experienced as disease and calamity. They are part of the constitution of the humans who inhabit and share that world.

Notes

1. It is worth mentioning that this idea of a 'crossed-over' state or process as being at the heart of theodicy and affliction is cognate at yet another remove with the Semitic religious practice of the Passover, celebrated at the same time of year as beliefs surrounding the Cross of Christ, the putative Jewish founder of Christianity.
2. See Heald (1999: 139) on the Bantu Gisu, and Whyte (1990: 102–3) for Bantu Marachi (also cited in Geissler and Prince 2010).
3. For a number of instances, see the cases in Parkin (1978: 153–58).
4. Ray Abrahams (personal communication, 1978).
5. For fuller discussion of the concept over time, see Parkin (1978), Hammer (1999), Dilger (2005, 2006) and Geissler and Prince (2010), where the concept of *chira* appears to have increasingly become a prominent synonym and explanation for the HIV/AIDS epidemic in both urban and rural areas.
6. Ray Abrahams (personal communication, 1978).
7. Compare the verb *ku-fanya*, 'to make or do'.

References

Ardener, E. 2007[1978]. 'Some Outstanding Problems in the Analysis of Events', in E. Ardener, *The Voice of Prophecy*, ed. M. Chapman. Oxford: Berghahn, pp.86–104.

Arnold, D. 1985. 'Medical Priorities and Practices in Nineteenth Century Bengal', *South Asian Research* 5(2): 167–86.

Atran, S., D. Medin and N. Roos. 2004. 'Evolution and Devolution of Knowledge: A Tale of Two Biologies', *Journal of the Royal Anthropological Institute* 10(2): 395–420.

Beckmann, N. 2009. 'Morality and Uncertainty: Living with HIV/AIDS in Zanzibar, Tanzania', D.Phil. dissertation. Oxford: University of Oxford.

Bösch, F. 1930. *Les Banyamwezi*. Münster: Aschendorff.

Crazzalora, J.P. 1938. *A Study of the Acholi Language*. London: Oxford University Press.

Croll, E., and D.J. Parkin. 1992. 'Anthropology, Environment and Development', in E. Croll and D.J. Parkin (eds), *Bush Base, Forest Farm: Culture, Environment and Development*. London: Routledge, pp.3–10.

Davis, C. 2000. *Death in Abeyance*.Edinburgh: Edinburgh University Press.

De Heusch, L. 1982[1972]. *The Drunken King, or the Origin of the State*. Bloomington: Indiana University Press.

——— 1985. *Sacrifice in Africa*. Manchester: Manchester University Press.

Devisch, R. 2007. 'Feeling and Borderlinking in Yaka Healing Arts', in R. Littlewood (ed.), *On Knowing and Not Knowing in the Anthropology of Medicine*. Walnut Creek, CA: Left Coast Press, pp.117–35.

Dilger, H. 2005. *Leben mit AIDS: Krankheit, Tod and Soziale Beziehungen in Afrika*. Frankfurt am Main: Campus.

——— 2006. 'The Power of AIDS: Kinship, Mobility and the Valuing of Social and Ritual Relationships in Tanzania', *African Journal of AIDS Research* 5(2): 109–21.

——— 2008. '"We Are All Going to Die": Kinship, Belonging and the Morality of HIV/AIDS Related Illnesses and Deaths in Rural Tanzania', *Anthropological Quarterly* 81(1): 207–32.

Douglas, M. 1954. 'The Lele of Kasai', in D. Forde (ed.), *African Worlds: Studies in the Cosmological Ideas and Social Values of African Peoples*. London: Oxford University Press, pp.1–26.

——— 1970. *Natural Symbols*. London: Barrie and Rockliff.

Evans-Pritchard, E.E. 1956. *Nuer Religion*. Oxford: Clarendon Press.

Forde, D. (ed). 1954. *African Worlds: Studies in the Cosmological Ideas and Social Values of African Peoples*. London: Oxford University Press.

Geissler, P.W., and R.J. Prince. 2007. 'Christianity, Tradition, AIDS, and Pornography: Knowing Sex in Western Kenya', in R. Littlewood (ed.), *On Knowing and Not Knowing in the Anthropology of Medicine*. Walnut Creek, CA: Left Coast Press, pp.87–116.

——— 2010. *The Land Is Dying: Contingency, Creativity and Conflict in Western Kenya*. Oxford: Berghahn.

Gluckman, M. 1958. 'Analysis of a Social Situation in Modern Zululand', Rhodes-Livingstone Institute Papers No. 28. Manchester: Manchester University Press.

Green, E. 1994. *AIDS and STDs in Africa: Bridging the Gap between Traditional Healing and Modern Medicine*. Boulder, CO: Westview Press.

———— 1999. 'Engaging Indigenous African Healers in the Prevention of AIDS and STDs', in R. Hahn (ed.), *Anthropology in Public Health: Bridging the Gaps in Culture and Society*. Oxford: Oxford University Press, pp.63–83.

———— 2000. *Rethinking AIDS Prevention: Learning From Successes in Developing Countries*. Westport, CT: Praeger.

Guthrie, M. 1967–1971. *Comparative Bantu: An Introduction to the Comparative Linguistics and Prehistory of the Bantu Languages*, 4 vols. Farnborough: Gregg.

Hammer, A. 1999 *Aids und Tabu: Zur soziokulturellen Konstruktion von Aids bei den Luo in Westkenia*. Münster: Lit Verlag.

Heald, S. 1999. *Manhood and Morality: Sex, Violence and Ritual in Gisu Society*. London: Routledge.

Janzen, J. 1992. *Ngoma: Discourses of Healing in Central and Southern Africa*. Berkeley: University of California Press.

———— 2008. 'Healing and Health Care', in J. Middleton and J.C. Miller (eds), *New Encyclopaedia of Africa*, Vol. 2. Detroit: Charles Scribner, pp.523–35.

Johnson, F. 1939 *A Standard Swahili-English Dictionary*. Nairobi: Oxford University Press.

Kisekka, M.N. 1973. 'The Ganda of Uganda', in A. Molnos (ed.), *Cultural Source Materials for Population Planning in East Africa*. Nairobi: East African Publishing House, pp.148–62.

Krige, J.D., and E.J. Krige. 1954. 'The Lovedu of the Transvaal', in D. Forde (ed.), *African Worlds: Studies in the Cosmological Ideas and Social Values of African Peoples*. London: Oxford University Press, pp.55–82.

Middleton, J. 1960. *Lugbara Religion*. London: Oxford University Press.

Mushanga, M.T. 1973. 'The Nkole of Western Uganda', in A. Molnos (ed.), *Cultural Source Materials for Population Planning in East Africa*. Nairobi: East African Publishing House, pp.174–86.

Parkin, D.J. 1973. 'The Luo of Kampala, Nairobi and Western Kenya', in A. Molnos (ed.), *Cultural Source Materials for Population Planning in East Africa*. Nairobi: East African Publishing House, pp.330–39.

———— 1978. *The Cultural Definition of Political Response: Lineal Destiny Among the Luo*. New York: Academic Press.

———— 1979. 'Straightening the Paths from Wilderness: The Case of Divinatory Speech', *Journal of the Anthropological Society of Oxford* 10: 147–60.

———— 1982. *Speaking of art: a Giriama impression*. Bloomington. African Studies Program. Indiana University.

———— 1985. 'Introduction', in D. Parkin (ed.), *The Anthropology of Evil*. Oxford: Blackwell, pp.1–25.

———— 1990. 'Eastern Africa: The View from the Office and the Voice from the Field', in R. Fardon (ed.), *Localizing Strategies: Regional Traditions of Ethnographic Writing*. Washington, DC: Smithsonian Institution Press, pp.182–203.

———— 1991. *Sacred Void: Spatial Images of Work and Ritual among the Giriama of Kenya*. Cambridge: Cambridge University Press.

———— 2000. 'Islam among the Humors: Destiny and Agency among the Swahili', in I. Karp and D.A. Masolo (eds), *African Philosophy as Cultural Enquiry*. Bloomington: Indiana University Press, pp.50–65.

———— 2007. 'In Touch without Touching: Islam and Healing', in R. Littlewood (ed.), *On Knowing and Not Knowing in the Anthropology of Medicine*. Walnut Creek, CA: Left Coast Press, pp.194–219.

Parkin, M.A., and D.J. Parkin. 1973. 'The Giriama of Coastal Kenya', in A. Molnos (ed.), *Cultural Source Materials for Population Planning in East Africa*. Nairobi: East African Publishing House, pp.274–88.

Southall, A.W. 1971. 'Cross-cultural Meanings and Multilingualism' in W. Whiteley (ed.), *Language Use and Social Change*. London: Oxford University Press, pp.376–93.

Taylor, C. 1992. *Milk, Honey and Money: Changing Concepts in Rwandan Healing*. Washington DC: Smithsonian Institution Press.

Turner, V.W. 1968. *The Drums of Affliction: A Study of Religious Processes among the Ndembu of Zambia*. Oxford: Clarendon Press.

Varkevisser, C. 1973. 'The Sukuma of Tanzania', in A. Molnos (ed.), *Cultural Source Materials for Population Planning in East Africa*. Nairobi: East African Publishing House, pp.234–48.

Wreford, J.T. 2008. *Working with Spirit: Experiencing* Izangoma *Healing in Contemporary South Africa*. Oxford: Berghahn.

Whyte, S.R. 1990. 'The Widow's Dream: Sex and Death in Western Kenya', in M. Jackson and I. Karp (eds), *Personhood and Agency: The Presentation of Self and Other in African Cultures*. Uppsala: Acta Universitatis Uppsaliensis, pp.95–114.

———— 1997. *Questioning Misfortune: The Pragmatics of Uncertainty in Eastern Uganda*. Cambridge: Cambridge University Press.

Whyte, S.R., and M.A. Whyte. 1981. 'Cursing and Pollution: Supernatural Styles in Two Luyia-speaking Groups', *Folk* 23: 65–80.

Chapter 9

'Holism' and the Medicalization of Emotion

The Case of Anger in Chinese Medicine

Elisabeth Hsu

If 'holistic' health care contrasts with 'medicalized', reductionist and therapy-oriented interventions, this chapter concerns a seeming paradox.[1] It claims that a social process of 'medicalization' made Chinese medicine 'holistic', namely the medicalization of the emotions. Rather than appraising holism as an aspect of embodiment, this chapter critiques it from the perspective of the body politic. In doing so, the chapter draws on a well-researched sociological concept, 'medicalization' (see, e.g., Foucault 1989), and transposes it into premodern times, as did others (e.g. McVaugh 1993), when discussing social processes that resulted in the expansion of medicine's jurisdiction.

The notion of balance that emerges from these discussions points to a morally mediated emotionality, that of moderation. The chapter thus engages with anthropological and historical research on the emotions, and with morality more generally. In particular, it draws on a historical sociology of the 'affective make-up' or 'psychic habitus' (as pioneered by Norbert Elias 1979, 1982) and the political history of emotional expression (as pursued by William Reddy 1997, 2001) when it compares the discussion of anger in two thematically related texts on medical practice.

The structure of the argument is as follows: feudal Chinese court society in the third and second centuries BC advocated 'moralities of moderation', as a medical case record from the period suggests. They disapproved of anger and considered it pathogenic. Moralized emotions of the kind were then, with their codification in the canonical medical literature, 'medicalized' during the Imperial period (after 221 BC). This medicalization resulted in anger being implicated into a string of hot/cold and hard/soft patho-physiological processes inside the body. The two texts examined in this chapter suggest that anger was first moralized and then medicalized, and in this way, hint at the possibility that so-called holistic health care is a result of the 'medicalization of the emotions'.

Background

While the theories of Chinese medicine have been discussed at length, particularly those grounded in 'correlative thinking', the contributions to this volume focus on medical practice. The thematic focus on practice draws attention to medical case materials that open up new possibilities for exploring how medical practitioners and their clientele speak about and handle their emotions. It rekindles debates that have long been abandoned but deserve a fresh look.

This chapter thus responds to Emiko Ohnuki-Tierney (1984: 75), who in the context of critiquing the concept of holism as a defining feature of East Asian medicines, claimed that the contemporary Japanese have no concept of emotional distress as a direct cause of illness. While her critique of holism remains valid in questioning whether psychodynamics underlie all somatic complaints, this chapter formulates a somewhat belated challenge to her claim that East Asian medicines are little concerned with emotional aetiologies. It makes no allusion to the current 'psycho-boom' (Kleinman et al. 2011), but argues, rather, that emotions matter not only to psychotherapists but to people in East Asia more generally, even if their verbal expression may not blatantly suggest this. In fact, as illustrated with vignettes from family and fieldwork experiences in socialist China, it would appear that the very essence of being Chinese can be associated with 'having emotions' (*you ganqing* 有感情).

To recapitulate: when Ohnuki-Tierney (1984) took issue with Arthur Kleinman's (1980) concept of the 'somatization of affect', she drew attention to the plural East Asian medical and religious practices that she called physiomorphic. Unlike her contemporaries, who focused on the traditional scientific theory of the five agents (*wu xing* 五行) and the (ir)rationality of correlative thinking, Ohnuki-Tierney was interested in nerves, blood types and the abortion of fetuses, and thereby initiated research into the kaleidoscope of East Asian healing. She called the magical aspects of these healing traditions physiomorphic, following Lévi-Strauss (1966: 221), who characterized magic as 'the physiomorphism of man' (as opposed to anthropomorphic religious thinking). Physiomorphic healing involved 'a complex process whereby metonyms, which symbolize causes, become metaphors for the imbalance of bodily forces' (Ohnuki-Tierney 1984: 87). Ohnuki-Tierney's interest in emotional healing evidently focused on those aspects of emotion that explained illness causation in the highly culturalized form that is any symbolic idiom.

Sivin (1987), by contrast, expands on the notion of somatization when he refers to correlative reasoning as a 'somatic language'. However, this somatic language may paradoxically have been created for expressing a 'psychologization of distress', as recent research suggests (Hsu 2010: 14). This research applied, like Kleinman (1980), sociological findings from the United States to China, namely that a somatization of affect among blue-collar workers contrasted with the psychologization of affect among white-collar workers. However, rather than using the observed sociological difference for an argument of cultural difference, as did Kleinman (1980), this recent research transposed the observed sociology of emotional expression in the contemporary USA to the China of the third and second centuries BC. Accordingly, doctors and patients of the upper social strata in feudal court society would have developed a vocabulary that psychologized affect.

Detailed textual research has suggested that in order to express emotional distress in medical language, physicians started reasoning in terms of two viscera, which, in turn, provided the foundation for the later standard form of correlative reasoning in terms of the 'five viscera'. These two viscera, which were the heart and the liver, gained prominence in medicine not primarily due to an increase in anatomical knowledge, as is generally assumed. Rather, at a time when people experienced emotional processes within a bipartite *yin yang* body (Hsu 2008), the *yang*-heart and the *yin*-liver were

199

introduced into medicine in order to allow for the 'psychologization of affect' in terms of a 'visceral language' (Hsu 2010: 14–15). This chapter takes the above a step further. Rather than reproducing the Cartesian mind/body dichotomy intrinsic to the terms somatization and psychologization, it probes to what extent these same historical processes are more accurately framed as contributing to a 'medicalization of the emotions'.

The focus is on anger in two thematically related texts from different periods. The first text belongs among the medical case records in the monumental first dynastic history, *Shi ji* 史記 [The records of the historian] (Takigawa 1932–34), completed around 86 BC. The second is a thematically related passage in a medical text, which enjoyed social recognition comparable, but not identical, to that of a 'classic' or 'canon' in European intellectual history, namely the *Huangdi nei jing* 黃帝內經 [Yellow Emperor's inner canon] (Ren 1986). The chapter ends with comparing a medical case record from presumably the second century BC (where anger is mentioned in a rubric about morality) with a surprisingly similar condition in the canonical medical text from presumably the first millennium AD of the Imperial period (where anger is discussed in terms of the scholarly medical hard and soft, hot and cold).

Beyond the Ecological Notion of Balance: 'Holism' and the Emotions

In early modern Europe, scholarly Asian medical practitioners were thought to follow the principles of a humoral pathology. The Jesuit missionaries of the sixteenth and seventeenth centuries, who reported on Chinese scholar-physicians, compared the four Greek elements – water, fire, earth and air – to the Chinese *wu xing* – wood, fire, earth, metal and water – and called them the 'five elements'. As Sivin (1987: 70–80) rightly notes, this translation has caused more confusion than clarification. *Wu xing* do not refer to stable matter, constitutive of the universe or of humans, as do the Greek elements or humours; nor can *xing* 行 be comprehended as fluids, into which humours have been translated in modern English. In Han China (206 BC to AD 220), *xing* referred to the gait, to forms of conduct and to activities, and in the light of this, convention today is to call the *wu xing* either the 'five phases' (Porkert 1974) or the 'five agents'

(Kalinowski 1991). *Xing* is a concept far removed from the Greek notion of humour as a constituent element of man.

It may have been primarily in the light of epidemiological considerations, perhaps for preventing infectious diseases, that the Chinese Imperial administration promoted reasoning in terms of the five agents which aimed at regulating the 'body ecologic'.[2] However, as stressed here, maintaining the body in balance need not merely mean living in accord with the seasons. It may also imply the avoidance of personal entanglement and moral transgression across social boundaries (Parkin, this volume). In other words, avoidance of excess need not centre on the ecological experiences of the seasonal cycle but may also apply to balance in social conduct.[3] Being balanced often invokes a moral and also an emotional dimension.

The medical anthropologists who emphasized the holistic aspects of East Asian medicines underlined doctrinal insistence on moderation and people's avoidance of emotional upset. Their understanding of holism centred on overcoming Cartesian dualism.[4] Margaret Lock (1980), for instance, referred to the emotions as 'internal causes'. Indeed, correlative thinking links them to the internal five viscera. Accordingly, anger arises in the liver, joy in the heart, fear and fright in the kidneys, sorrow and grief in the lungs, and worry in the spleen. Furthermore, the emotions are characterized as such by Chen Yan 陳言 (fl. 1174), who is today primarily remembered for his elaboration of an earlier, presumably medieval distinction between three different sorts of illness causation (see Sivin 1987: 273–90): the six kinds of excess (*liuyin* 六淫, also called *liu qi* 六氣) as external factors (*wai yin* 外淫),[5] the seven emotions (*qi qing* 七情) as internal factors (*nei yin* 內淫), and the factors that are neither internal nor external (*bu nei bu wai* 不內不外). Lock highlighted the close interdependence between visceral and emotional states in 'holistic' East Asian medicine and contrasted it with the mind/body dualism in biomedicine.

When Thomas Ots provided a phenomenological analysis of bodily perceptions that *zhongyi* (literally, Chinese medicine) doctors in the People's Republic of China relate to emotional distress, he did not contrast 'a Western dichotomized' with 'a supposedly holistic Chinese view of body-mind' (Ots 1990: 26). He commented that Western medical physicians also noted correspondences between emotional and somatic complaints, before he provided a long list of complaints which one could term somatic but which clearly connoted emotional distress in *zhongyi*. His study of 243 patients included 106 diagnosed as suffering from psychological distress, among whom the liver or heart was affected in more than two thirds of the cases. Evidently, not all viscera were affected equally, contrary to expectations that systematic correlative enumerations may evoke.[6] Ots's phenomenological outlook highlighted continuities between Eastern and Western and the so-called holistic and dualistic management of emotionality.

Zhang Yanhua (2007) has most recently provided a book-length account of how emotional distress is treated in Beijing hospitals. Her focus is on *qingzhi* 情志 (emotions) and her emphasis is specifically on 'stagnation' (*yu* 鬱) as a cause of emotional disorders. Accordingly, flowing and connecting (*tong* 通),[7] and the circulation of *qi* 氣, are prime concepts of well-being. However, *qingzhi* is a Westernized term for the emotions in comparison to the more colloquial *xinqing* 心情, which was commonly used during my visits to China in the 1980s, more commonly, in fact, than the better researched *renqing* 人情 (Yan 1996: 122–46; 2003: 139–41). Moreover, *yu* is a multivocal term that has not merely negative connotations. Neither *qingzhi* nor *yu* are relevant to the discussion of anger in early Chinese medicine.

It would appear that in the early modern medical literatures, in particular, flows and the circulation of blood and money became predominant (see Duden and Kuriyama, this volume), evidently with reverberations to the present day (Zhang 2007). Flows pervaded Chinese antiquity as well but perhaps they were not as ubiquitous as generally assumed. Madness, for instance, was related to rising *yang* that resulted in hot headedness (Hsu 2007b), and the earliest reliably datable medical treatise that takes different winds to be the cause of madness – winds that typically blow and flow – is a medieval Dunhuang manuscript (*c.* AD 649; see Chen 2002: 132–46). In the second century BC, neither the circulation of *qi* nor its stagnation were central to the discussion of anger. Rather, as we will see, the arousal of *qi* and its upward movement were an issue.

There is important research on *qing* 情 (Eifring 2004) and the emotions more generally (Santangelo 2009). Notwithstanding, Zhang's (2007: 46–51) discussion of concepts related to Confucian philosophy, such as *du* 度, approximated as 'degree/position', 'moderation' and *he* 和 'harmony', is directly relevant here. In particular her detailed discussion of *ganqing* 感情 (emotions) resonates well with the field experiences presented below.

Morally Mediated Emotionality

'To have feelings' (*you ganqing* 有感情) clearly has moral overtones. 'Anticipating the other's needs and acting accordingly without being explicitly told is most valued as a true manifestation of *ganqing*' (Zhang 2007: 60). It is accordingly less something one declares and says one 'has', than something that prompts one into a context-sensitive 'doing' (*xing* 行). Zhang's research reinforces Potter and Potter's findings on how emotionality was culturally encoded among Zengbu villagers who expressed love through 'work' (Potter and Potter 1990: 180–95).

Important for the line of argument here is that *you ganqing* is an aspect of the social person, if not the defining aspect of Chinese personhood. It can be employed as what Reddy (1997) calls an emotive that aims to (and sometimes does) transform a given situation. This became apparent to me through a statement with which some of my Chinese friends would assure me that I was one of them: 'You value emotions very much' (*ni hen zhongshi ganqing* 你很重視感情).[8] Since this comment was uttered sometimes completely unexpected, for instance in a group of friends who were enjoying a meal, and since it could not be related to a particular event, it is difficult to know what exactly prompted my interlocutors to say it. Notably, this comment was always made in a sociable moment, and not in a romantic or intimate context. On those occasions the word *ganqing* meant emotions that are morally sanctioned and appropriate, and that arise from 'a sensitive concern for others', as Elvin paraphrases the Confucian virtue *ren* 仁 (Elvin 1985: 165).

Another statement comes to mind: 'The Chinese are complicated' (*zhongguoren hen fuza* 中國人很複雜). This utterance clearly alludes to an essentialized Chinese psyche. It implies that certain forms of social interaction cannot be judged at face value. Sometimes this utterance alluded to complex personal entanglements that prompted someone to act inappropriately. It conveyed a sense that the reading of Chinese emotionality is a complex affair, deemed far more complicated than that of Europeans or North Americans. I repeatedly was told by Chinese how cunning and evil the Chinese are. No other people could emulate them in this evilness. Their psyche was complicated.

The above two statements provide a hint that contemporary Chinese consider the emotions an intrinsic aspect of sociality and refer to them often only in morally mediated ways. Incidentally, such talk in these personal field experiences was tied to situations that addressed, if not aimed to transform, my social identity. A morally appropriate emotionality was considered an intrinsic aspect of Chinese sociality. The display of strong emotions was generally not considered socially disruptive, as both Kleinman and the Potters noted in their classic ethnographies. However, the strong will of an impulsive ego (*tai zhudong* 太衝動) and passion in a love affair were considered *guodu* 過度, 'to go beyond the measure', whereby *du* is the Confucian virtue encountered above that admonishes one to be self-conscious of one's positionality in society.

Anger as Psychic Habitus: *Sheng Qi* and *Qi Shang*

In the section that follows, contemporary Chinese medical notions of balance are traced to 'moralities of moderation' in early Chinese medicine and to a subsequent 'medicalization of emotion' in canonical medical texts. Moralities of moderation advocate regular food intake, exercise, work, sleep and sexual patterns, and avoidance of excess, not least being emotional indulgences (Sivin 1987). They contrast with situations in Chinese and other societies, past and present, where feasting is celebrated and an excess of food and drink is cherished, where people mill around and engage in activities that are geared towards interactively intensifying their sensual and emotional life (Chau 2008).

Norbert Elias's historical sociology becomes relevant in this context as it sets out to explain long-term transformations of a stronger and more even-handed control of the emotions in the light of a long-term transformation in the 'mechanisms of feudalization' and 'state control' (Elias 1979, 1982). Elias compared medieval documents to early modern texts on etiquette in court life, which allowed him to identify changes in people's 'affective make-up'.

The first volume (Elias 1979) discusses table manners, attitudes to so-called natural functions like defecating and urinating, blowing one's nose, spitting, behaviour in the bedroom, relations between men and women, and changes in aggressiveness (*Angriffslust*). The second (Elias 1982) relates these changes in a person's psychic habitus to transformations in court society. Elias demonstrates how, because of an increasing division of labour among an aristocracy that started gathering around the king, the self became entangled in denser and longer chains of dependency. This in turn gave rise to habits in thinking that were more 'psychological' and 'rational', in that they required restraint from an impulsive assertion of the self and resulted in long-term calculations for indirect gains. Furthermore, restraint exerted by another's brute force was increasingly replaced by self-restraint as levels of shame and embarrassment became more pronounced and were internalized. Importantly, the knight's aggressiveness, which was celebrated in the Middle Ages (Elias 1979: 191–205), was no longer appreciated in the more urban court society of the French absolutist king.

The knight's aggressiveness that was cherished in medieval Europe shows traits of what some anthropologists in small scale societies have described as a form of anger – for instance, the now classic *liget* among the head-hunting Ilongot of the Philippines (Rosaldo 1980) or the 'homicidal furore *pii*' among Huaorani in the upper Amazon, paraphrased as 'courage, fearlessness, anger and force' (Rival 2005: 295). Anger is only in certain, culturally specific situations celebrated as such, and in these contexts not actually considered an 'emotion' but rather a 'vital principle' or 'creative energy', as Heald (1989: 69) suggests, who worked with the Gisu, egalitarian agriculturists in East Africa. However disparate the societies in question, in all these three cases, anger appears to be linked to an arousal of life energies, which are felt bodily. In this context it is worth noting that in colloquial contemporary Chinese, 'to be angry' is *sheng qi* 生氣, which literally means 'to generate *qi*' and which accordingly could be approximated as 'to generate life energy'. *Qi* is here an energy of arousal; it rises and makes one rise in anger.

Importantly, this anger that is creative energy is masculine. The fitful rage that Laura Rival (2005) describes is experienced only by Huaorani men. There is *pii nenga*, a felt energy and life force, which animates every human body, and *pii inte*, the fitful rage that, if sustained, will end in homicide; only men experience *pii inte*. Likewise, Michelle Rosaldo (1980) describes *liget* as an anger that overcomes young men and prompts them into taking heads; it is a sign of their masculinity and is appreciated particularly by their affinal kin. Similarly, Suzette Heald (1989: 58–59) contrasts the weaker *libuba*, that women and children feel, with *lirima*, 'the force behind the strength of character which makes men courageous and determined' in the extremely painful initiation ceremonies that young Gisu men have to undergo if they wish to marry and set up a homestead.

Again, it is interesting that the Chinese language contains hints of a positive attitude towards such masculine aggression. For instance, *gang* 剛, 'hardness', is associated in the *Book of Changes* with the male principle; *ruo* 弱, 'softness', is associated with the female principle (*Zhou yi* 周易, *qian* 乾 and *kun* 坤; Anon. 1980: 13, 17). *Gang* is also mentioned as a positive attribute of the liver in the *Shi ji* (Takigawa 1934: 34). Anger and aggression, to which by implication such hardness gives rise, are positively valued; justified anger is an attribute of the military general, to whose office the bodily functions of the liver are likened (*Su wen* 素問 8; Ren 1986: 38). The Chinese word *gang* seems to imply a notion of socially approved anger and aggression, which typically is masculine.

Elias stressed that the medieval knight's aggressiveness was lustful; his life should be brimful with this-worldly joy: '*Nul courtois ne doit blamer joie, mais toujours joie aimer*' (Elias 1979: 197). Elias thereby aimed to erase anyone's misconception nurtured by clerical documents from the Middle Ages that little value was given to the this-worldly life. Great was the joy of mutilating and killing other people, particularly the poor and defenceless. It was socially approved: 'War is a joyous thing!' (Elias 1979: 196). In Elias's description, emotional life was marked by intense piety, by the violent fears of hell that this piety caused, by guilt and strong feelings of penitence, by immense outbursts of joy and happiness, and by the sudden flaring up of hatred with uncontrollable force and belligerence (paraphrasing Elias 1979: 200). One loved life, celebrated bravery, loyalty and friendship, and faced death in 'enraptured' fashion.

Such aggressiveness was no longer appreciated in eighteenth-century France, and the impetuosity with which Duke of Montmorency led his people into death in battle against the king (Elias 1982: 279–80) comes across as sheer recklessness. Court society cultivated other forms of conduct and conflict resolution. In a similar vein, *amok*, a form of homicide, which for Malay men was the socially approved form of taking revenge if their honour had been violated, became known in cross-cultural psychiatry as a 'culture-bound syndrome', a 'morbid rage reaction' (Yap 1967: 177). The colloquial 'going berserk' has comparable overtones of disapproved social conduct, if one considers that berserker denotes 'A wild Norse warrior of great strength and ferocious courage, who fought on the battle-field with a frenzied fury known as the berserker rage' (*Oxford English Dictionary* 'berserk'). Masculine forms of displaying violence that once were honoured are in civilized society ridiculed or medicalized.

In pre-Imperial and early Imperial China we see the emergence of an idiom in medical language, *qi shang* (*qi* rises), that points to a comparable change in psychic habitus. One manuscript text from the second century BC, known as 'Mai shu' (The vessel/pulse book), notes that the sages keep their head cool, and their feet warm, so as to hinder *qi* from rising (see Zhangjiashan 247 hao Han mu zhujian zhengli xiaozu 2001: 244); another passage in this text provides the rationale for this medico-moral device: 'If *qi* moves, then there is grief' (*qi dong ze you* 氣動則憂), whereby 'grief' in this sentence probably refers in a generic sense to any excessively strong emotion (Hsu 2010: 40–41). Notably, the 'Mai shu' text speaks of *qi shang* 氣上 – rather than the creation of energy *sheng qi* – and *qi shang* is pathogenic.

Moralities of Moderation in Early Chinese Medicine

In the 105th chapter of the *Shi ji* (Takigawa 1934: 1–62), there are twenty-five medical case records of a physician attending to the nobility of Qi in eastern China, of which the first ten in particular throw light on court life in the third and second century BC. Each case concerns a different medical disorder, but in eight out of ten cases wine and/or women are given as the cause; in two cases it is the emotions. The case records evidently pointed to debauchery among the nobility of Qi. They contained data that could be used to formulate a critique of court life in the codified language that is any medical jargon. It is possible that for this reason these medical case records were integrated into Sima Qian's dynastic history, but that is another story (Hsu 2010: 57, 114 et passim).

These ten case histories (Takigawa 1934: 24–39) were recorded in a formulaic fashion. The linguistically marked three recurrent phrases each introduced a textual unit conveying information that can be interpreted as reporting on the 'name of the disorder', on its 'cause' and on 'the means whereby the diagnosis was made'. It was detective work to identify whether and how the diagnostic qualities recorded in the third textual unit correlated with the two others. Eventually, most diagnostic qualities turned out to be indexical of the semantic constituents (mostly well-known nosologies) in the names of the disorder (often compound words recorded in no other texts of medical history). However, for the causes of the eight disorders which pointed to debauchery, few parallels, and usually only tangential ones, could be found in the canonical medical literature. In the rubric on illness causation, the physician appeared to make lifestyle responsible for the patient's illness and put blame on morally unacceptable conduct.

Lustful life at court was disapproved of, and so were strong emotions and distemper. In Case 2, an infant in the king's family suffered from irritability (*shao you* 少憂); he vomited and rejected food and drink. In Case 6, a man from Qi contracted his illness from being in great anger (*nu* 怒), and in this condition indulging in women; he suffered from a wasting disorder (see Appendix). In Case 2, the heart was affected; in Case 6, the liver. These were the two viscera then located in the upper and lower part of a body divided into two parts by the diaphragm. It was in terms of this bipartite *yin yang* body that physicians in the third and second centuries BC seem to have accounted for strong emotions and emotional distress, as would suggest the following quote from a manuscript text, called 'Yin shu' (The book on guiding), that was unearthed from a tomb closed in the early second BC near Zhangjiashan (see Zhangjiashan 247 hao Han mu zhujian zhengli xiaozu 2001: 299):

The nobility contracts illness	貴人之所以得病者,
by way of not being harmonious in joy and anger	以其喜怒之不和也.
If one is joyful, then the *yang qi* augments	喜則陽氣多,
if one is angry, then *yin qi* augments	怒則陰氣多

Keeping the body in emotional balance was evidently an aspect of the 'moralities of moderation' cultivated in the feudal court life of the period. The above quote from the 'Yin shu' underlines the medico-moral stance of Cases 2 and 6 of *Shi ji* 105.

The Medicalization of Anger in Canonical Chinese Medical Texts

It is interesting that in his assessment of the medieval knight's aggressiveness, Elias emphasizes the lust for aggression and killing. Foucault's *Discipline and Punish* opens with what is – to our sensitivities – a similarly gruesome description of the quartering of a criminal. Foucault starts his analysis with the publicly displayed power of the classical sovereign in seventeenth-century France by arguing that the king's subjects were thereby made to comprehend it in all its physicality with all their senses (Foucault 1979: 3–6). Foucault's ensuing argument is well rehearsed: as government power becomes increasingly invisible, it is internalized by myriads of disciplined, docile bodies. This theme of invisible but internalized power also underlies Foucault's discussion of medicalization (Foucault 1989). It appears as though Foucault was inspired by Elias's study of the sociogenesis of the individual's 'affective household'.

The last three centuries BC were marked by China's unification and the building up of an Imperial bureaucracy. Where previously there had been disunity, contest and warfare between city states and small kingdoms, unification initiated a process of centralized state-building (Lewis 1990). During this period of enforcing bureaucratic structures of government, the well-known medical canons that advocated the regulation of an individual's emotional and bodily processes were commissioned and compiled (Ma 1990).

As seen in the previous section, anger was already considered illness-inducing in early Chinese medical texts, which may well record knowledge dating from pre-Imperial times, such as in the above cited passage from a Zhangjiashan manuscript of the early second century BC and Case 6 of *Shi ji* 105. Case 6 mentions anger in a rubric that is introduced by the recurrent phrase 'the illness was contracted by ...' (*bing de zhi*), which, as argued above, in all the first ten cases concerns an illness-inducing transgression against moralities of moderation.

In the canonical medical texts, however, anger became increasingly implicated in patho-physiologies of *wu xing* correlations. In doctrinal *Su wen* texts of the 'body ecologic', for instance, anger correlates with thunder and wind that predominate in spring and can be either life-initiating or illness-inducing. In *Ling shu* 靈樞 46

we find a description that has striking parallels to Case 6 of *Shi ji* 105. The text speaks of *gang* (hard) inner feelings, like anger, which it contrasts to a *ruo* (soft) outer appearance, and wasting flesh. It states that a person who has a thin skin and eyes that are firm, solid and deep-seated typically has raised eyebrows and a heart that is hard (*qi xin gang* 其心剛).[9] If a person has such hardness, then he will frequently be angry (*gang ze duo nu* 剛則多怒). Anger, the text continues, causes heat to rise into the chest, which, in turn, effects a wasting of the flesh and fat. The paragraph ends with the statement: 'This means that the person in question is violent and hard, but his flesh and muscles are soft' (Ren 1986: 388). Emotional hardness causes weakness in the flesh (see Appendix).

Case 6 and *Ling shu* 46 both concern an illness caused by anger, which manifests itself as a disorder where the flesh is wasting away. In Case 6 anger is mentioned among the indulgences of the nobility, which pertain to transgressions against an implicit morality of moderation. In *Ling shu* 46 it is intrinsic to hard/soft and hot/cold patho-physiological processes and has become implicated in a medicalized discussion of bodily processes. Anger as an emotion that is morally unacceptable has thus become an integral aspect of patho-physiology.

The sociality of the court nobility and the distemper and debauchery *Shi ji* 105 reports on in its first ten case histories is of a different order from that of the Imperial administration, which may have been geared towards the 'regulation of populations', a concern of government characterized by Foucault (2003) as one of the pillars of 'biopower'. Accordingly, the anger in Case 6 of *Shi ji* 105 is best comprehended as a transgression of the moralities of moderation that prevailed in feudal court life in pre-Imperial times. By contrast, the anger discussed in *Ling shu* 46 has become part of hard/soft and hot/cold patho-physiologies, and is perhaps best read as pointing to a disciplining of the body through a 'medicalization of emotion'.

Discussion

The medico-moral dimension of avoiding extremes comes into sharp relief through the study of anger in cross-cultural perspective. The anger that is comprehended as creative among the Ilongot, Gisu and Huaorani is in certain situations encouraged as an aspect of young men's masculinity. However, anger has also been moralized in other ways. Elias (1979, 1982) highlighted, particular to the materials discussed here, that feudal court societies in Europe developed a psychic habitus that reinterpreted the medieval knight's courage as reckless aggression. His study of how people's affective make-up can change in tandem with long-term transformations of government appears to have cross-cultural validity. In a strikingly similar vein, the Chinese colloquialism 'to produce *qi*', *sheng qi*, relates anger to the creation of energy, while 'rising *qi*' (*shang qi*) was in a scholarly medical second century BC text considered pathogenic.

Rather than culturalizing the emotions and becoming preoccupied with questions of their universalism versus cultural constructedness, this chapter has searched for other ways of accounting for cross-cultural continuities without downplaying specificities due to historical and socio-political differentiation. It highlighted cross-culturally found expressions of anger, celebrated as both courageous and creative, which are gendered. It also showed how, cross-culturally, feudal court societies that linked 'honour' or 'merit' to morals of moderation redefined such outbursts of anger as socially disruptive: either as reckless behaviour or as an illness-inducing event.

Accordingly, the basic understanding of keeping the body in balance in Chinese medicine historically would have arisen in the Chinese feudal court societies of the third and second century BC that disapproved of anger as socially disruptive. With the materials presented here, the argument could not be made that social stratification at the time was according to politico-ritual rank (rather than socio-economic class) along a gradient of increasing prestige, honour or 'merit' (see Hsu 2007a), but it could be shown that those upper ranks advocated moralities of moderation.

As the Imperial administration in charge of medical issues expanded its jurisdiction with the codification of the emotions as internal causes of illness, anger became even more integrated into medical jargon. If medicalization means the expansion of medical jurisdiction into many different domains of social life, and if the Imperial bureaucracy compiled medical texts that advocated moderation, it increasingly medicalized moral precepts advocating moderation. Accordingly, the so-called holistic Chinese medical treatment of emotional distress with the physicality of needles and herbs may have historically grown out of a psychic habitus of moderation in Elias's sense, and its subsequent medicalization in a Foucauldian sense.

This leads us to reflections on the notion of medicalization. In full awareness that Foucault himself said that the disciplining of the body that he discussed was simultaneously individualizing and totalizing in a way that has been unparalleled elsewhere (Foucault 1982: 213), it would appear that the Foucauldian notion of medicalization helps us explain how the language of emotions in Chinese medicine was transformed to such a degree so as not to be immediately recognizable as such. It allows us to reinterpret the processes of so-called somatization and psychologization, which reproduce dualistic thinking, in a way that is grounded in general sociological theory. The 'medicalization of emotion' in Imperial China would thus have consolidated the 'visceral language' created in feudal times for communicating emotional upset that was morally disapproved of. Reasoning in terms of *wu xing* – which is emblematic of correlative thinking and typically has been linked to a form of cognition – is perhaps more adequately comprehended as a medico-moral mode of managing emotionality.

Appendix

Translated excerpt of *Shi ji* 105, Case 6 (Takigawa 1934: 32):
Cao Shanfu of the ward Zhangwu in Qi fell ill. 齋章武裏曹山跗病
Your servant, Yi, examined his *mai* and said: 臣意診其脈曰
'It is a lung consumption. 肺消癉也
In addition there are chills and hot flushes'. 加以寒熱
Forthwith I informed the members of the household saying: 即告其人曰
'He will die. Incurable. 死不治
In accordance with what he needs, provide maintenance. 適其共養
A doctor should not treat this one'. 此不當醫治
The 'Model' says: 法曰
After three days, he will be in a state that matches madness. 後三日而當狂
In a frenzy, he will rise to walk about, desiring to run. 妄起行慾走

After five days, he will die'. 後五日死
He then died at the end of the predicted time period. 即如期死
Shanfu's illness was contracted from being in great anger, and in this condition indulging in women. 山跗病得之盛怒而以接內
The means whereby I recognized Shanfu's illness were that 所以知山跗之病者
when your servant, Yi, pressed onto his *mai*, *qi* [coming] from the lungs was hot. 臣意切其脈 肺氣熱也

Translation of *Huangdi nei jing Ling shu* 46 (Ren 1986: 388):
The Yellow Emperor said: 黃帝曰
As to the person prone to ail from consumption, how does one diagnose him? 人之善病消癉者，何以候之。
Shao Yu answered: 少俞答曰
'If the five viscera are all soft and weak, one is prone to ail from consumption'. 五藏皆柔弱者，善病消癉
The Yellow Emperor said: 黃帝曰
'How does one recognize the softness and weakness of the five viscera?' 何以智五藏之柔弱也
Shao Yu answered: 少俞答曰
'If there is softness and weakness, 夫柔弱者
there must be hardness and rigidity; 必有剛強
hardness and rigidity causes one to be frequently angered, 剛強多怒
as to the soft, it is easily harmed'. 柔者易傷也
The Yellow Emperor said: 黃帝曰
'How does one diagnose softness and hardness?' 何以候柔弱之與剛強
Shao Yu answered: 少俞答曰
'Such a person has a thin skin but the eyes are firm, solid and deep-seated, 此人薄皮膚而目堅固以深者
long, forthright, straight and haughty, 長衝直揚
his heart is hard. 其心剛
When it is hard, then he is frequently angered. 剛則多怒
When he is angry, then the *qi* rises and goes against the flow. 怒則氣上逆

213

In the midst of the chest it gathers and accumulates. 胸中蓄積
Blood and *qi* go against the flow and stagnate, 血氣逆留
they [stretch?] the skin and fill the flesh [such that] 臆皮充肌
the blood and vessels do not move, 血脈不行
and while rotating, become hot. 轉而為熱
When there is heat, then it consumes the skin and flesh, 熱則消肌膚
hence it turns into a consumption. 故為消癉
This means that the person in question is violent and hard, but his
flesh and muscles are soft'. 此言其人暴剛而肌肉弱者也。

Notes

1. This chapter has been in gestation for a long time, with different sections presented at the following conferences: EASA 2002, ASA 2003, EACS 2004, EASA 2006, RAI 2007 and ArgO-EMR 2008. I thank my audiences for their feedback, Frank Pieke for encouragement to experiment with Foucauldian concepts, and Peregrine Horden for his valuable comments on recent drafts.
2. On the 'body ecologic', which concerns 'the ways in which people perceive and interact with their natural environment', as an addition to the three research perspectives outlined as alternatives to the currently dominant Cartesian view of the body (Scheper-Hughes and Lock 1987), see Hsu (1999: 76, 78–83); as a framework for tracing the conceptual history of the 'theory' of *wu xing* to a cross-cultural ecological observation, the seasonality of illness, see Hsu (2007a); for the attempt to link the body ecologic to the body politic of Imperial China, see Hsu (2009). See also Rittersmith (2009) on the 'body ecologic' as a habitus of overseas Chinese.
3. In modern Chinese, for instance, *guo* 過 means 'to transgress', 'to be excessive', 'to be mistaken'.
4. Strictly speaking these medical anthropologists have conflated two concepts: 'dualism' is generally understood as the opposite of 'monism' (and East Asian medicines are not monistic, e.g. Hsu 2008), and 'holism' of 'reductionism' (*The Concise Oxford Dictionary*, s.v. 'monism', 'holism').
5. The six *qi* – *yin* and *yang*, wind and rain, dark and light (Sivin 1987: 55) – or *liu yin* 六淫, 'six excesses' – wind, cold, summer heat, damp, dryness and fire (Sivin 1987: 275–86) – share with the Ayurvedic three *dosha*s not only a comparable numerology of three (2 x 3 = 6) but also a similar etymology: *dosha* means 'mistake' and *yin* 淫 'excess'. This may explain why Leslie (1976: 4) believed there were 'six humours' in Chinese medicine, rather than referring to the five agents.
6. In the *Huangdi nei jing*, the correlations between the five/seven emotions and the viscera are notoriously unstable (Unschuld 2003: 231–34). In pre-Imperial China the heart was the seat of all cognition, perception and emotion (Csikszentmihalyi 2004).

7. 'Crane *qigong*' practitioners also generally spoke of the flow and blockage of *qi*, and of *yin* and *yang*, but Thomas Ots interpreted this as uninteresting, an incidence of 'well-trodden explanatory models of TCM [Traditional Chinese Medicine]'. Strangely, Ots depicts it as a great achievement of the ethnographer to elicit the statement, 'Yes, spontaneous *qigong* helps to free our *suppressed* emotion' (emphasis added). The person from whom Ots extracted this statement, however, did not consider it the usual 'style of argumentation' (Ots 1994: 126).
8. Between 1978 and 1989 I spent in total over three years in the People's Republic of China.
9. In *Ling shu* 46, the heart is *gang*; in *Shi ji* 105, Case 6, *gang* (hardness) is an attribute of the liver. Variations of the kind are frequent in Chinese medical texts.

References

Anon. 1980 [9th–2nd century BC] *Zhou yi* 周易 [The Changes of the Zhou]. References to *Zhou yi zheng yi* 周易正義 in Ruan Yuan 阮元 (ed.) [1816], *Shi san jing zhu shu* 十三經注疏 [Commentary to the Thirteen Canons]. Beijing: Zhonghua shuju. Vol. 1, pp.5–108.

Chau, A.Y. 2008. 'The Sensorial Production of the Social', *Ethnos* (special issue) 73(4): 485–504.

Chen Hsiu-fen. 2002. 'Medicine, Society and the Making of Madness in Imperial China', PhD thesis. London: Department of History, School of Oriental and African Studies.

Csikszentmihalyi, M. 2004. *Material Virtue: Ethics and the Body in Early China*. Leiden: Brill.

Eifring, H. 2004. *Love and Emotions in Traditional Chinese Literature*. Leiden: Brill.

Elias, N. 1979[1939]. *The Civilizing Process*, Vol. 1: *The History of Manners*. Oxford: Blackwell.

——— 1982[1939]. *The Civilizing Process*, Vol. 2: *State Formation and Civilization*. Oxford: Blackwell.

Elvin, M. 1985. 'Between Earth and Heaven: Conceptions of the Self in China', in M. Carrithers et al. (eds), *The Category of the Person: Anthropology, Philosophy, History*. Cambridge: Cambridge University Press, pp.156–88.

Foucault, M. 1979[1975]. *Discipline and Punish: The Birth of the Prison*. London: Peregrine.

——— 1982. 'Afterword: the Subject and Power', in H.L. Dreyfus and P. Rabinow (eds), *Michel Foucault: Beyond Structuralism and Hermeneutics*. New York: Harvester Wheatsheaf, pp.208–26.

——— 1989[1963]. *The Birth of the Clinic: An Archaeology of Medical Perception*. London: Routledge.

——— 2003[1976]. '17 March 1976', in *Society Must be Defended: Lectures at the Collège de France, 1975–76*. New York: Picador, pp.239–64.

Heald, S. 1989. *Controlling Anger: The Sociology of Gisu Violence*. Manchester: Manchester University Press.

Hsu, E. 1999. *The Transmission of Chinese Medicine*. Cambridge: Cambridge University Press.

———— 2007a. 'The Biological in the Cultural: The Five Agents and the Body Ecologic in Chinese Medicine', in D. Parkin and S. Ulijaszek (eds), *Holistic Anthropology: Emergences and Divergences*. Oxford: Berghahn, pp.91–126.

———— 2007b. 'The Experience of Wind in Early and Medieval Chinese Medicine', *Journal of the Royal Anthropological Institute* (special issue) N.S. S117–S134.

———— 2008. 'Outward Form (*xing* 形) and Inward *qi* 氣: The Sentimental Body in Early Chinese Medicine', *Early China* 32: 103–24.

———— 2009. 'Experiences of Personhood, Health, and Disease in China: Some Reflections', *Cambridge Anthropology* 29(3): 69–84.

———— 2010. *Pulse Diagnosis in Early Chinese Medicine: The Telling Touch*. Cambridge: Cambridge University Press.

Kalinowski, M. 1991. *Cosmologie et divination dans la Chine ancienne: Le compendium des cinq agents* (Wuxing dayi, VIe siècle). Paris: Ecole Française d'Extrême-Orient.

Kleinman, A. 1980. *Patients and Healers in the Context of Culture: An Exploration of the Borderland between Anthropology, Medicine, and Psychiatry*. Berkeley: University of California Press.

Kleinman, A., et al. 2011. *Deep China: The Moral Life of the Person, What Anthropology and Psychiatry tell us about China Today*. Berkeley: University of California Press.

Leslie, C. 1976. 'Introduction', in C. Leslie (ed.), *Asian Medical Systems: A Comparative Study*. Berkeley: University of California Press, pp.1–12.

Lévi-Strauss, C. 1966[1962]. *The Savage Mind*. Chicago: University of Chicago Press.

Lewis, M.E. 1990. *Sanctioned Violence in Early China*. Albany: State University of New York Press.

Ling shu 靈樞, see Ren Yingqiu.

Lock, M.M. 1980. *East Asian Medicine in Urban Japan*. Berkeley: University of California Press.

Ma Jixing 馬繼興. 1990. *Zhongyi wenxianxue* 中醫文獻學 [Study of Chinese Medical Texts]. Shanghai: Shanghai kexue jishu chubanshe.

McVaugh, M. 1993. *Medicine before the Plague: Practitioners and their Patients in the Crown of Aragon, 1285–1335*. Cambridge: Cambridge University Press.

Ohnuki-Tierney, E. 1984. *Illness and Culture in Contemporary Japan: An Anthropological View*. Cambridge: Cambridge University Press.

Ots, T. 1990. 'The Angry Liver, the Anxious Heart and the Melancholy Spleen: The Phenomenology of Perceptions in Chinese Culture', *Culture, Medicine, and Psychiatry* 14: 21–58.

———— 1994. 'The Silenced Body – the Oppressive *Leib*: On the Dialectic of Mind and Life in Chinese Cathartic Healing', in T. Csordas (ed.), *Embodiment and Experience*. Cambridge: Cambridge University Press, pp.116–36.

Porkert, P. 1974: *The Foundations of Chinese Medicine: Systems of Correspondence.* Cambridge, MA: MIT Press.

Potter, S.M., and J.M. Potter. 1990. *China's Peasants: The Anthropology of a Revolution.* Cambridge: Cambridge University Press.

Reddy, W.M. 1997. 'Against Constructionism: The Historical Ethnography of Emotions', *Current Anthropology* 38(3): 327–51.

——— 2001. *The Navigation of Feelings: A Framework for the History of Emotions.* Cambridge: Cambridge University Press.

Ren Yingqiu 任應秋 (ed.). 1986. *Huangdi neijing zhangju suoyin* 黃帝內經章句索引 [Concordance of the Yellow Emperor's Inner Canon]. Beijing: Renmin weisheng.

Rittersmith, A. 2009. 'Contextualising Chinese Medicine in Singapore: Microcosm and Macrocosm', *Journal of the Oxford Anthropological Society e* (N.S. – Online) 1(1): 1–24.

Rival, L. 2005. 'Soul, Body and Gender among the Huaorani of Amazonian Ecuador', *Ethnos* 70(3): 285–310.

Rosaldo, M.Z. 1980. *Knowledge and Passion: Ilongot Notions of Self and Social Life.* Cambridge: Cambridge University Press.

Santangelo, P. 2009. *Sentimental Education in Chinese History: An Interdisciplinary Textual Research on Ming and Qing Sources.* Leiden: Brill.

Scheper-Hughes, N., and M. Lock 1987. 'The Mindful Body: A Prolegomenon to Future Work in Medical Anthropology', *Medical Anthropology Quarterly* 1(1): 6–41.

Shi ji 史記 see Takigawa Kametaro.

Sivin, N. 1987. *Traditional Medicine in Contemporary China: A Partial Translation of 'Revised Outline of Chinese Medicine' (1972) with an Introductory Study on Change in Present-day and Early Medicine.* Ann Arbor: University of Michigan Center for Chinese Studies.

Su wen 素問, see Ren Yingqiu.

Takigawa Kametaro 瀧川龜太郎 (ed.) 1932–34. *Shiki kaichû kôshô* 史記會注考證 (Examination of the Collected Commentaries to the *Records of the Historian*). Toyo Bunka Gakuin, Tokyo.

Unschuld, P.U. 2003. *Huang Di Nei Jing Su Wen: Nature, Knowledge, Imagery in an Ancient Chinese Medical Text.* Berkeley: University of California Press.

Yan, Y. 1996. *The Flow of Gifts: Reciprocity and Social Networks in a Chinese Village.* Stanford, CA: Stanford University Press.

——— 2003. *Private Life under Socialism: Love, Intimacy, and Family Change in a Chinese Village, 1949–1999.* Stanford, CA: Stanford University Press.

Yap, P.M. 1967. 'Classification of the Culture-bound Reactive Syndrome', *Australian and New Zealand Journal of Psychiatry* 1: 172–79.

Zhang, Y. 2007. *Transforming Emotions with Chinese Medicine.* Albany: State University of New York Press.

Zhangjiashan 247 hao Han mu zhujian zhengli xiaozu 張家山二四七號漢墓竹簡整理小組 (eds) 2001. *Zhangjiashan Han mu zhujian (247-hao mu)* 張家山漢墓竹簡 (二四七號墓) [Bamboo Strips from the Han Tomb Zhangjiashan No. 247]. Beijing: Wenwu.

Chapter 10
Aiming for Congruence
The Golden Rule of Āyurveda

Francis Zimmermann

A common Sanskrit phrase summarizes the 'principle of balance' according to which contrary qualities compensate for one another: 'Contraries [are counterbalanced] by contraries' (*viparītā viparītaiḥ*).[1] Its meaning seems unambiguous to anyone familiar with Galenism in the West: more of this leads to less of that; it seems to be a matter of proportion. Advocating a different approach to Āyurvedic medicine, however, I would like to make a distinction between two different understandings of the concept of balance. When calculating in terms of degrees and quantities, to strike a balance means to reach a suitable ratio between two contrary components in a combination. When reasoning in terms of natures and qualities, however, balancing the contraries is no longer a matter of proportion but of adequacy. I would like to suggest that we should interpret the Āyurvedic doctrine regarding the transactions of humours in the living body with particular respect for this distinction. Assessing and balancing the humours, according to my reading of the classical texts, is a matter not of degree and ratio but of nature and congruence.

I shall take as an example the diagnosis and treatment of arthritis as they were practised in Kerala by my teacher, Vayaskara N.S. Mooss, in the 1980s. To illustrate the correspondence between a compound medicine and the humoral constitution of the patient, I shall describe the reverse symmetry between the discordant humours responsible for arthritis and the therapeutic properties of medicinal plants used in compounding *Dhanvantara taila*, 'the oil of [god] Dhanvantari', a most appreciated specific against arthritis and one of the bestsellers in contemporary Āyurvedic pharmacies. I will compare my ethnographic data collected in Kerala with my translations of relevant Sanskrit writings. Readers who would like to put the following discussion back in the context of the classical literature of Āyurveda should refer to Dominik Wujastyk's excellent *Roots of Ayurveda* (2003), which offers selected texts in translation with an accurate bibliography.

Health and Disease in a Congenial Soil

Traditional medicine benefits in India from the liberality of laws which enable competition between Hindu Āyurveda, Arabic medicine, Tamil alchemy, homoeopathy and 'allopathy' (the local name for biomedicine, taken as one tradition among many). Āyurveda draws its principles from the nature of the land, a tradition directly connected with the ecology. Kerala, at the south-west of the Indian peninsula, enjoys a humid tropical climate. Apart from the mountain range of the Ghats to the east (from where a number of medicinal plants are collected by the tribals to be commercialized in the plains and used in Āyurvedic pharmacy), Kerala mainly consists of an alluvial plain covered with rice fields and coconut groves. Lagoons and slow-winding rivers form a vast communication network called the Backwaters; banks covered with luxuriant vegetation offer enchanting landscapes to the eye, but one senses what hold parasitic diseases as well as rheumatism and arthritis have in this climate. Kerala people have traditionally enjoyed all kinds of spices in abundance. Cranganore (the oldest), Cannanore, Calicut, Cochin and Quilon (Kollam) are the main ports by which spices were routed for export at the height of the spice trade, in which, for about eighteen centuries, Kerala enjoyed a virtual monopoly. For we must add to our statistics of pepper, ginger and cardamom produced in its groves, forests and plantations a whole gamut of all the other spices like cinnamon, cloves and nutmeg, imported from various Eastern countries of origin, and then re-exported to the Mediterranean world.

Āyurveda appears to fit wonderfully with the context, as much ecological as commercial, of the land of spices. Rheumatisms, which are prevalent in this region of very heavy monsoon rains, respond to compound medicines made of a cocktail of spices. A pharmacology which develops the theory of spices responds to a physiology based on the theory of humours. Rains and winds are internalized in the form of three humours – Wind, Bile and Phlegm[2] – and spices are defined as specifics curing such and such humours. It is a doctrine of a pre-established harmony between illnesses and remedies.

The specific tradition of humoralism which will be evoked in this chapter was practised by a learned practitioner in South India in the early 1980s, and it is, so to say, a tradition ethnographically situated in a given soil; it graphically describes the alliance of wind (the monsoon winds) with water (the Backwaters of Kerala) for causing 'rheumatic diseases', an approximate translation of the category 'diseases due to Wind' (the humour). Medical discourse comes at the end of a long chain. At the point of beginning is the land, where the tradition is anchored in the vigour of its tropical wet climate, the prevalent illnesses (rheumatisms) and the flora corresponding to this climate (the spices). At the other end of the chain is the physician who prescribes cocktails of spices against rheumatisms, and, in doing so, harnesses the forces of the climate and the soil for the benefit of his patient.

In recalling cases of arthritis treated by Vayaskara Mooss, I shall try to show that, in the context of the classical doctrine of Āyurveda, not only the patient's body was to be restored to balance but also their speech and mind; that is to say, the whole person. Apart from being submitted to an elaborate cycle of evacuant medications, oil baths and massages, the patient was to follow a regimen of life and perform their daily duties in accordance with their own nature. You could neither see nor touch nor smell the subtle substances that had been vitiated and were to be restored to balance; they were not the same as blood nor skin although they were somewhat akin to the soft parts of the body. The existence of these imperceptible fluids thought to be the principles of physiology and the causes of disease were inferred from observation of the patient's rhythms and gestures, their attitudes and postures, and their performance and discourse. True, these vital fluids which we construe as humours were swept along complicated transactions. The arthritic patient was inundated by Wind (*vāta*); oily massages and enemas were applied to restrain this desiccating humour and restore the body's 'unctuousness' (*snehatva*). The basic imagery of flows and fluids tend to give the impression of an overall flux of continuous transactions. But we should resist this

220

presupposition and take notice of various clues pointing to a clearly discrete mode of reckoning. Inferences in diagnosis were made on the basis of discontinuities. Whenever gestures, performances and discourse seemed to be harmonious, an improvement was inferred in the state of the patient's humours; whenever the clinical gaze detected breaks, gaps, jerks and unevenness, one would suspect a deterioration. The underlying logic of humours in action was not that of a continuous and gradual variation in the patient's condition but that of breaks, gaps and abrupt reversals.

Arthritis and Gout: Imbalance and Disjointedness

All things in this world are divided into *saumya*, those 'of the nature of Phlegm', and *tīkṣṇa*, the 'acrid' like Bile. This is one of the tenets of Hinduism, the cosmic duality of Agni, the hot and dry sun, and Soma, the cold and wet moon, which is condensed into the medical pair of opposites, Bile and Phlegm. When fevers are classified from this angle, Wind, the third humour, is placed in a fundamentally versatile position:

> When Wind, due to its mediumistic power,
> Allies itself with Phlegm, we get cold fever;
> Burning fever, when it allies itself with Bile;
> And mixed fever, when [the three humours are] mixed.
>
> (*Aṣṭāṅgahṛdayasaṃhitā*, Nidānasthāna 2.48)

Wind is the Hindu equivalent of our animal spirits, an imaginary fluid endowed with *yogavāhitva*, a 'mediumistic power, the power to vehiculate (*vāhitva*) junctions (*yoga*)', the power to arrange any combination of humours and produce any particular 'temperament' (*prakṛti*) or 'intemperature' (*vikṛti*), by conveying the humours and saps thus combined to the minutest parts of the body.

A diagnostic correspondence was established in the early twentieth century between 'wind diseases' (*vātaroga*) and arthritis. A number of diseases well-defined in Western biomedical diagnostics seem to correspond to this Āyurvedic category only at the risk of anachronism and misinterpretation. In other words they seem to illustrate, exemplify and faithfully translate this exotic and polysemic phrase, wind disorders, at the risk of directing the diagnosis in the wrong direction. The nosological domain of wind disorders may be divided into three zones:

1. Arthritism, or rheumatic diathesis. This is the most relevant modern-medicine illustration of what wind disorders stand for in Āyurveda, namely gout and rheumatism. Rheumatoid arthritis (an inflammatory arthritis in which joints, usually including those of the hands and feet, are inflamed, resulting in swelling, pain and often the destruction of joints) and other types of inflammatory arthritis, like ankylosing spondylitis (inflammation of the spine and large joints, resulting in stiffness and pain). Such disorders are thought to result from imperfect digestion and the non-complete elimination of waste.

2. Sensorimotor polyneuropathies superadded to the malfunctioning of food digestion – in some cases of diabetes for example – and other peripheral neuropathies or damage to nerves other than the brain or spinal cord. In this category of Western diagnostics are included ankylosis (stiffness or fixation of a joint by disease or surgery), tetany (physiological calcium imbalance marked by the tonic spasm of muscles), neurological disorders like Parkinson's disease, muscular dystrophy, tumefactions and swellings, neuropathies of the limbs mostly due to infectious diseases (but this aetiology is unknown), which include tetanus, poliomyelitis.

3. Syndromes and accidents far removed from the ideal type of arthritis, which are construed as consequences of the desiccation of vital fluids. These include consumption, cachexia and the progressive wasting away of the body, especially from pulmonary tuberculosis, as well as miscarriage since the spontaneous expulsion of the foetus is thought to follow from the exhaustion of all internal unctuousness in the pregnant woman. This condition in a pregnant woman is most significant as an illustration of the existence of various facets of wind disorders and of the polyvalence of medicines like *Dhanvantara taila*, since this medicated oil (described below), apart from being a panacea in rheumatology, is specifically prescribed, to be taken internally mixed with food, in gynaecology to prevent miscarriage.

Contemporary Āyurvedic practitioners have been accustomed to subsume all these disorders, whatever their differences, under the reductionist category of 'rheumatic diseases', a misnomer of a translation of *vātaroga* which amounts to limiting the extension of the Sanskrit phrase and results in channelling our imagination into the first of the above-mentioned three semantic zones.

Reductionism is unavoidable since we must translate a set of polythetic syndromes into a set of unambiguous disease names. The choice of 'rheumatic diseases' as a conventional rendering of *vātaroga* has been dictated to modern practitioners by implicit presuppositions on the central position of humoralism in Āyurvedic medicine and on the central position of nerve impulse, that was construed as a fluid, and the concept of Wind (*vāta*) as a humour in Āyurvedic physiology. Rheumatology, the medical science dealing with rheumatic diseases, has become a model for the translation of traditional concepts into biomedical terms because it corresponds best to the ancient complex of ideas revolving around nerve impulse. Images of blockade are applied first to a physiological dialectics of balance and imbalance between the humours, and then to a physiological dialectics of conjunction and disjunction between the patient's body and their environment. The proper meaning of Sanskrit *āvaraṇa* is 'blockade', but, when applied to a physiological process it further connotes both imbalance and disjointedness.

The exacerbation and inflation of Wind – nerve impulse as a fluid flowing throughout the body – alternatively yields a 'decrease and depletion of the [other] humours' (*dhātukṣaya*) or the 'blockage', or better, 'blockade of one of the [humoral] channels [or networks]' (*mārgasyāvaraṇa*). The first case is that of arthritis, with loss of weight and anaemia; the second case is that of gout, which is a disease due to repletion (excessive amount of uric acid in the blood). In the latter case, the 'subtle nature' (*sūkṣmatva*) of Wind is the humour's weapon allowing it to rush and besiege the two other humours in their own *mārga*-s (channels or networks), thus exciting, exacerbating, inflating them. In medical terminology, Sanskrit *āvaraṇa* has shifted from the idea of a blockade (a military image) to that of a pervasion and overtaking (a physiological concept). The shift from an image to a concept, at the level of discourse, is but the reflection of a more fundamental shift from arthritis to gout in the nosological grid. Wind stuck in the joints blocks the blood vessels. Wind and blood, 'having pervaded one another' (*anyonyam āvārya*), jointly provoke the advent of gout, thus defined as a 'wind-and-blood' (*vātarakta, vātaśoṇita*) disease. The aetiology of wind-and-blood diseases reaches its highest point in the analysis of the 'various forms of *āvaraṇa* of Wind'.

Compound Medicines as a Mirror of the Patient's Humoral Condition

The Āyurvedic physicians whose remedies I have been studying in Kerala over the last three decades constitute a small scholarly elite immersed right from childhood in the recitation of classical texts of their discipline. Their pharmacopoeia crystallized very naturally into one of those formularies which in the old medical language of Europe used to be called 'antidotaries'. The *Sahasrayogam*, 'The thousand-and-one medicated compositions', an apocryphal text dating back to the seventeenth century at the earliest, is such a collection of compound medicines based on medicinal plants. It reproduces a selection of formulas culled from more ancient sources, which are written mostly in versified Sanskrit and for a minor part in a versified mixture of Sanskrit and Malayalam (the vernacular of Kerala). It gives recipes of electuaries, syrups and decoctions, medicated oils and ghees, enemas and sternutatories, plasters and collyriums, the preparation of which is so convoluted that they were only for use by specialists, and for a rich clientele. These compositions follow the principle of cure by opposites; they are essentially vegetable preparations, overdetermined as much by the concentration of numerous ingredients and adjuvants (polypharmacy) as by the diversity of the directions for use (polypragmasy, or multiplicity of uses).

Fats play a major role in Āyurvedic pharmacy, particularly sesame oil (*taila*) and ghee. Oil and ghee are the main carriers or excipients; they vehiculate throughout the body the mixture of savours and qualities of the medicinal plants with which they have been suffused by means of a series of coctions. The store at the disposal of the modern practitioner includes a hundred oils, some fifty ghees, and for the rest about four hundred remedies in different formats. The decoction of a paste of vegetable substances remains the basic technique in the preparation of oils and ghees.

Dhanvantara taila, for example, combines in principle forty-six vegetable ingredients with sesame oil and milk. The authoritative formula, which until the 1980s in Kerala was taught to the trainees through the study of *Sahasrayogam*, actually comes from Vāgbhaṭa's

Heart of Medicine (seventh century AD), known in Kerala as Vāhaṭa, *Aṣṭāṅgahṛdayasaṃhitā*, *Śārīrasthāna*, Chapter 2, verses 47–52.[3] In the course of a forceful process of normalization and legalization of Āyurvedic medicine and pharmacy, the name and textual identity, composition and therapeutic indications of *Dhanvantara taila* were registered in 1978 in the *Ayurvedic Formulary of India* (GoI 1978).

The original text in Sanskrit consists of six distichs. The first four distichs list the ingredients beginning with the leading one, mallow roots (*Sida rhombifolia*), indicate proportions and give clues to a proper processing of the medicine through an elaborate series of cooking and filtering operations. All glosses necessary for an accurate interpretation of the formula have been transmitted orally, and they are kept secret by the few pharmaceutical companies who nowadays manufacture the medicine. The two last distiches give the list of therapeutic indications which begins with, 'It cures all wind disorders; most esteemed [as a prescription] to pregnant women' (*sarvavātavikārajit | sūtikā ... pūjitam*). I quote these few words to confirm the above-mentioned detail in the multi-faceted nosology of Wind diseases. Apart from being a panacea in rheumatology, *Dhanvantara taila* is prescribed in gynaecology to prevent miscarriage, and this particular therapeutic indication was already known to the anonymous physicians who compiled Vāgbhaṭa's Heart of Medicine fourteen centuries ago.

The recipe, considered literally – 'Take (P1) mallow roots, (P2) barley grains, (P3) kernels of jujube ... and this cures (M1) rheumatisms', etc. – is the accumulation of several series of words: the decoction of a first paste made of fourteen medicinal plants (P1 to P14); sesame oil; the decoction of a second paste made of thirty-two specified plants (of which only twenty-six are actually used nowadays) (P15 to P46); milk; twelve names of illnesses, which represent the therapeutic indications for the remedy (M1 to M12).

It is clear that the combination of savours and qualities of ingredients P1 to P46 plus oil and milk – which can be enumerated as: P1 – sweet, cold, oily, restorative; P2 – pungent, cold, heavy, and so on – forms an architecture of savours and qualities opposite of those characterizing M1 to M12, which can also be enumerated as: M1 – pungent, astringent, light, and so on, since the principle is always to cure by means of opposites. Since P2 and M1 are pungent, compensations have to be made in processing the compound, so that the side-effects of P2 (barley), which is pungent and provokes Wind, will be alleviated by the bulk of other ingredients which, like P1 (mallow), are oily and calm Wind. These corrections are precisely what *saṃskāra*, 'cooking', adds to *saṃyoga*, 'combination'.

Various bitter and aromatic spices have been incorporated into both the pastes, but such cocktails cannot be composed without having a carrier and a buffer solution, in the pharmaceutical sense. The carrier and buffer solution used in Āyurveda is an oil that is meant to act as a connecting and lubricating agent, to temper and buffer the acridity of the mixtures and to carry their quintessence through the body channels, when this oil has been duly impregnated with spices and other powerful vegetable substances through a lengthy series of cookings. Due to its docility to mixtures (as a solvent) and to its powers of diffusion, sesame oil is particularly 'insinuating' (*vyavāyin*). Sesame oil shares with the humour Wind (its intimate enemy) a mediumnic power as a medium which has already been mentioned:, it possesses *yogavāhitva*, the power to vehiculate (*vāhitva*) combinations (*yoga*) of humoral qualities and medical properties, and consequently it facilitates connections between the mixture of substances in the medicine and the multifaceted pathological syndrome in the patient. To conclude, the composition of *Dhanvantara taila* mirrors the humoral constitution of the rheumatic patient for whom this particular medicated oil was selected, but inverting it as it is composed according to the rule which prescribes cures by opposites.

The Art of the Learned Physician

My teacher in Kerala, Vayaskara N.S. Mooss (1912–1986), a celebrated physician, botanist and Sanskrit scholar, was a true proponent of the 'pure' Āyurvedic tradition, *śuddhāyurveda*. His consultation room was furnished with an imposing teak desk and metallic cabinets containing precious books – Sanskrit texts, and a first-rate English library of medical botany. Several armchairs were provided for visitors, since a patient seldom came alone but more often with a member of their family or a friend. In the line of classical practice, diagnosis, the assessment of the patient's *prakṛti*, the patient's 'nature' or 'temperament', resulted from conversation. The physician never touched the patient. Prescriptions were written down on headed notepaper. The physician was essentially a Sanskrit scholar; the core of his art was the written prescription, replete with Sanskrit technical terms and phrases. In former days (that is, up to the turn of the twentieth century), prescriptions were engraved on a *cadjan*, a piece of palm leaf. A vivid description of a consultation held by my teacher's grandfather, Vayaskara Aryan Narayanan Mooss, is to be found in the *Travancore State Manual*:

> He was visible for about four hours daily (6 AM to 10 AM) and he listened to what every patient had to say, quietly and attentively. No word was lost on him, for he was all attention. He was a most thoughtful man and had a wonderful memory. One visitor after another narrated his story to his heart's content and the only interruption which was offered to the web of narrative from each visitor was the questionings by the Musu. When he had finished listening to the whole lot of the visitors of the day, he looked at his pupils or disciples who attended on him by turns, and pointing out [sic] to each patient he quoted the text which was to be prescribed in the particular case. He gave only the initial words of the text. The pupils immediately wrote out the full text of the prescription ... The written *cadjan chits* [engraved palm leaves] of prescription were placed before the Musu and he would hand them over himself one by one to the patients concerned ... It may be stated that the Musu and his visitors would all sit on the floor of an open front verandah of the Illom [the Nambudiri family compound], while those who would not sit with him would stand in the yard, or if they were of an inferior caste outside the enclosure, but all were before him in view and he would talk to all who had come. (Nagam Aiya 1906: Vol. 2, p.554)

The disciples were trained in selecting, quoting and applying versified and lengthy recipes taken from Vāhaṭa's *Aṣṭāṅgahṛdayasaṃhitā*. Classical Āyurveda was a form of scholasticism. A specific feature of this tradition in Kerala, however, was that the most authoritative practitioners had traditionally retained a great proficiency in one particular field of practical knowledge: the taxonomy, combination and processing (that is, cooking) of medicinal plants. The reasons for the privileging of medical botany are to be found in the local ecology. Drains and ducts in the paddy fields, and images from the vegetable kingdom such as the network of veins in a green leaf, the rising of the sap and the milky exudations of resinous trees provide models for the body image (Trawick 1995). The idea prevails of a continuity from plants to men; saps (*rasa*), medicinal properties (*auṣadha-guṇa*) and processes of cooking and coction – by the sun, on the kitchen fire, and through the seven organic fires transforming chyle into blood, blood into flesh, and so on – remain the same all along the chain of living beings. Instead of anatomy, the physician makes use of a combinatory system of saps and properties.

Fully fledged cures alternate the administration of evacuants (mainly purgatives) with gentle massage and drugs associated with a set of images like unctuousness, sap, milk, semen and *ojas* or 'the quintessence of vital fluids', among which oils and lubricants play the essential role of buffers to compensate for the violence of evacuants (Zimmermann 1992). *Dhanvantara taila* is such a drug, and a wise physician will decide between external applications such as oily massages, baths, showers and affusions of oil upon the skin to permeate its seven layers, which are the usual modes of administration of medicated oils, or a potion, a teaspoon let us say, to be swallowed with some drink or rice. In the latter case, *Dhanvantara taila* is several times refined and re-impregnated with additional quantities of all its ingredients. This 'procedure of repetition' (*āvartanavidhi*) or re-medication, which increases its value as a vehicle and a buffer, may take many days and nights, each additional turn adding one day and night to the procedure. The marketing of such a precious medicated oil, 'one-hundred-and-one times re-cooked', points to the powers of unctuousness and its ability to clear up the channels and nourish the body fluids and tissues; health is nothing but intimate smoothness and outward plumpness.

Hygiene and pharmacy have generated a wealth of descriptive phrases, the statistical and semantic study of which is telling. Take the words used, for example, to describe diseases due to the vitiation of Wind (*vāta*), in the aetiology and pathology of *vātaroga*, *vātarakta*, and the like. The same stock of verbal roots is resorted to again and again, from which various adjectives and verbal nouns are derived. The body is bent like a bow and verbal roots abound that say so: *NAM-*; *ā-YAM-*, which gives *āyāma*, 'stretching, bending, crooking', and *antarāyāma*, *bahyāyāma*, *vraṇāyāma*, various forms of paralysis or rheumatism; *KUÑC-*, hence *sandhyākuñcana*, ankylosis. The body is stiffened, rigidified, and the muscles are contracted: *STAMBH-*, *ā-KṢIP-* (hence *ākṣepa*, convulsion), and so on. All these verbs and their derivatives are employed to specify and qualify the idea of hardness – bending, convulsing, blocking – and are to be subsumed under one or another of the twenty 'sensory qualities' (*guṇa*) which connote stiffness, harshness, hardness, sharpness or solidness. These constitute a fixed set of images which are not only used to describe patients' complaints but also used as inferential tools to deduce from the complaints the invisible circulation of Wind (the humour) besieging the other humours in the depths of the body's vessels. A fundamental shift of meaning needs to be taken into account: words that at first were images soon become concepts, according to a figure of speech which is known in Europe as catachresis, and in India by the Sanskrit word *svasaṃjñā* (Zimmermann 1989: 134). Wind, for example, in the sense of gas causing flatulence in the bowels, is an image, a visual representation of stiffness, from which is inferred the existence in the body of a pathogenic entity, namely the humour Wind. Breaking wind is an image; the humour Wind as a pathogenic principle at the root of all neurological diseases is a concept; and the linguistic shift from wind (image) to Wind (concept) is a catachresis.

At first the vocabulary centred upon the theme of hardness plays a descriptive role, but soon it becomes explanatory. The emphasis has shifted from description to explanation. This technical vocabulary is not only applied to the outside appearance of the body but is also used in a more abstract way, as a metalanguage, to put forward an aetiology. Wind in the channels is submitted to a kind of siege or blockade, *āvaraṇa* (from *ā-VṚ-* 'to surround, invest, obstruct'). Its course is 'obstructed' (*āvṛta*) by an excess of one or the two other humours, or of one of the *dhātu*-s (constituents), or of *mala*-s (impurities). Hence Wind as a fluid becomes hard, stiff, indurated.

Learned practitioners in the 1980s still were experts in the handling of 'combinatory rules' (*tantrayukti*), a system of inferential reasoning which blended the logic of diagnosis with the linguistics of figures of speech. To them, humoral balance was the felicitous result of the art of *Yukti*, the art of establishing 'congruent junctions' (*samayoga*). The art of *Yukti*, a combinatorics of some sorts, bears upon words, phrases, stereotypes and figures of speech, not to mention an artificial and preconceived scheme of fixed phrases recurring throughout Sanskrit medical texts. Such a linguistic, logical and poetic play on words cannot take place but in the context of diglossia, because a down-to-earth vernacular is needed to counterbalance the artificiality of the learned language. Scholars should turn to the vernacular from time to time, in order to

229

illustrate, to contextualize and to bring the Sanskrit discourse down to everyday life. Āyurvedic consultations, as I was still able to see in the 1980s, were conducted in turns on the Sanskrit and vernacular levels of language. In my teacher's consultation room, Malayalam was studded with Sanskrit citations, and conversely, the Sanskrit descriptions of diseases were encapsulated in prescriptions teeming with Malayalam names of drugs.

A whole 'book' (*sthāna*) is devoted to the art of 'estimates [of specific situations]' (*vimāna*) in the medical collections, and the *Vimānasthāna* in the 'Compendium of Caraka' opens with an enumeration of the various facets and criteria to be taken into account when adjusting the treatment to a given case:

> After collecting, for a given disease, the details of its [generic] aetiology, prodromes, symptoms, homologies (*upaśaya*), statistics, prevalence, regular forms and variants (*vidhi-vikalpa*), severity and duration, the task of a conscientious physician (*avahitamanasā... bhiṣajā*) is to reckon an estimate (*mānam*) [relevant in this individual patient's case] of his humours (*doṣa*), the medicines he takes, the local environment and the current season, his state of strength, the state of his bodily seven tissues (*śarīrasārā*), his diet, his congenial dispositions (*sātmya*), his psychic make-up (*sattva*), his constitution (*prakṛti*) and his relative youthfulness, as treatment depends on our devising an accurate estimate of all these specificities. (Caraka, *Vimānasthāna* 1.3)

In keeping as close as possible to the original phrasing, this translation aims to bring out the underlying idea of disjunctions and conjunctions between the different realms or spheres of lived experience: homologies, permutations, timings and so on. Reading a little further we come across the 'principle of contraries' alleviating one another. Metabolism occurs between the three humours constitutive of the body's physiology and the six saps absorbed through regimen and diet:

> In metabolic exchanges between humours and saps inside the body (*rasa-doṣa-sannipāte*), those saps which contain exactly identical qualities (*samāna-guṇāḥ*) or broadly identical qualities (*samāna-guṇa-bhūyiṣṭhā*) to a given peccant humour will aggravate it, and those saps of exactly contrary qualities (*viparīta-guṇāḥ*) or broadly contrary qualities (*viparīta-guṇa-bhūyiṣṭhā*) to a peccant humour will alleviate it. (*Vimānasthāna* 1.7)

One can easily recognize here what taxonomists would describe as a polythetic classification of humours, saps and sensory qualities. Let

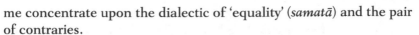

me concentrate upon the dialectic of 'equality' (*samatā*) and the pair of contraries.

Aetiology, prodromes, symptoms and other categories of signs belonging to the monograph of a particular disease are listed, as above, in chronological order following the progression of the disease. 'Causes' (aetiology) are the signs detectable before the onset; there is no question of causality as we understand it today, but only of antecedent signs. Then come prodromes, or precursory signs. Symptoms proper are manifested in full in the stage of maturity. 'Homologies' (*upaśaya*), which raise the issue of congruence, addressed in the following pages, are recorded when therapeutics takes command. And so on and so forth. This semiology of disease is meant as a guide to action for the practitioner. The reckoning of signs forcibly leads towards the dispensing of treatment, and it is so constraining that, in difficult cases, the principle according to which diseases should have contrary remedies is turned the other way round. Since remedies, in principle, are efficacious against diseases whose humoral character is contrary to them, all failures of treatment will be proof that the diagnosis was false, while any success may be reckoned as a kind of therapeutic diagnosis (Zimmermann 1989: 122).

To Conclude on the Concept of Congruence

'Equality' (*samatā*) in Āyurvedic medicine does not exactly mean balance in the sense of an 'equilibrium' (although this is the regular translation and the general idea involved) but should more precisely be construed as 'congruence'. Ideas of equality, and more generally of agreement, appropriateness, conformity or congruence (Sanskrit *sātmya, upaśaya, ucitatva*, and so on), have prevailed in Āyurvedic medicine, where humours and the medicinal properties of drugs constitute various sets of contrary powers that must be counterbalanced by each other. Thus Caraka defines the human body as *sama-yoga-vāhin*, 'the vehicle of congruous articulations' (*Śārīrasthāna* 6.4). Medicine is the art of establishing harmonious *yoga* or *saṃyoga*, 'junctions' or 'articulations', between man and his environment, through the prescription of appropriate diets and regimens. The moral significance of such a definition of the body is made perfectly clear by a few mythological stories which, for

231

the most important diseases, provide a religious aetiology. It is the case for *rājayakṣman*, 'the kingly consumption', which results from overexertion, profligacy and all sorts of disarticulated behaviour, such as repressing the natural urges or eating incompatible foods. The aetiological story is that of the god Candra, who was so excessively attached to Rohiṇī that he completely exhausted his semen – in other words, all his vital fluids, all his *sneha*, the 'unctuousness' of his body (Caraka, *Cikitsāsthāna* 8.4). Equality, balance and congruous articulations are meant for the conservation and restoration of these precious fluids.

That is the context in which the following eulogy of the body should be understood, which occurs at the beginning of a chapter devoted to the aetiology of *rājayakṣman*:

> An intelligent man should measure his strength and proportion his actions to it, because the body consists in summoning up one's strength, and man is someone who has the body for his root (*balasamādhānaṃ hi śarīraṃ śarīramūlaś ca puruṣa iti*).
>
> One should avoid acts of violence (*sāhasaṃ karma*), thus protecting one's life. For it is while living that man obtains the desired results of action. [This is a striking formulation of the Hindu ethic of non-violence, which is self-centred and used as a means of fulfilling one's wishes] ...
>
> An intelligent man should devote himself especially to those bodily [disciplines] which yield *yogakṣema*, a quiet and prosperous life (*śārīreṣv eva yogakṣemakareṣu prayateta*) ...
>
> Leaving aside everything else, one should cherish the body. For, when the body vanishes, for embodied beings it means that all vanishes [that is, all the four aims of human life, all *puruṣārtha*-s, to quote Cakrapāṇi's commentary]. (Caraka, *Nidānasthāna* 6.4–7)

The human body is the point of intersection where different orders of things overlap: physical forces and moral values, physical strength and the desired results of action.

A few words to conclude on the ontological status of humours in Āyurveda: Remember the distinction made between images and concepts, and the subtle shift from the vivid imagery of fluids to inferences on the existence of pathogenic entities. Humours are images (exudations, putrefactions of organic liquids); humours are concepts (principles invoked in physiology and pathology), and more precisely, humours are categories in a taxonomy of qualities (hot and cold, dry and wet) and processes (blockade, convulsion). Humours are arrays of correlated attributes predicated on biological entities in medical discourse to describe sensory qualities and the physiological processes that are under the influence of these sensory qualities. They belong with language and discourse. Compound medicines are made up of qualities (sensory attributes); physiological processes (verbs) are qualified by attributes (adjectives); and attributes are glossed by processes. In that sense, humours are medical categories, restricted to medical discourse, but they do not constitute ontological domains.[4]

In Hindu cosmology at large, the three humours represent three ontological realities, which are respectively wind (for Wind), fire (for Bile) and water (for Phlegm). When medical practice is put into the context of Hindu cosmology, the polarity of Agni (the sun or fire) and Soma (the moon or water) takes command. Accordingly, humoralism does have ontological dimensions. But in daily practice, the conventional names of the humours as well as any names, adjectives and verbs belonging to the technical terminology of medicine and pharmacy are devoid of any ontological implication. When used in the context of pharmacy and medical practice, they simply constitute a terminology. The Āyurvedic physician draws on this terminology where he finds attributes and categories to be used in diagnosis and therapeutic action.

Thus in daily practice, or in the weak or naive version of humoralism (the hot/cold syndrome), as if it were the result of a process of degradation and popularization of the scholarly tradition, the humours have been stripped of their ontological complexity and conflated with the sensory qualities. The hot/cold syndrome is more or less synonymous with the dialectics of Bile and Phlegm, thus reduced to its core golden rule: aiming at congruence.

Notes

1. All translations from Sanskrit are my own; nuances and code switching between the different linguistic repertoires involved in the medical discourse of learned practitioners play a fundamental role in the following analysis.
2. The capital letter is consistently used hereafter to indicate the name of a humour – Wind, Bile, Phlegm.
3. For a general introduction to Vāgbhaṭa, see Wujastyk (2003). For an elaborate analysis of *Dhanvantara taila* in French, see Zimmermann (1989).

4. The distinction between linguistic categories and ontological domains is borrowed from cognitive psychology (Zimmermann 2003).

References

GoI. 1978. 'The Ayurvedic Formulary of India, Part I'. New Delhi: Department of Health, Ministry of Health and Family Planning, Government of India.

Nagam Aiya, V. 1906. *The Travancore State Manual.* Trivandrum: Travancore Government.

Trawick, M. 1995. 'Writing the Body and Ruling the Land: Western Reflections on Chinese and Indian Medicine', in D. Bates (ed.), *Knowledge and the Scholarly Medical Traditions.* Cambridge: Cambridge University Press, pp.279–96.

Wujastyk, D. (ed. and trans.). 2003. *The Roots of Ayurveda: Selections from Sanskrit Medical Writings.* London: Penguin.

Zimmermann, F. 1989. *Le discours des remèdes au pays des épices: Enquête sur la médecine hindoue.* Paris: Payot.

——— 1992. 'Gentle Purge: The Flower Power of Ayurveda', in C. Leslie and A. Young (eds), *Paths to Asian Medical Knowledge.* Berkeley: University of California Press, pp.209–23.

——— 2003. 'Bodily Humors in the Scholarly Tradition of Hindu and Galenic Medicine as an Example of Naive Theory and Implicate Universals', in G. Sanga and G. Ortalli (eds), *Nature Knowledge: Ethnoscience, Cognition, and Utility.* Oxford: Berghahn, pp.262–71.

❖ Chapter 11
Harmony or Hierarchy?
The Mindful Body and the Sacred Landscape in Tibetan Healing Practices

Patrizia Bassini

In this chapter I examine the notion of balance in Tibetan healing following three lines of enquiry. In order to explain these levels, I start by using Millard's (2010) identification of two different types of knowledge: first, the paradigmatic mode of knowledge, which makes vast reference to Tibetan medical texts; second, the narrative mode of knowledge, which emphasizes people's life events that articulate suffering. To these two modes of knowledge I add a further important process that shapes human experience and this is to be found at the level of practice.

Scholarly Tibetan medical knowledge has traditionally been practised in monastic institutions and clearly explains how imbalance between the human and the divine realm can cause disorders, and outlines ways in which patients can 'rebalance' their relationship with the offended divine landscape and hence regain vitality and strength. By contrast, in actual practice and from a domestic or home-based perspective, among Tibetan lay people this 'rebalancing process' appears to be more like a state of permanent imbalance. Henceforth, through my analysis, I want to investigate whether in actual practice we can speak of balance in the Tibetan healing context.

The way I understand and use the term body in this essay may require some clarification. The concept of body is used in the

German sense of *Leib* rather than *Körper* (Ots 1994: 117). *Leib* draws attention to the inherent awareness, identity-infused and knowledgeable aspect of the body, whereas *Körper* designates the human biological vessel, or *Gefäß* in German.

If we progressively descend into the depth of the analysis from paradigmatic and narrative modes of knowledge to knowledge based on the observation of practices in the field, we come to realize that notions of equilibrium and harmony become increasingly problematic. Perfect cosmological explanations that help understand the aetiology of illnesses are confronted with, as Tucci put it, 'Tibetan lives in a permanent state of anxious uneasiness' (Tucci 1970: 172). Can we talk of harmony in a context where people perceive the divine landscape surrounding them as capricious and bloodthirsty and engage in endless numbers of rituals to ward off harm from evil forces?

The ethnographic material presented below was collected over an eighteen-month period between 2002 and 2005 among Tibetans in the Tibetan Autonomous Prefectures of Golok and Tsholho, Qinghai, China.[1] Names of people and places have been duly changed or omitted in order to preserve anonymity in a still very sensitive political region.

The Body in the Tibetan Medical Canon

The aim of this section is to explain the working of the body according to the paradigmatic mode of knowledge in Tibetan medicine and show how the notion of balance is a fundamental tenet for the preservation of good health.

According to Meyer (1992), the scholarly tradition of Tibetan medicine, compared to the Greek, Indian and Chinese medical traditions, began relatively late, in the seventh century AD. This corresponds to the period of the reign of King Songtsen Gampo, who introduced a system of writing to Tibet and invited doctors from neighbouring countries to translate, under his patronage, medical texts from their respective traditions into Tibetan. These events clearly explain the profound influence of the Indian and Chinese medical traditions on Tibetan medical concepts and practices: the system of channels running through the body, for instance, is undoubtedly of Indian origin, whereas the classification of internal organs, the examination of the pulse, and the practice of moxibustion are based on Chinese medicine.

During the second half of the eighth century, a divine aura was conferred on Tibetan medicine by the saint Padmasambhava, who is credited with the establishment of Buddhism in Tibet and the inception of the cult of the Medicine Buddha, Bhaisajyaguru. According to these sources, the Four Tantras of Tibetan medicine, the *Gyushi* (*rgyud bzhi* རྒྱུད་བཞི), were handed down from Vairocana, the disciple of Bhaisajyaguru.[2]

The *Gyushi* condenses disorders into 404 specific types of illnesses (see Meyer 1992). There are 101 light illnesses, which do not necessarily need treatment by a Tibetan doctor (*em chi* ཨེམ་ཆི); 101 serious illnesses, which are not curable without the treatment of medicines; 101 illnesses that are caused by the intervention of spirits and demons, and which not only require medicines and treatments provided by Tibetan doctors but also the religious rituals performed by monks to appease supernatural malignant forces; and lastly, 101 untreatable illnesses, which are caused by karmic predestination and are curable neither by doctors nor by a high religious authority (*rin po che* རིན་པོ་ཆེ).

According to this illness aetiology, many disorders are to a large extent entwined with moral tenets that regulate social life. In Tibetan Buddhist thinking, life alone is the manifestation of the accumulation of defilement in past lives, and this also applies in the case of illness. Indeed, according to the Tibetan medical canon, at the source of every illness there are three main causes or human defilements: desire (*'dod chags* འདོད་ཆགས), anger (*zhe sdang* ཞེ་སྡང), and ignorance (*gti mug* གཏི་མུག). Moral conduct, which integrates regular religious practice, is therefore fundamental for the preservation of health and good fortune.

According to this mode of knowledge there is a clear link between the individual, the social order and the environment. Conflict and imbalance between these spheres have serious bearings on one's future well-being and fortune. Thus, the individual is not conceived as a finite entity but is in constant dialogue with surrounding elements. This concept also finds validation in the laws that govern bodily constitution based on the seven bodily constituents (*lus zungs bdun* ལུས་ཟུངས་བདུན): chyle (*zas kyi dwangs ma* ཟས་ཀྱི་དྭངས་མ), blood (*khrag* ཁྲག), flesh (*sha* ཤ), fat (*tshil* ཚིལ), bone (*rus pa* རུས་པ), marrow (*rkang mar*

ཀང་འམར།), and semen (*khu ba* ཁུ་བ). These tissues are engaged in constant interaction and metamorphosis. Unlike Western understandings of bodily functioning, according to Tibetan medicine, good health does not merely depend on the functional performance of our internal organs but on the substances moving from one to the other, in the above sequence.

The wonderful Tibetan medical paintings collected in Parfionovitch, Dorje and Meyer (1992), originally produced between 1687 and 1703, summarize Tibetan understandings of human anatomy and medical knowledge. Anatomical representations map out the location of organs, veins and energy centres in the human body. Human anatomy was very well known to Tibetans due to burial practices that prescribe the dismemberment of the body of the deceased; however, the illustrations suggest that this medical system, in contrast with Western biomedicine, is oriented towards function rather than the meticulous identification of organs in the body. In fact, the physiology of this medical system is based, as in Ayurveda, on the seven tissues. In similar vein, illness arises when wind (*rlung* རླུང་), bile (*mkhris pa* མཁྲིས་པ) and phlegm (*bad kan* བད་ཀན།) become unbalanced.

In sum, when we analyse the working of the body at a paradigmatic level we see that a healthy body is a body in balance. If Tibetan people ward off supernatural malignant forces imminent in the surrounding landscape by observing moral and religious practices, the dynamics between wind, bile and phlegm – which can be respectively identified with the three fundamental Buddhist defilements: desire, anger and ignorance – will not be disturbed and can preserve their healthy balance.

Tibetan Illness Narratives

This section summarizes some of the illness narratives offered by my Tibetan interlocutors in Qinghai to illustrate whether at this level of inquiry we can still speak about balance in relation to people's bodies, health and the divine landscape that surrounds them.

Figure 11.1 is a visual representation of the 'semantic network' (Good 1977) that characterizes the phenomenon of heart distress (*snying nad* སྙིང་ནད།) in Qinghai. Of course there may be crossovers between the clusters in the representation, therefore Figure 11.1

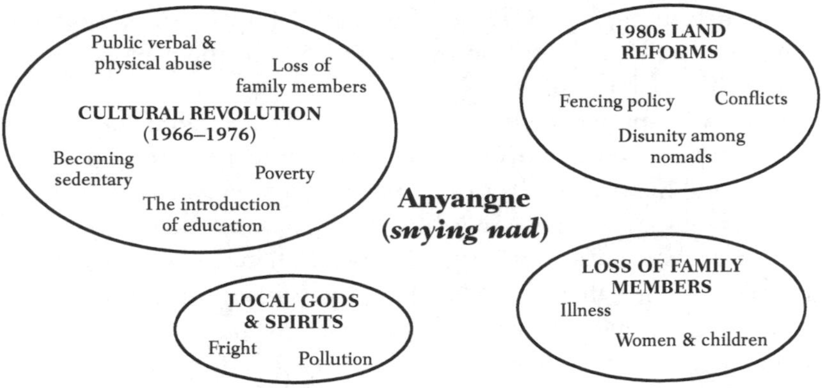

Figure 11.1. Shared histories give rise to *anyangne* (*snying nad* སྙིང་ནད།).

needs to be understood as a heuristic device intended to summarize the connections participants made between life events or causes and outcomes.

Tibetans linked heart distress as well as other illnesses to their personal and shared history. Patients often closely related their illnesses to experiences of historical vicissitudes of the last twenty to fifty years. Many cases I came across regularly touched upon issues such as the suffering that resulted from abuse and forced labour during the Cultural Revolution, land disputes, the loss of family members, and extreme poverty.

Tibetan nomads were also forced by government policy to become more sedentary and to send their children to school, causing in this way profound and radical changes to their lifestyle and social arrangements. In the 1980s there were suddenly many land disputes amidst nomads due to a policy of the division and fencing of tracts of land. Crossing the Tibetan grasslands with herds and accessing water sources became increasingly difficult, causing division and animosity among nomads.

Heart distress, in particular, was also connected to discourses of bereavement. A good number of the women I encountered during my investigation in Golok, Qinghai, had lost one or more children in the first years of life. Women were at greater risk of mortality after delivering their babies because of frequent *post partum* infections. Other Tibetans linked their heart condition to the spiritual realm:

they believed they had offended the local divinity by sleeping in the mountains and, as a result, drew pollution onto themselves, which manifested itself as illness.

From the analysis of these narratives the emerging theme was that Tibetan people in Qinghai clearly connect physical distress, particularly heart distress, to emotions about personal and shared histories. Figure 11.2 summarizes the symptoms that patients of heart distress reported during my investigation in Golok. Participants described feeling their heart 'pushing up' (*snying rlung stod 'tshang* སྙིང་རླུང་སྟོད་འཚང་), a piercing pain in the heart (*snying la gzer rgyag pa* སྙིང་གཟེར་རྒྱག་པ་), the heart being squeezed (*snying btsir ba* སྙིང་བཙིར་བ་), and they also experienced shaking ('*dar ba* འདར་བ་), sadness (*skyo ba* སྐྱོ་བ་), and difficulty sleeping (*gnyid dka' ba* གཉིད་དཀའ་བ་). It is also important to stress that among medical treatments such as Tibetan herbal remedies, moxibustion (*me btsa'* མེ་བཙའ་), bloodletting (*rtsa gtar* རྩ་གཏར་) and bloodletting and moxibustion combined (*gtar bsreg* གཏར་བསྲེག་), Tibetans resort to ritual healing too.

If not daily, regular practices include divination, fumigation rituals (*bsang* བསང་), ablutions (*khrus byed pa* ཁྲུས་བྱེད་པ་), rituals of ransom (*rgyal zlog* རྒྱལ་ཟློག་), yearly fumigation and ablution rituals (*sa bdag yul khrus* ས་བདག་ཡུལ་ཁྲུས་), pilgrimage (*gnas 'jal* གནས་འཇལ་), and more commonly prostration (*phyag 'tshal ba* ཕྱག་འཚལ་བ་) and circumambulation (*bskor ba* བསྐོར་བ་). What Figure 11.2 shows is that many participants look at the divine realm as an important cause of their heart distress. This view is also relevant to understanding popular aetiologies of other

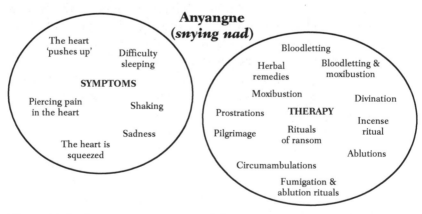

Figure 11.2. *Anyangne*: symptoms and therapy.

illnesses. This became increasingly evident when I observed how much time and effort and how many means are employed in religious practice. As I shall also show below, for Tibetans in Qinghai, physical and emotional health is indeed profoundly entrenched in the spiritual sphere.

The large number of rituals that participants engage in to cleanse themselves from pollution (*grib* གྲིབ) shows how the period of the Cultural Revolution, up until the beginning of the 1980s, was perceived as polluting for them. Indeed, as many studies have previously shown (e.g., Shicklgruber 1992; Daniels 1994; Karmay 1998; Ramble 1998; Huber 2002; Rozario and Samuel 2002; Mills 2003), many Tibetan people view pollution as a so-called 'root cause' of illness (*nad kyi 'byung gzhi* ནད་ཀྱི་འབྱུང་གཞི) and regularly perform rituals to prevent or repel it.

In one case, a Tibetan man declared that he took a lama to perform cleansing rituals at the same spot where he fell off a yak during the time he was condemned to forced labour by Communist Party members. Another lama who had been compelled to take a wife clearly expressed the concern that such an action would bear negative consequences for his karma, proving that the time of the Cultural Revolution was indeed perceived as polluting. Indeed, during this time, Tibetan people in Qinghai were not able to practise their rituals and as a consequence they continue to carry the negative karmic trace accumulated during those years, which needs to be disposed of through intensive ritual practice.

At the level of illness narratives, the propitiation of divine beings present in the landscape is also an important mode for preventing harm to one's health and fortune. However, what comes across already at this stage is that people do not seek balance but rather have to submit to a hierarchical religious order that compels them to pacify unforgiving, aggressive and malicious forces surrounding them. This will become even more apparent in the next section.

Ritual Practice and the Four Seasons

Tibetan people in Qinghai relentlessly attempt through ritual to control the damaging impact, which arises from polluting human activity, on their health and fortune. Table 11.1 presents some of the rituals in which Tibetan people engaged during my fieldwork.

Table 11.1. Rituals performed by participants.

Ritual	Type of ritual	Specialist	Purpose	Benefits
Divination	Instrumental	Lama	Seek advice for decision-making on health, business, travel, etc.	Protection, assurance that one has taken the right decision and cannot incur divine reprisal.
The householder's fumigation ritual	Instrumental, soteriological	Senior male in the household	Seek protection and help in eliminating pollution.	Empowerment, and accumulation of merit.
Rituals of ransom	Instrumental	Lama and other members of the monastic order	Repulsing the demon afflicting the patient with heart distress.	'Peace of mind' and better sleep.
Ablutions	Instrumental	Lama	Purification through water ritual.	Protection and empowerment.
Fumigation & ablution rituals	Soteriological, social and instrumental	Lama	Yearly community-based purification through water ritual.	Protection, empowerment, accumulation of merit, cement social bonds.

These practices play a fundamental role in upholding people's physical and emotional well-being. Like most rituals that attempt to cure illness, the purificatory rites presented in this table are mainly instrumental.[3] Divination, *Jieldoch* (*rgyal zlog* རྒྱལ་ཟློག, a ritual of ransom) and *Chishepa* (*khrus byed pa* ཁྲུས་བྱེད་པ, ablution) are mostly geared towards attaining protection and removing pollution. Besides its instrumental function, the householder's daily fumigation rite (*bsang* བསང་), which I explore in detail below, also has a soteriological purpose: it aims at accumulating merit to improve one's karma. Finally, the ritual of *Sadechyulchi* (*sa bdag yul khrus* ས་བདག་ཡུལ་ཁྲུས) has a social component besides instrumental and soteriological goals.

Through the examination of appropriate ethnographic material, I will illustrate the rituals Tibetan people engage in on a daily and seasonal basis and show how peoples' bodies are connected to a landscape populated by a great number of divine beings. This sacred landscape has the power to bestow fortune but also to inflict illness on supplicants. Protection from harmful influences is only attainable by submitting to a religious hierarchy through ritual practice and moral behaviour.

As Table 11.2 shows, ritual practice takes place throughout the year. Besides showing how pervasive ritual practice is in Tibetan life on the grasslands, this calendar also illustrates how close the relationship is between Amdo Tibetan bodies and the surrounding sacred landscape. Starting in November, many nomads – men and women, children and adults – stream to the monastery (*dgon pa* དགོན་པ) and spend one-hundred days in prayer (*dgun chos* དགུན་ཆོས). Their prayers have of course different purposes depending on individual circumstances, but all those I observed focused on appeasing or gaining the favour of the gods of the landscape that surrounds them. There are further religious festivities that run for the week preceding the full moon in February, March and April. During spring, new sheep and yaks are born and nomads take particular care of their new livestock. Just before the summer, nomads shear their yaks. The wool is woven by women during summer to make new tents. Starting in May, for two months everyone is involved in the collection of the caterpillar fungus or *yartsa* (*dbyar rtsa dgen 'bu* དབྱར་རྩ་དགུན་འབུ). This is usually the time when the monks have their holiday and are free to return to their families. While the monks are taking care of the homestead, all family members are free to concentrate on the

Table 11.2. The yearly cycle in the grasslands.

Yearly cycle	Nomads	Nomad doctors	Religious cycle
JANUARY	Prayer meetings (*dgun chos* དགུན་ཆོས།) in *gonpa* (*dgon pa* དགོན་པ།). These last 100 days.	Prayer meetings in *gonpa*. These last 100 days. Concentration on patients' consultations.	Prayer meetings in *gonpa*. These last 100 days.
FEBRUARY	Losar/Tibetan New Year	Losar/Tibetan New Year Concentration on patients' consultations.	Religious festivity from half moon to full moon
MARCH	New sheep are born	Concentration on patients' consultations.	Religious festivity from half moon to full moon
APRIL	New Yaks are born	Concentration on patients' consultations.	Religious festivity from half moon to full moon
MAY	Collection of caterpillar fungus Yak shearing time	Collection of caterpillar fungus Collection of medicinal plants	Monks leave monastery for a holiday. They look after their family's homestead while the family members collect caterpillar fungus.
JUNE	Collection of caterpillar fungus	Collection of caterpillar fungus Collection of medicinal plants	Monks leave monastery for a holiday. They look after their family's homestead while the family members collect caterpillar fungus.

Table 11.2. The yearly cycle in the grasslands (*continued*)

Yearly cycle	Nomads	Nomad doctors	Religious cycle
JULY	Movement to summer camps Nomad women weave tents with yak wool and milk yaks to produce cheese and butter.	Collection of medicinal plants	'Mountain Shower' (first half of the month) Temple dance (end of the month)
AUGUST	Nomad women weave tents with yak wool and milk yaks to produce cheese and butter. Sheep shearing time.	Collection of medicinal plants	
SEPTEMBER	At the end of September nomads move back to their winter camps.	Collection of medicinal plants	
OCTOBER	Nomads sell yaks and sheep.	Movement to winter camps	
NOVEMBER	Prayer meetings in *gonpa*. These last 100 days. Kill yaks for consumption.	Prayer meetings in *gonpa*. These last 100 days. Concentration on patients' consultations.	Prayer meetings in *gonpa*. These last 100 days.
DECEMBER	Prayer meetings in *gonpa*. These last 100 days.	Prayer meetings in *gonpa*. These last 100 days. Concentration on patients' consultations.	Prayer meetings in *gonpa*. These last 100 days.

collection of *yartsa*. They often travel far to the higher hills to pick the best *yartsa*, found above 4,000 metres in cold and well-drained lush grasslands. Meanwhile, the *yartsa* season has become a fundamental source of revenue to help sustain the nomads for the rest of the year.

When the *yartsa* season ends at the beginning of July, *Sadechyulchi* takes place. This religious ritual focuses on appeasing the earth spirits and involves performing ablutions for the participants with consecrated water from a local river. This is also the time when nomads move to their summer camps with their tents, where they will remain until the beginning of October. The summer is a very joyful period when many colourful grassland flowers perfume the air. During this time numerous species of flowers and plants are collected for medicinal purposes. Men shear the sheep and women are busy milking yaks. The milk is then turned into butter or cheese. At the end of September the nomads start to move back to their winter camps and sell part of their livestock. Ritual and secular life move in tandem: taking from the land through human action but also regularly appeasing the sacred forces imminent in this divinely imbued ecology.

The Householder's Fumigation Ritual

Using Ake Tombi's case, I will illustrate the integral role of ritual practice in the preservation and promotion of health. *Bsang* (purifying smoke) is one of the most common home-based rituals among Tibetans and shows quite clearly the close relationship between Amdo people's well-being and the sacred landscape they inhabit.

Ake Tombi was a retired 56-year-old widower living in Tsholho. People told me that his first wife, who gave him two daughters and one son, died many years ago. He had married a second time in recent years but, according to locals, soon after the marriage his new wife had run away to Lhasa, taking with her all the bridewealth, which included coral and all the expensive Tibetan garments Ake Tombi had bought her. Despite his age, Ake Tombi was still very energetic and took great care of his appearance, as well as his house and motorbike, which he polished frequently.

Ake Tombi lived alone in a large traditional Tibetan house that consisted of a series of rooms that stretched along two of the four high rammed-earth walls that enclosed a beautiful garden. By local standards he was a wealthy man, thanks to his government position, which he held until retirement at the age of fifty-three, and his Communist Party membership. Ake Tombi lived in the older part of the house. The central reception room displayed large pictures of Mao Zedong. The newer part of the house, on the other hand, displayed large pictures of Lhasa and all the places of worship that surround the holy city. Ake Tombi repeatedly told us about his recent trip to Lhasa and how he had spent 30,000 yuan in five weeks. In this part of the house there was also a *lhakhang* (*lha khang* ལྷ་ཁང་།, temple). As tenants in his house for about three months, my husband, daughter and I were able to observe many of his daily routines. We rented two large rooms in the newer section of the house.

The Cultural Revolution had started while Ake Tombi was still at school. Dissatisfied with staying at home in a village situated in a valley along the Machu (*rma chu* རྨ་ཆུ།, Yellow River), he decided to enrol in the Red Army on 5 November 1969. He was sent to Golok to fight the Tibetan nomads' ongoing uprising against Chinese occupation, being one of the many Tibetans who fought their own people. When I asked him about the circumstances in Golok at that time, he replied that many nomads were starving. Frequently, he had witnessed how in desperation nomads would literally throw themselves onto the rubbish they found in town in order to search for food.

During his time in the army, Ake Tombi became literate in Chinese and new opportunities opened up for him. He was soon promoted, and in 1975, at the end of six years in the army, he returned to Tsholho, where he was given the position of village leader. Later he was offered better and more prestigious positions within government that allowed him to travel extensively throughout China, and he visited places such as Beijing and Shanghai.

Nevertheless, Ake Tombi had been and still was very dedicated to practising his Buddhist daily rituals. He told us that in his youth during the Cultural Revolution he practised secretly and burned his offerings to the deities inside a pot in his own home. When reminded that according to Communist Party propaganda religion was 'poison' and therefore prohibited, he replied that there was a difference between theory and practice, and that, if he did not receive a salary (about 2,000 yuan a month) from the Communist Party, he would certainly not serve them. In other words, the main reason why he

247

had joined and remained a member of the Communist Party was the financial benefit.

Ake Tombi started practising Buddhist rituals intensively after an episode during his time in the army. He told us that he fell sick after he had shot an eagle. He could no longer eat and vomited all the time. After some time without any improvement in his condition, he decided to consult a lama. The lama told him that the killing of the eagle was the source of his illness and that he had to perform rituals in order to appease the displeased deities who had turned away from him. Indeed, many Amdo Tibetans reported becoming ill as a result of hunting wildlife in the mountains. Wild animals are viewed as belonging to the local gods inhabiting the landscape, and killing them prompts divine anger.[4] Since that incident, Ake Tombi became extremely devoted to his daily ritual practice, which aimed, as he explained, to gain the protection of the family deity, the mountain deities of his county, Amye Machen and the protective deity of Lhasa.

Ake Tombi started every day by carrying smoking juniper to every room of his house. This was to purify the house before he summoned the deities to receive his offerings, which he placed in the *sangkong* (*bsang khung* བསང་ཁུང་།, cone-shaped incense burner) in his garden. Pleasing the deities was very important, he commented, because they helped keep pollution away from the household and the family. The ritual had a very worldly and pragmatic orientation. Indeed, Ake Tombi remarked that he prayed for his family's health, prosperity and longevity.

Every morning in front of the *sangkong*, Ake Tombi sprinkled some drops of *changkar* (*chang* ཆང་།, lit. alcohol; *dkar* དཀར།, lit. white; usually made of barley) and scooped out of a bag his offering, which consisted of a mixture of herbs, mainly juniper.[5] He then placed this in the incense burner while pronouncing the following prayer:

> Cho ma hum, Cho ma hum, Cho ma hum [homage to the deities],
> I am calling to make my offering to lama Yidam [tutelary deity], Chuawu [hero], Khandro [female enlightened being], Chijongsongma [protective deity],
> The guardian deity of the locality and the saviour of mankind Gongmajelmo,
> The main god holder of the locality Sochjichpa who gives advice on wisdom,

Lamoshevdrong, landlord of this locality and his deity Chualgon
[protective deity of Lhasa],

Our mother Chualdanlhamo [protective deity of the Gelugpa sect, the
speaker's family deity],

Amyemachen [mountain deity in Golok],

Amyewayang [local mountain deity],

High Cheperdzagen [local mountain deity], wherever I go, wherever I
stay, may my fortune increase, whatever I do I may become successful,

Whatever matter I engage in, may all have an easy path and please protect
me,

Please.[6]

The prayer reveals a sense that a person's well-being is at stake.
Through the ritual the boundaries of the self expand to include the
whole house. Well-being is preserved primarily through ritual practice
rather than therapy, which is an important clue to understanding
more general popular attitudes to illness prevention in Amdo. By
appealing to the sacred landscape, the supplicant's surrounding
ecology is imbued with the divine and henceforth protected from
malicious influences.

Only after pleasing the deities did Ake Tombi perform *tshaser* (*tsha
gsur* ཚ་གསུར་), an offering to the spirits. This ritual consisted in offering
food to the dead who had not yet been reincarnated. The offering
was burned on the floor near the gate of the house. Ake Tombi told
us that he performed this ritual every morning out of compassion.
Still, this ritual had a soteriological function that aimed at attaining
positive karma for the next life. Spirits, Ake Tombi explained, were
like beggars asking for a donation: if displeased they might harm
people in anger. In his *lhakhang* Ake Tombi also performed thirty
prostrations every morning. Only then he sat down to have his
breakfast and, before drinking his milk tea with butter, he offered
some drops to the four cardinal points.

Upon performing these rituals, he said that he felt the deities
coming to him like a breeze through his hair and, for a few instants,
his body would be almost paralysed. With the performance of these
rituals his sleep had improved, he had good dreams and could light-
heartedly tackle anything during the day without worries. Provided
he performed these rituals, he added, the food he ingested could not
harm him. As a matter of fact, he said that he was able to eat half a
kilo of butter in the morning as well as meat without experiencing

any digestive problems. This was all due to the practice of his daily rituals, he told us. However I never saw him eating that much butter.

Religious practices were fundamental for a good recovery too. Ake Tombi added that medical treatment was more efficacious combined with religious practice. This is why one had first to refer to a lama for religious counselling and to invoke the deities to secure oneself divine protection, and only then did one refer to a doctor or a hospital. In other words, rituals helped prepare the path to recovery and make the body more receptive to treatment. Ake Tombi explained that he used to have heart distress (*snying nad* སྙིང་ནད), high blood pressure (*khrag rtsa mtho ba* ཁྲག་རྩ་མཐོ་བ) and gall bladder disease (*mkhis nad* མཁྲིས་ནད). Although his gall bladder still gave him sporadic problems because he ate too much butter, since he intensified his daily ritual practice he had managed to recover from heart distress and high blood pressure.

As proof of his health and of the divine favour he enjoyed, he also remarked that in the months we spent at his house my daughter, my husband and I got ill several times whereas he had been healthy throughout. Later I suspected that Ake Tombi's comment was also a way of indirectly criticizing the young generation – especially my Tibetan husband – for losing touch with their Tibetan Buddhist heritage, blaming us for our illnesses because we had not performed any rituals. The implication was that if we were to engage in ritual practice we would also benefit from being included in the sacred landscape. He, however, never considered the possibility that our illnesses may have been due to us not being locals (especially my daughter and I) and therefore not being accustomed to the regional diet and lack of sanitary facilities.

Ake Tombi learned the fumigation ritual from his parents. Usually the senior male member in the household performs this ritual on behalf of the whole family but when he is away a senior female member is an acceptable substitute.[7] In his mind, the fate of Ake Tombi's family was positive because they had made many generous offerings to the deities and to Buddhist institutions. According to Ake Tombi, poor people stayed poor because they did not make many offerings: one ought to be generous with the deities to benefit from their blessings in this and the next life.

Ake Tombi explained that his son, for instance, did not perform religious rituals. Therefore, in the event of Ake Tombi's death the deities might not favour him any more, leading to misfortune for the family. When I asked him why his son was not practising, Ake Tombi responded that his son, the only boy after two sisters, had had a very comfortable and easy childhood. He had always been pampered by his parents. He also refused to go to school and only managed to get a government job through the father's network of relations. Indeed, all Ake Tombi's children had secured themselves well-paid government jobs.[8]

Besides demonstrating that fighting for the Cultural Revolution and being a Communist Party member does not compromise people in Amdo from being good Tibetan Buddhists, Ake Tombi's case also clearly depicts the rationale behind the choice and the pattern of seeking medical care among the people I talked to in Qinghai. In contrast to the biomedical model of disease aetiology, Tibetan patients in Qinghai seek answers to questions such as 'why now?' and 'why me?' in their present and past lives, which may have upset the protective influence of deities. By this rationale, sinful behaviour draws pollution, which manifests itself as illness or misfortune.

In Ake Tombi's case the eagle that he shot during army service can also be interpreted as symbolizing the Tibetan resistance in Golok. Indeed, as Makley reports, 'many old Tibetan party members [in Labrang] ... now quietly sought the karmic guidance of tulkus and worked hard to accumulate good merit' (Makley 2007: 133). The violent repression of the Tibetan resistance during the time of the implementation of the socialist agenda in Qinghai is perceived by many Tibetans, including Communist Party members, as very polluting. This explains why many Tibetans who are Communist Party members are amongst the most fervent in their religious practice.

Tibetan patients in Qinghai often interpreted illness as a manifestation of something more profound, something that goes beyond the body and reaches out for meanings in the Tibetan religious cosmology. This explains why so many refer to their lamas for divination. The lama determines the exact causes and prescribes a pattern of treatment often based on religious practice. Then medical care is sought as a complementary treatment to cure the 'inflammation' or 'disease' but not the 'illness' itself. Indeed, according to Ake Tombi, health is a demonstration that the deities are pleased with one's behaviour, whereas illness arises as a consequence of offending the divine beings in the landscape. Although he knew that eating too much butter was not healthy, Ake Tombi did not feel that his health was threatened as long as he practised his religious rituals.

Through the examination of the most common rituals performed by people I knew in Qinghai, the analysis of the practices that accompany the different seasons on the Tibetan grasslands, and the investigation of the particular case of fumigation ritual, we can see more clearly that rather than seeking to achieve a state of equilibrium with the surrounding landscape, Tibetan people in Qinghai attempt to re-establish 'order' by means of ritual practice.

Only through submission to Buddhist religious divine beings and rich offerings geared at ingratiating divine favour are patients able to prevent harm to their health and fortune. In this context, therefore, Tibetans understand and rationalize their experience of health and illness in accordance with an ordered coexistence with the sacred landscape that surrounds them. Therefore, at the level of practice we can see how rituals also help reinstate a hierarchical order, one which was disturbed by defiling human actions.

Conclusion

Although historical events as well as social, political, economic and ecological circumstances constitute the triggers for the onset of disorders in the body in popular discourse, the often unspoken underlying cause of illness and misfortune remains the divine landscape of people's most immediate surroundings. In Tibetan thinking the sacred landscape is not an intangible abstraction, to which supplicants adhere as an act of faith, but a daily concern observable and experienced in the surrounding sacred landscape, which needs to be attended to through rituals in order to preserve health, order and prosperity. If the anthropological gaze is restricted to paradigmatic forms of knowledge and lay narratives, the fundamental role of the sacred landscape in lay perceptions, interpretations and experiences of health and illness may remain undetected.

I therefore contend that by moving our examination of the notion of balance through three levels – paradigmatic, narrative and practice – to examine people's relationship with the sacred landscape in the context of Tibetan healing, we realize that, in contrast to the paradigmatic mode of knowledge, which advocates a balanced lifestyle, at the level of practice people attempt to restore harmony, health and order by submitting to a religious hierarchy. Therefore, as Hsu argues elsewhere in this volume, balance does not necessarily describe a state of equilibrium between different parts arranged symmetrically, being of equal importance and carrying the same weight. Indeed, my findings indicate that ordinary Tibetan people attempt to generate harmony by becoming part of a hierarchical order in the religious as well as in the social sphere.

Appendix

Ake Tombi's prayer:

mchod o ma a ho, mchod o ma a ho, mchod o ma a ho

༈།། མཆོད་ཨོ་ཨ་ཧོ༔ མཆོད་ཨོ་ཨ་ཧོ༔ མཆོད་ཨོ་ཨ་ཧོ༔

mchod bla ma yi dam dpa' bo mkha' 'gro chos skyong srung ma

མཆོད་བླ་མ་ཡི་དམ་དཔའ་བོ་མཁའ་འགྲོ་ཆོས་སྐྱོང་སྲུང་མ།

yul lha gzhi bdag pho mgo nag gi skyabs re sa gnas skyong gong ma rgyal mo

ཡུལ་ལྷ་གཞི་བདག་ཕོ་མགོ་ནག་གི་སྐྱབས་རེ་ས་གནས་སྐྱོང་གོང་མ་རྒྱལ་མོ།

lha snying yul 'dzin gyi ye she bya zhub gshog drug pa

ལྷ་སྙིང་ཡུལ་འཛིན་གྱི་ཡེ་ཤེས་ཞབས་དྲུང་ཚང་གི་བརྟེན་པ།

sa 'di'i sa bdag gnas bdag bla mo zhabs drung tshang gi bsten pa'i chos skyong srung ma dpal mgon

ས་འདིའི་ས་བདག་གནས་བདག་ལ་མོ་ཞབས་དྲུང་ཚང་གིས་བསྟེན་པའི་ཆོས་སྐྱོང་སྲུང་མ་དཔལ་མགོན།

ma gcig dpal ldan lha mo

མ་གཅིག་དཔལ་ལྡན་ལྷ་མོ།

a myes rma chen

ཨ་མྱེས་རྨ་ཆེན།

a myes ba yan

ཨ་མྱེས་བ་ཡན།

bcud par rdza rgan mthon po sogs kyis nga song sa'i sa nas kha las dar ba dang bsdad sa'i sa nas don bya 'grub pa

བཅུད་པར་རྫ་རྒན་མཐོན་པོ་སོགས་ཀྱིས་ང་སོང་སའི་ས་ནས་ཁ་ལས་དར་བ་དང་བསྡད་སའི་ས་ནས་དོན་བྱ་འགྲུབ་པ།

bya ba bcos bcos tshang ma lam bzang bo zhig la 'gro bar mgon skyabs gnang bar mkhyen

བྱ་བ་བཅོས་བཅོས་ཚང་མ་ལམ་བཟང་པོ་ཞིག་ལ་འགྲོ་བར་མགོན་སྐྱབས་གནང་བར་མཁྱེན།

mkhyen

མཁྱེན།

Notes

1. Fieldwork was carried out as part of my doctoral research (see Bassini 2007). A departmental studentship from the Institute of Social and Cultural Anthropology, combined with a fee waiver by St Cross College and funding from the John Fell OUP Research Fund at the University of Oxford, were critical to the research this chapter is based on. My gratitude also goes to Elisabeth Hsu for her invaluable comments on my work and her encouragement over the years.
2. Tibetan-language terms are presented using the Wylie system for Tibetan orthographic transliteration, followed by the corresponding Tibetan script.
3. The classification of 'instrumental', 'soteriological' and 'social' types of rituals derives from Gellner (2001).
4. See also Karmay (1998: 25), wherein there is the story of a village that chose its headman on the basis that on several occasions he had hunted wildlife in the mountains but had never lost the local gods' favour.
5. For a detailed list of substances that are offered during the *bsang* ritual to the deities, see Karmay (1998: 403–4).
6. This is my translation of the prayer. The original wording is given in the Appendix.
7. Karmay states that 'in certain regions, such as Amdo, the [*bsang*] ritual is the prerogative of men, whereas in Central Tibet women may also perform it' (Karmay 1998: 380).
8. In the most recent news I received from Ake Tombi (summer 2007) I was informed that he was getting married again at the age of fifty-eight. His new wife was a young local farmer.

References

Bassini, P. 2007. 'Heart Distress and Other Illnesses on the Sino-Tibetan Frontier: Home-based Tibetan Perspectives from the Qinghai Part of Amdo', D.Phil. dissertation. Oxford: Institute of Social and Cultural Anthropology, University of Oxford.

Daniels, C. 1994. 'Defilement and Purification: Tibetan Buddhist Pilgrims at Bodhnath, Nepal', D.Phil. dissertation. Oxford: Institute of Social and Cultural Anthropology, University of Oxford.

Gellner, D.N. 2001. *The Anthropology of Buddhism and Hinduism: Weberian Themes*. Oxford: Oxford University Press.

Good, B. 1977. 'The Heart of What's the Matter: The Semantics of Illness in Iran', *Culture, Medicine and Psychiatry* 1: 25–58.

Huber, T. 2002. 'Ritual Revival and Innovation at Bird Cemetery Mountain', in T. Huber (ed.), *Amdo Tibetans in Transition: Society and Culture in the Post-Mao Era*. Leiden: Brill, pp.113–45.

Karmay, S.G. 1998. *The Arrow and the Spindle*. Kathmandu: Mandala Book Point.

Makley, E.C. 2007. *The Violence of Liberation: Gender and Tibetan Buddhist Revival in Post-Mao China*. Berkeley: University of California Press.

Meyer, F. 1992. 'Introduction: The Medical Paintings of Tibet', in Y. Parfionovitch, G. Dorje and F. Meyer (eds), *Tibetan Medical Paintings: Illustrations to the Blue Beryl Treatise of Sangye Gyamtso (1653–1705)*. London: Serindia Publications, pp.2–13.

Millard, C. 2010. 'Illness Narratives and Idioms of Meaning in Two Tibetan Medical Clinics', in S. Craig, M. Cuomu, F. Garrett and M. Schrempf (eds), *Studies of Medical Pluralism in Tibetan History and Society*. Halle: International Institute for Tibetan Buddhist Studies, pp.61–110.

Mills, M.A. 2003. *Identity, Ritual and State in Tibetan Buddhism: The Foundations of Authority in Gelukpa Monasticism*. London: Routledge Curzon.

Ots, T. 1994. 'The Silenced Body – The Expressive Leib: On the Dialectic of Mind and Life in Chinese Cathartic Healing', in T.J. Csordas (ed.), *Embodiment and Experience: The Existential Ground of Culture and Self*. Cambridge: Cambridge University Press, pp.116–36.

Ramble, C. 1998. 'The Classification of Territorial Divinities in Pagan and Buddhist Rituals of South Mustang', in A.-M. Blondeau (ed.), *Tibetan Mountain Deities: Their Cults and Representations*. Vienna: Verlag der Österreichischen Akademie der Wissenschaften, pp.123–43.

Rozario, S., and G. Samuel. 2002. 'Tibetan and Indian Ideas of Birth Pollution: Similarities and Contrasts', in S. Rozario and G. Samuel (eds), *Daughters of Hāritī: Childbirth and Female Healers in South and Southeast Asia*. London: Routledge, pp.182–208.

Schicklgruber, C. 1992. 'Grib: On the Significance of the Term in a Sacro-Religious Context', in S. Ihara and Z. Yamaguchi (eds), *Tibetan Studies*. Narita: Naritasan Shinshoji, pp.189–212.

Tucci, G. 1970. *The Religions of Tibet*. London: Kegan Paul.

What Next?

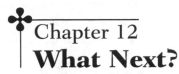

Chapter 12
What Next?
Balance in Medical Practice and the Medico-moral Nexus of Moderation

Elisabeth Hsu

The medical traditions discussed in this volume became known, first, by the term humoral pathologies and, later, as the Great Traditions of medicine based on the technology of literacy. More recently, they have been studied as reflective of cognition grounded in so-called correlative thinking, or microcosm–macrocosm homologies. Such characterization of the medical learning in question dates to the heyday of the rationality debate. When world history saw the consolidation of the former colonies' independence, it was a matter of national pride to celebrate scripture-based 'medical systems' as traditional sciences. Research interests of a very different era are reflected in this volume with its focus on practice and its guiding theme of keeping the body in balance.

Balance is currently a catchall term. In the cognitive sciences and sensorial anthropology, it refers to the human being's fine-tuned readjustment to ever-changing postures, and this proprioceptive experience is considered to provide the basis for concept formation and metaphor. In ecology, balance intimates complex interdependencies between organisms with different growth rates, and in the social anthropology of small-scale societies, likewise, balance expresses trust in reciprocity even if the universe appears unstable. In this volume, which is concerned with medical practice in stratified societies, balance implies a notion of regulation and moderation.

Illness may be experienced as an affliction, which ritual exorcism or medicinal antidotes can expel. Or, life energies may be depleted, and treatment consists of replenishing them. Accordingly, the treatment rationale for restoring the body to balance may consist of expelling afflictions or boosting depletions. A moderate lifestyle is thought to maintain the balance and prevent further disorders. The medico-moral nexus of moderation explicitly admonishes people to avoid oscillating between the two extremes of plenty and dearth, feast and frugality. It disapproves of alternations between excess and insufficiency.

It is well known that the literate medical traditions of Europe, the Middle East and Asia advocate balance (e.g., Young and Leslie 1992), which is often best explained in ecological terms (e.g., Zimmermann 1987) and those of the body politic (e.g., Alter 2005). Similar all-encompassing cosmologies of balance have been described for pre-Columbian Mesoamerica (Ortiz de Montellano 1990). However, in societies where neither seasonal change nor literacy is pronounced, medical practice can also be directed at keeping the body in balance. Parkin (this volume) points to medico-moral sanctions of sexual transgression among the Luo, and Bantu-speaking peoples more generally, and Geissler (1998) discusses these peoples' unwillingness to develop a concept of eliminating disease and their insistence on a cosmology of human–environment interdependencies. This volume includes for those analytic reasons – that notions of balance guide medical practice not only in humoral medicine – contributions from a wider geographic spectrum.

The ethnophysiological idea that 'worms are our life' reminds us that medicine often deals with hands-on problems of the everyday. Geissler (1998) implies a pragmatic stance: if people had other living conditions, other eating habits and effective de-worming medication, their medical cosmology would not celebrate human–environment inter-relatedness and balance to the same degree. In other words, medical notions of balance need to be evaluated not merely from the perspective of morality and kinship ideologies (Parkin, this volume) but also in regard to daily life technologies (Geissler 1998).

Furthermore, it is important to keep in mind that efforts at restoring a body to balance are often endorsed, side by side, with practices grounded in other therapeutic logics. Situational considerations matter, such as the choices available at a given time and place. Ontologies matter no less: if 'flows' keep the body in balance, a 'gathering' indicates imbalance. If 'coolness' is morally valued, hot-headedness indicates imbalance. Concepts of balance are tightly intertwined with many different cultural logics and socio-political climates. Where biomedicine emphasizes equilibrium and homeostasis, Mexican mothers experiment with a more dynamic concept of balance (Messer, this volume). This dynamic understanding of balance emerges clearly from the combination in this volume of anthropological, textual and historical research.

As already intimated in the Introduction, the studies presented in this volume range from the ancient worlds of the Mediterranean and East Asia through the Middle Eastern and European Middle Ages to early modern Germany and Japan, colonial and modern India, and contemporary Tibet, Mexico and Kenya. The volume also presents different ways of theoretically framing research on canonical and vernacular medical case records, on the languages of morality in and outside the consultation room, on shades of medical practice implicating the dimension of both commercial incentive and political recognition, and on domestic practices involving both prayer and herbal remedies.

As the volume ends with a question – What next? – an attempt is made to prepare the ground for future research through a critical reappraisal of some of the terminology inherited from earlier debates. In particular, future researchers are encouraged to move away from a fixation on medical theory towards investigating medical practice. Furthermore, they may benefit from widening the study of the cognitive (as opposed to the emotional) to that of cognition and emotion as part of a continuum. Finally, they may be inspired to include in research into different epistemologies also that of other ontologies.[1]

The Great Traditions

Twentieth-century research did away with the term humoral pathologies. Leslie (1976) featured the 'Asian medical systems' as Great Traditions. Porkert (1974) spoke of a medicine of systematic correspondences (grounded in inductive and synthetic as opposed to the Western scientific deductive, analytic thought) and Sivin (1987, 1995) emphasized microcosm–macrocosm analogies. These three characterizations were implicitly linked to a fourth one, literacy as a technology.

Leslie (1976) drew on Redfield's dichotomy between the Great and Little Traditions that opposed the 'reflective few' to the 'unreflective many' and those 'cultivated in schools or temples' to the 'unlettered' (Redfield 1956: 41–42). At the time, this dichotomy had already been critically reviewed. Tambiah's ethnographic study of spirit cults in northern Thailand countered Redfield by reinforcing the well-known South Asianist view that for villagers there was only one tradition. Accordingly, the 'static and profoundly *a-historical*' Great Tradition was 'a fabrication of anthropologists which they have bequeathed to the modern Indian consciousness' (Tambiah 1970: 370–71). Kapferer's response to this was that an indigenous concept, which had the function of creating social difference, had been turned into an analytic concept. The 'typification of everyday life' into Great and Little Traditions was 'largely a construction of the middle class'; it was 'an integral part of a symbolic language of class and status' and a 'cultural language of domination ... in which class and status find their particular structuring' (Kapferer 1983: 45). Kapferer pointed out that the proponents of the concept as well as its critics had failed to recognize this.

Alternatives have since been proposed. Bates (1995) spoke of 'scholarly medical traditions', thereby typifying them in respect of the social context in which they were practised: among scholar-physicians in stratified societies. One could object to this that a fairly recognizable conceptual toolkit (such as reference to hot and cold) pervades medical practice in all social strata (see Bassini, Messer, this volume). However, as argued in what follows, despite the similarities in conceptual toolkits across different social strata, the scholarly medical rhetoric is distinctive, intimating the indirectness of speech in polite society.

The treatises that Emilie Savage-Smith (this volume) has translated from Arabic convey well the scholarly understanding of the complex interdependencies that kept the medieval Islamic body in balance. Reasoning was in these Arabic treatises often in terms of an 'ethno-physics', where the physical form mattered, apart from the colours and smells of different fluids (usually not one of the four humours). For instance, it mattered whether an organ was compact or hollow, or porous and light, whether it was tilted one way or the other, and what the relation was between the part and the whole. Notions of balance drew on a distinctive schema of reasoning in consideration of different eventualities. They certainly would testify to 'accomplished medical theory' in Farquhar's (1994: 212) model which differentiates between three types of medical discourse – accomplished theory, symptom management and folk medicine – along a gradient from a very extended to an increasingly shorter form of the clinical encounter. In a related but different project, where Hsu (2000a) explored how three different types of medical authority assert themselves through different forms of rhetoric, Chinese scholar-physicians were found to insist on a flowery rhetoric that drew on polysemic, and not merely vague, word meaning (polysemic word meanings are concrete and distinctive in one situation but can be entirely different in another one). The prevalence of polysemic words in learned medical contexts was explained through 'patrimonial' structures and what Weber called 'traditional authority'. If one embeds the scholarly rhetoric in its sociality, instead of providing a decontextualized account of a semantic toolkit, it is indeed distinctive.

Zimmermann's classic study of the Ayurvedic concepts of dry and wet, *jangala* and *anupa* (Zimmermann 1987: 10–95), had much earlier made the case that polysemic word meanings prevail in those scholarly medical traditions, which, implicit in his account, clearly developed in contexts of patrimonial authority. In this volume, based on a decades-long friendship with a genteel Ayurvedic scholar-physician, Francis Zimmermann can also be interpreted as showing that in social settings marked by traditional authority people tend to take recourse to polysemic words. He discusses how the scholarly medical concepts of wind and wind disorders selectively absorbed shades of Western medical knowledge, and also conveys a sense of the unspoken but implicit and illocutionary in the physician's conversation with and treatment of the patient. The scholar-physician's language is shown to express an aesthetics of distinction.

In summary, even if the semantics of the words that are used are similar across different social strata, learned medicine draws on a distinctive rhetoric in medical practice. By attending to the appreciation of taste in medical practice, one can also provide an

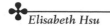

alternative explanation for the apparent pervasiveness of 'correlative thinking' in scholarly medical traditions, as we will see next.

'Correlative Thinking'

According to Farmer, Henderson and Witzel (2000) 'correlative thinking' prevails in all natural philosophies that emerged, often in tandem with the world religions, during a certain historical period (between 1000 BC and AD 1000) in the stratified, urbanized ancient civilizations. Indeed, for many medical historians, correlative thinking is an intrinsic aspect of humoralism and scholarly medical traditions. Farmer, Henderson and Witzel (2000) consider thinking in terms of correlations typical of a style of cognition, wedged between what they call magical and causal thinking, on the trajectory of humankind's neurobiological progression.

Most anthropologists and historians of the Greek, Islamic and Asian medical traditions have not taken note of the evolutionist argument of Farmer, Henderson and Witzel. However, even in those traditions that can be termed humoral, physicians are not always interested in humoral correlations, nor are these medical traditions as correlative in their different genres of medical reasoning as the centuries-old focus of Western scholarship on humoral correlations would make one believe. This is one of the key messages this volume intends to convey (e.g., King, Savage-Smith, Jones, Attewell, this volume), not least, by underlining how kaleidoscopic an assemblage learned medical practice is.

While recent research, which feeds into postmodern and post-colonial studies, has studied mostly pluralistic healing interventions (e.g., Hinrichs 1998), some anthropologists and historians continue to investigate the systemic correspondences of the four humours, three *dosha*s, and five agents. They have discussed them mostly in the light of their temporality. Agren (1986), for instance, suggested correlative thinking draws the physician's attention to synchronous events. Let us add to this cognitive style a sensorial dimension, such as pulse diagnostics as a tactile body technique. It is currently practised in most learned medical traditions. In Siddha medicine, practitioners are trained to make their pulse merge with that of their patients (Daniel 1991). In other words, it generates a sense of synchronicity between patient and practitioner. Although practitioners in Chinese medicine have a more analytic approach, in that they have a concept of calibration and contrast their own breathing and pulse with that of their patients (Hsu 2000b), they too do attend to the present. Touch makes present (Mazis 1979); it also makes present one's feelings of interdependence (Merleau-Ponty 1962: 316). While palpating the pulse, the attention of the patient and practitioner is on the synchronic and situational. Tactility attends to feelings and the atmospheric, to the subtle and its potentials. Where language creates narrative, and tends to search for the cause of the illness through identifying blame in the patient's past, the insistence of relying on tactility in diagnostics stresses the importance of engaging with the present. The diagnosis of a distinguishing pattern (*bianzheng lunzhi* 辯證論治), much like the formulation of what Nichter called an 'illness taskonomy' (Nichter 1991: S268–9), outlines a strategy for medical interventions that is attuned to the socially adequate in the present situation.

Correlative thinking thus becomes a distinctive learned medical way of attending to the present, a habitus of the physician, so to speak (Bourdieu 1989), which certainly is socially effective, and also physically felt. It need not always be expressed in the classical languages of Sanskrit, Greek or Arabic, as Attewell (this volume) highlights with regard to Yunani physicians' struggle for recognition in colonial India. In Uttar Pradesh's emergent bourgeoisie, treatises on 'correlative thinking' were also published in the vernacular Urdu, for instance.

The above examples may help explain the continued re-enactment of correlative thinking by medical doctors, who sought social recognition and distinction. They draw on insights from sociology, phenomenology and medical anthropology, and aim to explain the habit of reasoning in terms of correlations through the social, ritual and bodily-felt medical effects that it produces. Instead of focusing on cognition in a narrow way, the above explanation for the scholarly medical indulgence in correlative thinking highlights continuities between cognitive, perceptual and emotional processes.

The focus on body techniques, and their effectiveness, involves comparing and contrasting learned medical preference for the subtleties of pulse palpation with shamanic ritual. According to Desjarlais (1996), shamanic ritual aims to re-engage patients in their life-worlds through causing presence with drums and cymbals, or what de Martino (1988: 70) earlier theorized as the 'redemption of presence'. Cognitive processes of thinking in terms of correlations are thus intertwined with the affective ones caused by tactile, proprioceptive and auditory body techniques. Cognitive as well as affective processes (Damasio 1996) become in this way relevant to the study of correlative thinking. The pulse diagnostic touch and the flowery rhetoric that emphasizes correlations in the manifestly present, in the complexion, in the skies and airs, the voice, odours and other subtle changes, draws attention to the present in a way that is better suited to the maintenance of a refined taste among the upper social strata than the shaman's notoriously 'noisy' drama.[2]

The comparison with shamanic ritual should not devalue sophisticated medical rhetoric, which throughout the last few centuries has sought recognition as a scientific language. The phenomenology of healing can also be applied to Western medicine and its reliance on technologies that cause presence. The popular technologies developed during the nineteenth century for visualizing physiological processes, much discussed in the history of science (e.g., de Chadarevian 1993), receive in this way an alternative explanation for their effectiveness: a brief glance at a curve, say, a fever curve, would certainly be sufficient for the hospital doctor's Foucauldian gaze to establish itself and take control of the situation. This phenomenological perspective on medical treatment as a social process does not diminish the curve's scientific virtue as a technique of objectification.

Duden's research on the fluid body addresses the question of temporality too, but Duden (this volume) emphasizes the diachronic dimension intrinsic to flows. In a fluid body, she argues, the present is always an aspect of the past that is flowing to the future. The present is part of a narrative that begins in the past and goes into the future (or, occasionally, vice versa). Accordingly, any attentiveness to the tactually felt rhythm of pulsations implies an interest in a temporal sequence. In a fluid body the past is implicated in the present, and medical treatment involves more than merely generating a synchronous oneness between patient and practitioner. Duden does not invalidate the suggestion that learned medical treatment, just like shamanic ritual or biomedical fever curves, comprises practices geared toward a redemption of presence. Yet she signals that future research must attend in a nuanced manner to ways in which medical treatment engages linguistic and bodily techniques in its construction of temporalities.

Literacy as a Technology

If correlative thinking is not merely appreciated as a form of scientific knowledge but also as a therapeutic principle that causes presence, literacy as the technology that makes possible such systematizing intellectual enterprises calls out for a reappraisal too. Technologically, literacy has been singled out as a defining aspect of the Great Traditions and of the ancient civilizations. Accordingly, much of Western scholarship assumes that the emergence of scholarly medical texts was possible primarily due to written information storage. Writing has been understood to stabilize, accumulate and systematize knowledge in contrast to the oral transmission of knowledge that would be more fluid due to memory loss and improvisation (e.g., Goody 1977).

Parkin has long queried the 'somewhat doubtful criterion of scriptural texts as being at the basis of a Great Tradition' (Parkin 1990: 195). In his appraisal of the ethnography of eastern Africa, he redefined Great Traditions as 'overarching' and Little Traditions as 'vernacular', thereby redefining Redfield's concept (and stripping it of its above-mentioned questionable criteria): 'Africa has, then, regional patterns which variously draw on Africa-wide concepts as well as local variants recognized by the people themselves' (Parkin 1990: 185). Parkin's discussion was not of medicine but concerned the social anthropology of Africa, which he accused of a twofold bias: a literacy–orality bias, in that the 'view from the office' was privileged over the 'the voice from the field'; and the bias that drew ethnographers increasingly to Asia with its 'vaunted Great Traditions', away from Africa which supposedly had none (Parkin 1990: 195).

While Parkin reproached anthropologists for reproducing a deep-seated bias against sub-Saharan Africa as less civilized, he espoused Goody's concept of 'literacy as technology' that codifies knowledge and makes it more rigid: 'Overarching assumptions, often vigorously reworked through a range of cognate cultures, are actually more dynamically involved in shaping the local level ideas and practices precisely because they are not committed to a written and possibly less flexible form' (Parkin 1990: 185). Parkin also continues to adhere to Goody's view in his contribution to this volume, where he discusses some of the features specific to these African non-literate overarching traditions. Recent research in line with Parkin (1990) has redefined the Great and Little Traditions in terms of tensions between national and regional, local and global, personal and standardized forms of knowledge and practice (e.g., Attewell, Messer, Jones, this volume).

Ethnobotanists have also cautioned against literacy as technology of knowledge accumulation in studies which demonstrated that 'illiterate' children of an indigenous people who live in a natural environment recognized and knew more plant species than 'literate' children from a built-up environment (e.g., Zent 2001). To be sure, case studies of this kind do not refute Goody (1977), who would claim that more plant knowledge is stored in a literate tradition than can be contained in any oral tradition. However, they raise the question of whether, if knowledge is stored in libraries but not in the minds of the people, one can still speak of a living tradition. Furthermore, it queries what kind of knowledge can be written down and stored in this form. Jones (this volume) specifically attends to the levels of literacy that a physician's clientele may have had. He also explores the extent to which the complexities of correlative reasoning were superseded by simple situation-specific devices, such as the prescription of one antidote to one poison in the context of the Black Death. He makes no direct links. There are many grades and shades of orality and literacy, there is no linear trajectory from one to the other.

The trend today is to explore orally transmitted shamanic 'texts' and to focus on practice in what have been singled out as literate medical traditions. 'Knowing practice', as Farquhar (1994) stressed, involves invoking the written text in medical practice with situation-specific virtuosity and flexibility rather than through a rigid application of a written formula. Lineage-specific texts make sense often only in regard to situationally acquired and orally transmitted tacit knowledge (Scheid 2007). The socialities in which scriptural knowledges are transmitted differ (Hsu 1999), as do Western scientific cultures of producing 'objectivity' (Daston and Galison 2007).

Literacy as a technology matters but not as the only one. Recent scholarship has shifted the focus away from literacy as a technology to literacy as a culturally specific practice of aesthetics. Future research may follow suit.

Microcosm–macrocosm Homologies

With the lifestyle principle of 'balance' as the theme of this volume, we have made an effort to shift the focus of research away from literacy as the defining criterion of the medical learning in question. By asking how balance is maintained and restored in preventive care and therapeutic practices, the chapters explore to what extent a medico-moral nexus of moderation defines medical practice outright. Are there thematic continuities to medical practices in geographical regions that a focus on literacy has so far overlooked? The thematic focus on 'balance in medical practice' thus involves a widening of research from medical texts to ontological matters of medical practice.

This prompts us to revisit a widely assumed epistemological similarity between all the learned medicines, namely the microcosm–macrocosm homology. No doubt any learned medical archive is large enough to include texts that invoke microcosm–macrocosm homologies. Thus, there are passages in Chinese canonical medical texts that liken eyes to stars and vessels to rivers, as there are in Greek ones. Without denying this, Western scholarship was perhaps not always entirely aware of the problems comparative studies entail (Lloyd 1996), and appears to have given undue attention to such discussions, by characterizing them as 'the staple of the medical literature', explicitly stating that 'they aimed not to accumulate empirical fact but to drive home symbolically two underlying points' (Sivin 1987: 57). In this vein, European astro-medical homologies of body and cosmos have been contrasted with the Chinese microcosm–macrocosm analogy of the person, society and universe, although one is dualist and the other triadic (Sivin 1995). The point has been that both are symbolic and culturally constructed.

The following paragraphs discuss two different triadic microcosm–macrocosm homologies in Chinese medicine. They demonstrate very clearly that research focusing on texts describing homologies leads to the impression that learned, as opposed to non-literate, traditions have important similarities. By contrast the study of medical practice and everyday technologies is also likely to find important continuities with the non-literate. Moreover, as we will see, by focusing merely on epistemologies one does not do justice to the different ontologies implicated in learned medical practices.

269

According to the *locus classicus* of Han dynastic pulse diagnostics (*Su wen* 20), the *yin yang* 陰陽 dyad 'heaven and earth', and 'man', form a triad (*tian di ren* 天地人), whereby 'man' is mentioned last in this triad but conceived as being positioned between heaven and earth. The contemporary Chinese pulse diagnostic method, which may well have been the predominant one since medieval times, is confusingly called by the same name, *san bu* 三部. It consists of a linear vertical alignment of the positions *cun guan chi* 寸關尺 along the wrist in analogy with the vertically aligned viscera in a tripartite body.[3]

The one name *san bu* for these pulse diagnostic methods is confusing because they are based on rather different triadic microcosm–macrocosm homologies. It stresses their symbolic similarities at the expense of attending to differences in their practice. It overlooks that *cun guan chi* may be an ancient concept, while their vertical alignment in equal intervals at the wrist may be due to an innovative medieval pulse diagnostic body technique. This innovative technique may have been to use one's fingertips to feel the arterial heartbeat, *qie mo* 切脈. In fact, *qie mo* may not have been practised since antiquity, as is generally assumed (e.g., Kuriyama 1999: 23–60). Rather, there is evidence to suggest that *qie mo* marginalized other techniques during the medieval era, and in particular one mentioned in a manuscript text unearthed from a grave closed in 168 BC, namely *xun* 循 'to stroke'. This *xun* was probably done with one's palms (tentative translation of *zhong shou* 中手 in *Su wen* 20), probably along the forearm (Unschuld 1985: 88), and it is likely to have been undertaken for determining whether the qualities of the skin were *yin*-cold or *yang*-hot (Hsu 2008).

Why should the three fingers – index, middle finger and ring finger – be vertically aligned along the wrist, with the index positioned closest to the hand? Verticality shapes Tibetan social life on the mountain: in their experience of transhumance up and down the river gorges, in their tripartite house architecture and in other artistic expressions. There is a consensus on this (e.g., Blondeau and Steinkeller 1996; Ramble 1996). Accordingly, the vertically aligned three positions used for taking the pulse with one's finger tips on the wrist, homologous with the vertically aligned viscera in a tripartite body, point towards a Tibetan provenance of this body technique. This triadic microcosm–macrocosm homology contrasts with the Han dynastic triad that consists of a *yang* heaven and a *yin* earth, and includes as the third element the resultant relationship between the two, the *yin yang* of mankind.

The above example illustrates nicely that where an insistence on homologies in medical reasoning celebrates epistemological continuities between different scholarly medicines, a focus on practice, and the body techniques involved, highlights fundamental cultural differences. While Chinese medical reasoning in antiquity seems to have been much preoccupied with *yin yang* interdependencies, namely the hard and soft, hot and cold, rough and smooth, and the like, Tibetan physicians were presumably more interested in the arterial heartbeat. Evidently, Western research has put undue stress on the cultural constructedness of different scholarly epistemologies. This has happened at the expense of research into ontological questions of medical practice.

Messer and Bassini (this volume) both provide rich ethnographic accounts of how people draw on ontologically different practices in everyday life. Messer takes an approach that emphasizes common sense when she highlights how people start to experiment with medication guided by hot/cold considerations. People creatively generalize hot/cold reasoning to make sense of both age-old conceptions of spiritual attack or soul loss, and also of newly introduced biomedical treatments. They do so although the medical practices themselves are grounded in entirely different ontologies. Bassini, who also focuses on everyday care, highlights how a subordination to the divine, which the sedentary Amdo Tibetans she worked with experience as everywhere in the landscape, is integral to an otherwise quite pragmatically oriented life in accord with the seasons.

Messer's and Bassini's contributions both demonstrate that fundamental ontological differences underlying medical practice can be integrated into medical reasoning that is grounded in strikingly similar hot/cold epistemologies. Bassini's particular attention to the seasonal cycle, and the implicit knowledge contained in it, which is that some illnesses are seasonally patterned, points furthermore to aspects that all learned medical traditions appear to share. As is demonstrated in the following section, they probably have an ontological foundation.

The Ecological Notion of Balance in Learned Medical Traditions

Instead of foregrounding the themes of humours, literacy and rationality, and in place of making microcosm–macrocosm homologies the staple that is common to learned medical epistemologies, the thematic focus on balance in medical practice points out common ontological concerns. While this section discusses notions of balance in the light of ecological considerations and those of body politics, the following will explore balance in the light of the socialities of those people who enjoy an elevated politico-ritual status and entertain a medico-moral nexus of moderation.

Balance often implies a lifestyle in accord with the seasons and coalesces around recommendations for seasonally appropriate conduct given in numerologies of four (as in four humours), three (as in three *doshas*) and five (as in five agents, *wu xing*) in the Greek, South Asian and East Asian traditions respectively. An attempt is made in this section to explain why this ecological outlook may have become so prominent. Empirical facts of geographical latitude matter, but so do forms of government: the bureaucracies of these societies financed and staffed the codification of learned medical practice.

No one would doubt that the prevalence of certain disorders is seasonally patterned, but today the recognition of such patterning tends to be relegated to the domain of common sense and tacit knowledge. Clinical handbooks – such as *Harrison's Principles of Internal Medicine* (Longo 2012) – have no heading on the 'seasonality of disease', but general practitioners nevertheless tend to diagnose coughs, flu, rheumatic pain, manic depression and the like because it is the season for them to occur. In this respect, contemporary practitioners' diagnostic skills may not be much different from those of ancient practitioners, in that they are statistical and derived from the frequency with which the condition is seen on any given day.

The classical Greek word *chulos* or *chumos* means juice, but nevertheless became associated with the four seasons that mark the Mediterranean climate (King, this volume). In a similar vein, the Sanskrit word *dosha* designates a mistake but the three *doshas* became emblems of the South Asian experience that the year has three seasons (Zimmermann 1989). In literary Chinese the word *xing* 行 refers to gait, movement, conduct and behaviour, and since antiquity the Chinese speak of four seasons (*si shi* 四時). So why should the five agents, *wu xing* 五行, be associated with the four seasons *si shi*? Like the four humours and the three *doshas*, the concept of *wu xing* is not etymologically related to the the word for season. However, it is a cross-culturally valid, ethno-anemological observation that a change in wind direction brings seasonal change (Pandya 2007). In ancient China the spatial dimension was quinary: it comprised the four cardinal directions and a centre that was imbued with ritual and political prerogative (Wang 2000). As the spatial dimensions were heavily theorized among court retainers, such as the much revered astronomers cum astrologers, a social historical consideration may explain why court physicians started to refer to seasonal change in terms of the changes in wind direction: it allowed them to make use of the same quinary terminology as used by other court retainers, and thereby enhance their status (Hsu 2007). In this way, *wu xing* may have become the idiom in which court physicians kept the body in seasonal balance.

It is the case that living in seasonal accordance was a matter already advocated in pre-Imperial feudal times. However, this medico-moral stance appears to have become particularly pronounced in Imperial China (Hsu 2009). If governmental intervention significantly affected the course of epidemics (Rosenberg 1992), the Chinese Imperial administration, which endorsed the medical doctrine of living in seasonal accord, can be interpreted as a government interested in the prevention of epidemics and the regulation of populations. Despeux (2001) argued along such lines when she linked the emergence and instant spread of the doctrine of correlative reasoning in terms of the five circulatory phases and the six seasonal influences (*wuyun liuqi* 五運六氣) to the governmental efforts during the Song dynasty (AD 960 to 1279) at dealing with epidemics.

The notions of balance in learned medical practice in China and elsewhere, accordingly, would have been, first, ecologically motivated and, secondly, politically promoted by an administration presumably interested in the regulation of populations. It would appear that this ecological notion of balance, rather than microcosm–macrocosm homologies, can be singled out as overarching characteristic of learned medical ontologies.

However, this is not the end of the story. There are other ways of keeping the body in balance, which relate to a medico-moral nexus of moderation. They are not restricted to the above measures of body politics taken by bureaucracies which appear to have been interested in protecting populations from the epidemic frequency of seasonal illness occurrences.

The Medico-moral Nexus of Moderation

In his discussion of *chira*, David Parkin (this volume) explores Bantu terms meaning 'transgression'. *Chira* is an illness of affliction, in so far as a witch can afflict you with it. However, in another sense it is an illness that arises from transgression within a medico-moral universe of moderation. According to the Luo medico-moral universe, one should avoid emotional entanglement, exert self-restraint and refrain from sexual licentiousness. In contrast to the way of life that consists of feasting for a few days and fasting for weeks and months (Dietler and Hayden 2001), moderation should be the main feature of social conduct of any adult Luo. The notion of balance invoked here alludes to a moral and emotional dimension, rather than an ecological one. It presupposes a sedentary sociality where food security appears to be given, at least among adult Luo men.

To be sure the moralities of moderation advocated in medical texts that trace their legacy to Hippocrates and Galen do not exclusively pertain to ecological considerations. Like the Luo, they also preach moderation and self-restraint. They discourage indulgences in food and drink, sexual pleasures and strong emotions. Illness will ensue not only after exposure to the natural elements but also after excessive feasting.

In Galenic medicine, but seemingly not in Luo medical lore, emotional life is implicated in the discussion of fluids and their multiple possibilities for transformation (for instance, from phlegm to yellow bile, to black bile, to blood). Dosage matters: mandragora was used in love potions, but not without risks. It was known that, depending on the dosage, it would treat spasms or insomnia, or induce delirium. The outcome of medical treatment depended on fluid transformations, variations in dosage, endless combinations of remedies, and many more factors, apart from dietetic and seasonal considerations. King (this volume) enumerates complex interdependencies that constitute learned medical dilations on pathological imbalances. They are dizzying and echo the multiple vicissitudes of an entangled Luo emotional life.

Hsu (this volume) also draws attention to an emotional dimension in medical reasoning when she argues that the 'holism' for which esoterics today praise Chinese medical interventions paradoxically derives from a medicalization of moralized emotion. She compares two texts where outbursts of anger were considered to cause a wasting disorder: one mentions anger in the context of discussing morally disapproved behaviour, the other is a medical text that correlates hardness in character (inside the heart) with softness and weakness of the flesh (in its external appearance). Hsu considers morals of moderation to have marked notions of self-worth among members of elevated politico-ritual rank (or 'merit') in pre-Imperial China. She posits that only later, in Imperial China, did such moralized emotionality became medicalized.

Parkin invokes morals of moderation in his discussion of social transgression and emotional entanglement; Duden in hers of a woman's emotional capriciousness; and Hsu in respect of anger that is socially disapproved. Moderation is advocated to regulate sexual transgression, fickle unpredictability and energetic eruption, and an undue reliance on the powers of the self is discouraged. However, these morals of moderation should not be mistaken as implying any sort of equality between genders or different age groups or members of different social strata. Morals of moderation generally do not pertain to an ethics of egalitarianism. Keeping the body in balance may actually imply maintaining morally approved asymmetrical relations.

Although Kuriyama (this volume) centres on money rather than on the emotions, his contribution feeds not merely into the question 'what is a humour?' but also into 'what is meant by balance?' The imperative to ensure the flow of money in Edo Japan is in his analysis tightly linked to the social obligation of giving credit and, vice versa, to heartfelt indebtedness. The merchant's concern with maintaining the flow of money and thereby fuelling commerce and trade deems as selfish and greedy any intention to accumulate goods. The morality of moderation advocated here is less against boundary transgression and self aggrandizement through aggression as it is against stagnation and the accumulation of a shared substance or agency that through its flow makes up life.

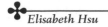

Moralities of moderation were upheld by well-respected Japanese merchants and their guilds, Luo elders, feudal Chinese and the German physician Johann Storch in his treatment of Baroque ladies. They share with each other perhaps less socio-economic class belonging than a ritually defined socio-political rank that grants them social prestige, 'merit' or 'honour'. The medico-moral nexus of moderation thus grants social prestige to members of a ritually defined, socially esteemed, if not political, rank. The medico-moral motto of keeping the body in balance may thus ultimately reinforce ritually, socially and politically given asymmetries in a stratified society. To what extent it emerges in historical periods where social stratification develops pronounced 'feudalistic' traits cannot be conclusively answered on the basis of the materials presented in this volume.

What Next?

The above has cleared the ground for future research by reminding us that the very concept of the literate Great Traditions emerged in response to questions raised by the rationality debate. The discussion in this collection, by contrast, has centred on medical practice. It has highlighted that problems of the everyday, body skills, and experiential dimensions of personhood matter as much as do regional ecologies and the socio-political histories. The medico-moral precepts discussed in this volume invoke balance in the sense of moderation (as opposed to an oscillation between extremes) and combine a sense of dignity with self care (as opposed to emotional entanglement, selfish greed or disruptive affect) in a vocabulary of ever-changing fluid interdependencies (as opposed to static norms of homeostasis and equilibrium).

Accordingly, issues pertaining to cognition can be linked to a sociology of taste. Correlative reasoning can be appreciated not only as a premodern science, but also as a therapeutic device that some find aesthetically pleasing. Elevated social status need not be derived from the technology of being literate, nor may it pertain as much to socio-economic class as to politico-ritual rank. Notions of honour and merit may well be contained in maxims of medical practice, and a sense of distinction can be gained from participation in a medico-moral nexus of moderation. Keeping the body in balance probably has little to do with the French revolutionaries' notion of equality between free brethren nor with Rousseau's primordial egalitarianism. Balance, it would appear, is maintained often through facilitating asymmetrical but mutually complementary relations.

Notes

1. The ideas presented here emerged in conversation with the contributors to this volume and some of Oxford Anthropology's current research students, among them, Kate Fayers-Kerr, Tara Kelly, Elizabeth Rahman and Alejandro Reig. I also wish to thank the three anonymous reviewers and the co-editor for their encouraging comments.
2. Upper-class clientele do seek shamanic treatment (e.g., Walraven 2006), but this tends to be depicted as a 'last resort' and supposedly happens only occasionally, and often furtively.
3. The qualities of the *mai* (vessels) at the *cun* (inch) position on the wrist close to the hand, which physicians palpate with their index, indicate the condition of the heart and lungs in the chest, i.e. the upper parts of the body; those of the *guan* (gate) position, which physicians palpate with their middle finger, indicate the condition of the spleen and liver that are located in the middle of the body's trunk; and those of the *chi* (foot) position on the wrist, which is farthest away from the hand and closest to the elbows, which physicians palpate with their ring finger, indicate the condition of the kidneys and gate of life in the abdominal parts of the body.

References

Ågren, H. 1986. 'Chinese Traditional Medicine: Temporal Order and Synchronous Events', in J.T. Fraser et al. (eds), *Time, Science and Society in China and the West*. Amherst: University of Massachusetts Press, pp.211–18.

Alter, J. 2005. *Asian Medicine and Globalization*. Philadelphia: Pennsylvania University Press.

Bates, D. (ed.). 1995. *Knowledge and the Scholarly Medical Traditions*. Cambridge: Cambridge University Press.

Blondeau, A.M., and E. Steinkeller (eds). 1996. *Reflections of the Mountain: Essays on the History and Social Meaning of the Mountain Cult in Tibet and the Himalaya*. Vienna: Verlag der Oesterreichischen Akademie der Wissenschaften.

Bourdieu, P. 1989[1984]. *Distinction: A Social Critique of the Judgement of Taste*. London: Routledge.

Damasio, A.R. 1996[1994]. *Descartes' Error: Emotion, Reason and the Human Brain*. London: Papermac.

Daniel, V. 1991. 'The Pulse as an Icon in Siddha Medicine', in D. Howes (ed.), *The Varieties of Sensory Experience: A Sourcebook in the Anthropology of the Senses*. Toronto: University of Toronto Press, pp.100–10.

Daston, L.J., and P. Galison. 2007. *Objectivity*. Brooklyn, NY: Zone Books.

de Chadarevian, S. 1993. 'Graphical Method and Discipline: Self-recording Instruments in Nineteenth-century Physiology', *Studies in the History and Philosophy of Science* 24(2): 267–91.

De Martino, E. 1988[1972]. *Primitive Magic: The Psychic Powers of Shamans and Sorcerers*. Lindfield: Unity.

Desjarlais, R. 1996. 'Presence', in C. Laderman and M. Roseman (eds), *The Performance of Healing*. London: Routledge, pp.143–64.

Despeux, C. 2001. 'The System of the Five Circulatory Phases and the Six Seasonal Influences (*wuyun liuqi*), a Source of Innovation in Medicine under the Song (960–1279)', in E. Hsu (ed.), *Innovation in Chinese Medicine*. Cambridge: Cambridge University Press, pp.121–65.

Dietler, M., and B. Hayden (eds). 2001. *Feasts: Archaeological and Ethnographic Perspectives on Food, Politics, and Power*. Washington, DC: Smithsonian Institution Press.

Farmer, S., J.B. Henderson and M. Witzel. 2000. 'Neurobiology, Layered Texts, and Correlative Cosmologies: A Cross-cultural Framework for Premodern History', *Bulletin of the Museum of Far Eastern Antiquities* 72: 48–90.

Farquhar, J. 1994. *Knowing Practice: The Clinical Encounter of Chinese Medicine*. Boulder, CO: Westview Press.

Geissler, P.W. 1998. 'Worms Are Our Life' Parts 1 and 2, *Anthropology and Medicine* 5: 63–79, 133–44.

Goody, J. 1977. *The Domestication of the Savage Mind*. Cambridge: Cambridge University Press.

Hinrichs, T.J. 1998. 'New Geographies of Chinese Medicine', *Osiris* 14: 287–325.

Hsu, E. 1999. *The Transmission of Chinese Medicine*. Cambridge: Cambridge University Press.

––––––– 2000a. 'The Spiritual (*shen*), Styles of Knowing, and Authority in Chinese Medicine', *Culture, Medicine, and Psychiatry* 24: 197–229.

––––––– 2000b. 'Towards a Science of Touch' Parts 1 and 2, *Anthropology and Medicine* 7(2): 251–68, 7(3): 319–33.

––––––– 2007. 'The Biological in the Cultural: The Five Agents and the Body Ecologic in Chinese Medicine', in D. Parkin and S. Ulijaszek (eds), *Holistic Anthropology: Emergences and Divergences*. Oxford: Berghahn, pp.91–126.

––––––– 2008. 'A Hybrid Body Technique: Does the Pulse Diagnostic *cun guan chi* Method Have Chinese-Tibetan Origins?' *Gesnerus* 65: 5–29.

––––––– 2009. 'Experiences of Personhood, Health and Disease in China: Some Reflections', *Cambridge Anthropology* 29(3): 69–84.

Kalinowski, M. 1991. *Cosmologie et divination dans la Chine ancienne: Le compendium des cinq agents* (Wuxing dayi, VIe siècle)/ Paris: Ecole Française d'Extrême-Orient.

Kapferer, B. 1983. *A Celebration of Demons: Exorcism and the Aesthetics of Healing in Sri Lanka*. Bloomington: University of Indiana Press.

Kuriyama, S. 1999. *The Expressiveness of the Body and the Divergence of Greek and Chinese Medicine*. New York: Zone Books.

Leslie, C. (ed.). 1976. *Asian Medical Systems: A Comparative Study*. Berkeley: University of California Press.

Lloyd, G.E.R. 1996. *Adversaries and Authorities: Investigations into Ancient Greek and Chinese Science*. Cambridge: Cambridge University Press.

Longo D.L. et al. (eds) 2012. *Harrison's Principles of Internal Medicine*. 18th edition. New York: McGraw Hill.

Mazis, G.A. 1979. 'Touch and Vision: Rethinking with Merleau-Ponty, Sartre on the Caress', *Philosophy Today* 23(4): 321–28.

Merleau-Ponty, M. 1962[1945]. *Phenomenology of Perception*. London: Routledge.

Nichter, M. 1991. 'Use of Social Science Research to Improve Epidemiologic Studies of and Interventions for Diarrhea and Dysentery', *Reviews of Infectious Diseases* 13(supplement 4): S265–71.

Ortiz de Montellano, B.R. 1990. *Aztec Medicine, Health, and Nutrition*. New Brunswick, NJ: Rutgers University Press.

Pandya, V. 2007. 'Time to Move: Winds and the Political Economy of Space in Andamanese Culture', *Journal of the Royal Anthropological Institute* (special issue) 13: S91–S104.

Parkin, D. 1990. 'Eastern Africa: The View from the Office and the Voice from the Field', in R. Fardon (ed.), *Localizing Strategies: Regional Traditions of Ethnographic Writing*. Edinburgh: Scottish Academic Press, pp.182–203.

Porkert, P. 1974. *The Foundations of Chinese Medicine: Systems of Correspondence*. Cambridge, MA: MIT Press.

Ramble, C. 1996. 'Patterns of Places', in A.M. Blondeau and E. Steinkellner (eds), *Reflections of the Mountain: Essays on the History and Social Meaning of the Mountain Cult in Tibet and the Himalaya*. Vienna: Verlag der Oesterreichischen Akademie der Wissenschaften, pp.141–53.

Redfield, R. 1956. *The Little Community and Peasant Society and Culture*. Chicago: University of Chicago Press.

Rosenberg, C.E. 1992. *Explaining Epidemics and Other Studies in the History of Medicine*. Cambridge: Cambridge University Press.

Scheid, V. 2007. *Currents of Tradition in Chinese Medicine 1624–2006*. Seattle: Eastland Press.

Sivin, N. 1987. *Traditional Medicine in Contemporary China: A Partial Translation of Revised Outline of Chinese Medicine (1972) with an Introductory Study on Change in Present-day and Early Medicine*. Ann Arbor: University of Michigan Center for Chinese Studies.

——— 1995. 'State, Cosmos, and Body in the Last Three Centuries B.C.', *Harvard Journal of Asiatic Studies* 55(1): 5–37.

Tambiah, S.J. 1970. *Buddhism and the Spirit Cults in North-east Thailand*. Cambridge: Cambridge University Press.

Unschuld, P.U. 1985. *Nan-ching: The Classic of Difficult Issues*. Berkeley: University of California Press.

Walraven, B. 2006. 'Ghost Catchers in Contemporary Korea', *Sungkyun Journal of East Asian Studies* 6(1): 1–30.

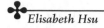

Wang, A.Q. 2000. *Cosmology and Political Culture in Early China*. Cambridge: Cambridge University Press.

Young, A., and C. Leslie (eds). 1992. *Paths to Asian Medical Knowledge*. Berkeley: University of California Press.

Zent, S. 2001. 'Acculturation and Ethnobotanical Knowledge Loss among the Piaroa of Venezuela: Demonstration of a Quantitative Method for the Empirical Study of Traditional Ecological Knowledge Change', in L. Maffi (ed.), *On Biocultural Diversity: Linking Language, Knowledge, and the Environment*. Washington, DC: Smithsonian Institution Press, pp.190–211.

Zimmermann, F. 1987 [1982]. *The Jungle and the Aroma of Meats: An Ecological Theme in Hindu Medicine*. Berkeley: University of California Press.

——— 1989. 'Mousson (Anthropologie)', in *Encyclopaedia Universalis*, Vol. 15. Paris: Encyclopaedia Universalis France S.A., pp.857–61.

Index